Nursing the Acutely Ill Adult

D0165559

Nursing the Acutely Ill Adult

Priorities in Assessment and Management

2nd edition

Edited by

David Clarke

Alison Malecki-Ketchell

 palgrave

First edition 2011
Second edition published 2016 by
PALGRAVE

Palgrave in the UK is an imprint of Macmillan Publishers Limited,
registered in England, company number 785998, of 4 Crinan Street,
London, N1 9XW.

Palgrave Macmillan in the US is a division of St Martin's Press LLC,
175 Fifth Avenue, New York, NY 10010.

Palgrave is a global imprint of the above companies and is represented
throughout the world.

Palgrave® and Macmillan® are registered trademarks in the United States,
the United Kingdom, Europe and other countries.

ISBN 978–1–137–46551–1 paperback

This book is printed on paper suitable for recycling and made from fully
managed and sustained forest sources. Logging, pulping and manufacturing
processes are expected to conform to the environmental regulations of the
country of origin.

A catalogue record for this book is available from the British Library.

A catalog record for this book is available from the Library of Congress.

Contents

List of Tables

List of Figures

Preface to the Second Edition

The first edition of this text was well received by colleagues working in this area; it was adopted as a core text in many undergraduate nursing programmes in the United Kingdom and also had an international readership. In addition, the text was utilised by many students undertaking post-qualifying programmes of education in acute and critical care nursing. Encouraged by the positive feedback of students and fellow educators we have prepared this second edition which we hope will prove to be just as useful across a wide range of programmes. The core concerns of the book have not changed; nurses continue to play a key role in providing effective and patient-centred health services. However, it is clear that following a number of investigations reporting significant concerns in respect of the quality and standard of healthcare, patient safety in the acute phase of care has now assumed even greater importance in most hospital settings.

The knowledge and skills of nurses have come under considerable scrutiny in this area of practice. There is recognition that nurses in all clinical areas must be able to competently undertake rapid, structured assessment and respond appropriately to their findings. This includes recognising when additional or more intensive monitoring is necessary or recognising that urgent referral to other members of the multidisciplinary team is required. Since the publication of the first edition there have been developments in both the use of early warning score tools and tablet and smartphone technology to ensure rapid recording and transfer of assessment and monitoring information. In addition, the use of care bundles is more common in some areas of acute and critical care, for example in relation to sepsis care and management. We have included reference to these developments in this new edition. In updating and revising the chapters in the book we have taken account of the feedback we received and have added two new chapters, one focused on understanding sepsis and another focused on acute stroke, both important areas of contemporary nursing practice. Clinical guidelines continue to be revised as new evidence emerges; wherever possible we have included new guidance and new evidence but it is inevitable that further change will occur during the lifespan of the book. Clear links to sources of guidelines or evidence have been provided in each chapter in order that readers will be able to ensure they can access current evidence.

Although acute care nursing practice continues to develop, nurses will always need to provide care which is both compassionate and competent; so, at one and the same time, nursing care must be sensitive to the needs of individuals and families but must also demonstrate a high level of skill, knowledge and understanding. It is clear that the patient is not cared for in isolation and the importance of sensitive, timely and accurate information provision to families is crucially important in acute and critical illness. In the book we have encouraged chapter authors to identify the kinds of information which needs to be communicated to patients and their families and to highlight the importance of this aspect of nursing practice.

The new edition maintains our position that in nursing the acutely ill adult competence in vital signs recording alone is insufficient. In acute care settings, nurses must have and be able to utilise knowledge of pathophysiology and disease to underpin their technical skills; that is, apply theory in their everyday practice. All nurses working in these settings must be able to undertake a structured assessment of the acutely ill individual and prioritise the patient's needs accordingly. Assessment is a continuous process and so it is essential, as part of ongoing monitoring, that nurses can recognise subtle changes in the patient's condition and understand and interpret the significance of such changes. Closely linked to this understanding and interpretation is the ability to recognise the actions which must follow in order that the changes identified do not lead to rapid deterioration and unnecessary loss of life.

We have retained the case study approach to understanding and managing common presentations in adults with acute illness as this has proved effective in providing nurses with the knowledge, understanding and skills required to systematically assess acutely ill individuals. In this second edition we seek to challenge nurses to develop a critical thinking approach to prioritising the nursing and medical interventions required to effectively manage a range of commonly presenting acute illnesses. We remain confident that nurses working in acute and critical care settings can rise to that challenge.

David Clarke and Alison Malecki-Ketchell

Notes on the Contributors

Pamela Beaumont PGCert BSC RN

Pamela works as a stroke specialist nurse on the Stroke Unit at Airedale General Hospital. Pamela's clinical experience includes over 30 years working within various medical units as ward sister, and later, discharge liaison nurse. Pamela is now clinical lead nurse for stroke at Airedale and is responsible for the clinical assessment and management of patients, nurse education within the unit, and audit and stroke service development within Airedale NHS Foundation Trust.

Mark Bevan PhD RN

Mark is Senior Lecturer, Faculty of Health and Life Sciences, Northumbria University, where he teaches and researches in renal care and advanced practice. His current research focus is on the use of electronic alerts in acute kidney injury prevention and non-attendance for treatment by dialysis-dependent patients.

David Clarke PhD RN

David is a lecturer and researcher in stroke care in the Institute of Health Sciences and Lead for the Post Graduate Certificate in Stroke Care at the University of Leeds. David's research is focused on interdisciplinary working in inpatient stroke care with his current research funded by the National Institute of Health Research, Health Services and Delivery Research, and Research for Patient Benefit programmes.

Michelle Clayton MSc RN

Michelle has been involved in caring for liver patients for more than 20 years. She balances clinical work with teaching a successful liver course for registered nurses. Michelle is the Lead Committee Member of the British Liver Nurses' Forum and is passionate about improving care for people with liver disease.

Elizabeth (Liz) Cleave MSc RN

Elizabeth has been a lecturer in cardio-respiratory and acute care in the School of Healthcare at the University of Leeds since the early 1990s. Her clinical background is within acute respiratory care and she has also held a clinical liaison role in cardio-respiratory areas.

Beverley Gallacher MSc RN

Beverley has been teaching biological science and pathophysiology to healthcare students at the University of Leeds since the mid-1990s. Prior to this she was a registered general nurse on a variety of surgical wards for nine years. Before entering nursing she obtained an undergraduate degree in biology at the University of York, UK.

Ian Goulden MSc RN

Ian Goulden is Pathway Leader for Adult Critical Care and Neuroscience, and Programme Leader for the MSc in Advanced Practice at the School of Healthcare at the University of Leeds, UK. His subject expertise and research interests include adult acute and critical care, adult neuroscience and end of life in critical care.

Paula Mayo MA RN

A registered nurse, Paula became a lecturer in the 1990s to share her commitment with others and to enhance practice with students, colleagues and wider communities. She has spent the last 17 years developing a professional interest in diabetes and is highly motivated and committed to improving the lives of people with diabetes.

Julie Jackson MSc RN

Julie's clinical experience includes renal medicine and critical care, both in the UK and overseas. She has worked in the University of Leeds as a lecturer practitioner and now works as a lecturer in adult nursing.

Alison Malecki-Ketchell MSc RN

Alison has been a lecturer since the mid-1990s and both her subject expertise and research interests are in acute and cardiac care. Alison's clinical background is as senior sister in cardiology and coronary care, and she has maintained close links with clinical practice throughout her teaching career. Alison is currently working towards a PhD at the University of Leeds.

Peter O'Donnell MSc RN

Peter is a nursing lecturer in the School of Nursing at the University of Bradford. He has a background in high dependency and intensive care nursing both in Australia and the UK. Peter teaches acute care nursing skills across undergraduate and postgraduate programmes.

Julia Maz DMed Sci RN

Julia is a lecturer in adult nursing at the University of Leeds. Julia completed a professional doctorate at the University of Sheffield. Her research interests lie predominantly around both the acute and chronic sequelae following spinal injuries. Julia's nursing practice saw her specialising in musculoskeletal and ultimately spinal injury care.

Catherine Waskett MSc MA RN SCPHN (HV)

Catherine is an adult critical care nurse and health visitor by background and has been employed as a lecturer in higher education for 15 years. Currently working in the School of Nursing at the University of Sheffield, Catherine is involved in teaching both undergraduate and postgraduate students in public health, neuroscience and critical care as well as advanced physical assessment and clinical decision-making skills for advanced practitioners.

Acknowledgements

The authors and publishers wish to thank the following organisations for granting permission to reproduce copyright material in this book:

Tables i.2 'Description of need' and i.3 'Features of a high-quality critical care service relating to assessment and management of accurately ill individuals' on pp. 4–7 are adapted from the Department of Health, under the Open Government Licence v.1.0.

Table i.4 'Key recommendations to improve the care of patients who were considered to be at risk of deterioration or who were deteriorating' on p. 9 from The National Patient Safety Agency under the Open Government Licence v.1.0.

Figures 1.2 'National Early Warning Score (NEWS), 1.3 NEWS Observation Chart', 1.4 'NEWS Thresholds and Triggers', and 1.5 'Outline Clinical Response to NEWS Triggers' on pp. 37–40 are reproduced from: Royal College of Physicians *National Early Warning Score (NEWS): Standardising the Assessment of Acute-Illness Severity in the NHS*. Report of a Working Party (London: RCP, 2012). Available from: www.rcplondon.ac.uk/resources/national-early-warning-score-news.

Figure 1.6 'Assessment and Communication: SBAR' on p. 41 reproduced with permission from NHS IQ (NHS England Sustainable Improvement).

Table 5.1 'Recommendations for management of transient ischaemic attack' on p. 123 reproduced with the permission of the National Institute for Health and Clinical Excellence. Adapted from CG:68 Stroke: *Diagnosis and Initial Management of Acute Stroke and Transient Ischaemic Attack* (TIA) (London: NICE, 2008). Available from www.nice.org.uk/CG68.

Figure 5.5 'Lobes of the brain' on p. 119 has been released as part of an open knowledge project by Cancer Research UK.

Figure 5.6 'Motor and sensory regions of the cerebral cortex' on p. 120 reproduced from: Blausen.com staff. 'Blausen gallery 2014'. Wikiversity Journal of Medicine. doi: 10.15347/wjm/2014.010. ISSN 20018762.

Figure 5.7 'Primary sensory cortex (homunculus)' on p. 121 reproduced from: Anatomy & Physiology, Connexions website. http://cnx.org/content/col11496/1.6/, Jun 19, 2013.

Figure 6.15 'Coronary angioplasty and stent insertion' on p. 168 reproduced with permission from: the National Heart, Lung, and Blood Institute (part of the National Institutes of Health and the US Department of Health and Human Services).

Figure 9.2 'The layers of the gastrointestinal tract' on p. 261 reproduced from Wikimedia Commons: https://commons.wikimedia.org/wiki/File:Layers_of_the_GI_Tract_english.svg.

INTRODUCTION

The Importance of Nursing Assessment in Acute Care

David Clarke

> Observation tells us the fact, reflection the meaning of the fact ... The trained power of attending to one's own impressions made by one's own senses, so that these should tell the nurse how the patient is, is the sine qua non of being a nurse. (Nightingale, 1907: 254–5)

This quotation is from a very different era in nursing practice, but in it Florence Nightingale made the important point that observation of patients and interpretation of the observations made required skills which were an essential part of what it was to be a nurse. It is clear that the range and type of patient observations made today has increased in number and sophistication, largely due to advanced technologies and the increased frequency with which nurses now encounter acutely ill adults. Skilled observations, undertaken as part of initial and ongoing patient assessment, remain central to nursing practice; their importance in effective management of acutely ill individuals is widely recognised. Providing prompt and appropriate assessment, treatment and management for the acutely ill adult represents a very large part of the day-to-day activity of nursing and medical staff within hospitals in the United Kingdom (Armitage et al., 2007; Jevon and Ewens, 2012; Royal College of Physicians (RCP), 2012). In addition, many acutely ill adults are initially assessed and treated by rapid response, outreach or hospital at home teams, or by an advanced nurse practitioner in their own homes. Patient assessment is a fundamental part of nursing practice but it is by no means a basic skill; it requires integration of knowledge and understanding in clinical practice. A more recent quotation from a key report helps set the context for the focus and content of this text. In his 2013 report *Improving the Safety of Patients in England* (National Advisory Group on the Safety of Patients in England, 2013: 4),

Don Berwick identified as one of his key messages to senior government ministers and NHS executives that they should:

Place the quality and safety of patient care above all other aims for the NHS.

This important message was meant not just for those responsible for the future direction and management of the NHS, but also for those who are responsible for patient care on a day-to-day basis; nurses are central to that care provision. In this second edition of *Nursing the Acutely Ill Adult* our purpose remains to identify priorities in patient assessment and management in acute care situations and, through detailed discussion of these, to develop knowledge and understanding of the meaning and significance of the signs and symptoms seen in a range of commonly occurring acute illness presentations. Nurses equipped with this knowledge and understanding have the capacity to ensure patient safety is an integral part of acute care nursing practice.

This introductory chapter will:

- Define key terms, including acute illness and critical illness.
- Briefly review factors which have influenced the development of acute and critical care services and highlighted the need for nurses to develop skills in assessment and management of the acutely ill patient.
- Outline the guidance available to support and inform nursing assessment and management of the acutely ill adult.

The terms 'acute' and 'critical care' will be used throughout this text. Table i.1 provides definitions of these and some other commonly used terms.

Background

The importance of skilled assessment and monitoring of acutely ill patients in hospital has been recognised for many years but gained increasing attention following the publication of a number of key policy documents in the early 2000s. These included *Comprehensive Critical Care* (Department of Health (DH), 2000a) and *Quality Critical Care: Beyond Comprehensive Critical Care* (Critical Care Stakeholder Forum (CCSF), 2005). These publications identified considerable variability in the quality of service provision across the United Kingdom and established the principle that patient care should be based on the level of need identified rather than which speciality

Table i.1   Glossary of terms

Acute care	The care provided to patients experiencing serious acute illness which is often accompanied by a rapid and progressive deterioration in their condition, and which requires urgent assessment to determine the level of care required. This will normally require frequent monitoring and reassessment of need. Acute illness can complicate existing chronic illness.
Critical care	The care provided to patients who require intensive monitoring and/or the support of failing organs. These patients are found throughout the hospital, many in general wards, but the sickest are cared for in dedicated areas such as intensive care and high-dependency units (Critical Care Stakeholder Forum (CCSF), 2005).
Assessment	Assessment requires systematic observation and targeted questioning in order to gather and interpret physical, physiological, psychological and social data which will contribute directly to establishing a clinical diagnosis and determining the level of care required by an individual. A number of guided systems used in acute assessment including ABCDE, AVPU, primary and secondary surveys will be reviewed in Chapter 1.
Competence	Competence is more than the ability to perform specific tasks; it includes capability which incorporates the acquisition and use of core skills in acute and critical care, the ability to assimilate underpinning knowledge and understanding, and development of the critical thinking skills needed to apply this knowledge and understanding to clinical practice. (Adapted from Eraut, 1994)
Collaboration	Collaboration means to work together, that is to act jointly to define and achieve a common purpose. In the context of acute and critical care this means to work alongside colleagues from medicine and other health professions in gathering, interpreting and acting upon assessment data; monitoring responses to interventions; and, importantly, reporting changes in a timely manner.
Care bundles	'A "care bundle" refers to a collection of processes used to care effectively for patients and involves putting together several evidence based elements of care (approximately 3–5 practices) that are essential to improving outcomes.' (CCSF, 2005: 30)

or part of the service the patient might be admitted to. The *Comprehensive Critical Care* report (DH, 2000a) recognised the simple fact that acute and critically ill patients were not only to be found in intensive care and high-dependency units. If signs of deterioration in acute and critically ill individuals are to be recognised and acted upon appropriately, it is essential that nursing and medical staff in all settings have the necessary knowledge and skills to accurately monitor vital signs, interpret the findings of this monitoring and then provide, or seek early assistance to access, the level of intervention and care required. To aid health professionals in providing effective care and the right level of monitoring, the *Comprehensive Critical Care* report recommended a simple four-level system to classify patients according to need (Table i.2).

The report highlighted the fact that in the absence of comprehensive services, early recognition of change or deterioration in health status may not occur and opportunities to prevent avoidable deaths may be lost (McQuillan et al., 1998; DH, 2000a). Later research and reports from the National Patient Safety Agency (NPSA) (2007) and the National Confidential Enquiry into Patient Outcome and Death (NCEPOD) (2009, 2012) confirmed these claims and provided continuing evidence that identification of acutely ill patients who were at risk and in need of urgent intervention or referral to critical care services was frequently delayed and sometimes missed altogether (Seward et al., 2003; Young et al., 2003; NCEPOD, 2009, 2012).

Table i.2 Description of need

Level	
0	Patients whose needs can be met through normal ward care in an acute hospital.
1	Patients at risk of their condition deteriorating, or those recently relocated from higher levels of care, whose needs can be met on an acute ward with additional advice and support from the critical care team.
2	Patients requiring more detailed observation or intervention including support for a single failing organ system or post-operative care and those 'stepping down' from higher levels of care.
3	Patients requiring advanced respiratory support alone or basic respiratory support together with support of at least two organ systems. This level includes all complex patients requiring support for multi-organ failure.

Source: Department of Health (2000a).
Reproduced under the Open Government Licence v1.0.

Central to the changes proposed in 2000 was the requirement to bring about improvements in systematic assessment of need using the Department of Health's classification system (Table i.2) to ensure that appropriate intervention and management could be provided rapidly (DH, 2000a). Achieving such improvements in assessments in acute and critical care relied heavily on nurses and other health professionals developing a sound understanding of the pathophysiology underlying common disease presentations, and on these professionals being able to competently apply that understanding when working with individual patients in clinical practice.

The *Comprehensive Critical Care* report (DH, 2000a) mirrored other NHS policy documents published at that time in seeking to increase the quality and effectiveness of care and in shifting the focus from organisation of care based on professionally determined speciality services to recognising and responding to the needs of patients (DH, 1999; DH, 2000b). The policy requirement was for a 'whole systems' approach to modernisation of services to ensure acute and critical care provision was not bounded by location, but was comprehensive and spanned all specialities (DH, 2000a). This included establishing critical care outreach and support services and introducing changes in training to share critical care skills and ensure direct care staff had the competence and knowledge to recognise and act appropriately upon signs and symptoms of deterioration or of increasing dependency and level of need. These services, together with acute care teams, are now well established in most hospitals in the UK. Nurses played a key role in implementing, monitoring and evaluating the effectiveness of these changes (CCSF, 2005; Manley and Hardy, 2006). The modernisation programme sought change at all levels, including establishing networks between groups of NHS and primary care providers to share expertise and good practice and improve the integration and effectiveness of pre-hospital, within-hospital and post-discharge acute and critical care services (DH, 2000a). Whilst the recommendations for training of qualified nursing and medical staff were fairly clear, the report did not comment on the fact that nurses in pre-registration and specialist post-registration training also needed more focused preparation to work in modernised health services where staff at all levels would be expected to be competent in assessment of the level of need. However, a later report from the Department of Health's Modernisation Agency (2003) identified that the education being provided at that time did not adequately prepare nurses and other healthcare providers to assess and manage the critically ill; this was particularly the case where care was being provided outside of designated critical care departments.

The *Quality Critical Care* report (DH, 2005) confirmed that between 2000 and 2004 significant development of comprehensive critical care services occurred. However, the report also noted that service improvements were not uniform, for example some hospitals had well-established outreach teams and others had not set up such teams. In addition, whilst the overall number of critical care beds had increased by 35 per cent between 2000 and 2004, critically ill patients were still being transferred between hospitals and the number of urgent operations being cancelled due to lack of critical care capacity was not being reduced. At the same time as critical care beds had increased, the overall number of hospital beds had fallen and the number of inpatients defined as acutely ill had increased (National Confidential Enquiry into Patient Outcome and Death (NCEPOD), 2005). The *Quality Critical Care* report (CCSF, 2005) made a series of recommendations to ensure that comprehensive critical care services continued to develop and improve; these were aimed at commissioners, service providers, education providers and individual professionals. The key features which have particular relevance for this book are identified in Table i.3.

The main aim of the *Quality Critical Care* report (CCSF, 2005) was to encourage organisations to build on the successes achieved since 2000 and maintain the momentum in order to ensure that critical care services continued to improve and become firmly integrated into primary and secondary care services. The successful implementation of all of the features of high quality services identified in Table i.3 depends on skilled nursing staff being able to coordinate assessment activity with medical and other health professional colleagues and being able to undertake appropriate ongoing monitoring, including using track and trigger systems (see below and Chapter 1).

A Continuing Concern with Assessment of Acutely Ill Individuals

The publication of reports from the National Institute for Health and Clinical Excellence (NICE, 2007) and the National Patient Safety Agency (NPSA, 2007) further highlighted the fact that despite significant improvements in organisation of acute and critical care services since 2000, concerns remained about the knowledge, understanding and competence of nurses and other health professionals in recognising early and developing signs that a patient is 'at risk'. Where health professionals are enabled to develop the required competence the evidence shows that morbidity and mortality can be reduced (Bellomo et al., 2004; Priestley et al., 2004; NICE, 2007).

Table i.3　Features of a high-quality critical care service relating to assessment and management of acutely ill individuals

Key feature	Explanation
Patient-centred care	Treating patients as individuals is fundamental and requires that they are the focus of care and that their identified needs should dictate the care provided. Keeping the patient at the centre of the care pathway requires flexible service provision (National Advisory Group on the Safety of Patients in England, 2013).
Evidence-based care, monitoring and evaluation	Regular monitoring and evaluation of care informs clinical decision making. Where good evidence of effectiveness of specific clinical interventions exists, care should be informed by such evidence. One key area of use of best evidence identified to support comprehensive critical care was the introduction of 'care bundles'. This approach was also identified as a central element of service improvement by the NHS Modernisation Agency (2003). The approach is endorsed by the RCP (2012) and NHS England (Patient Safety First, NHS England, 2015).
Early warning systems and outreach systems	The widespread introduction and use of 'track and trigger' systems on general wards, together with intervention tools, was identified as necessary. For example see the discussion in Chapter 1 on early warning scoring systems (Morgan et al., 1997; Goldhill and McNarry, 2004; RCP, 2012).
An appropriately trained and competent workforce, and staff empowerment, support and development	The *Quality Critical Care* report noted the importance of ensuring that staff working outside of critical care areas were competent in the recognition of critical illness. However, despite many other recommendations the report provided no specific guidance in this area. The discussion of the need for standardised programmes focused only on work-based training and did not comment on the need for changes in pre-registration undergraduate nursing education programmes, nor on the level of preparation required for post-registration or continuing professional development (CPD) programmes in acute and critical care.
24-hour access to multidisciplinary teams	The *Quality Critical Care* report noted the obvious importance of having access to a multidisciplinary team with the right skills, knowledge and experience in acute and critical care. However, it also emphasised the need for team members to develop a culture of respect for all disciplines, and for the team to engage in shared learning and be prepared to both challenge and support colleagues in order to enhance the effectiveness of patient care.

Source: Adapted from Department of Health, 2005. Reproduced under the Open Government Licence v1.0.

The NPSA (2007) report clearly identified the detrimental effects that can result when such competence has not been acquired. Such knowledge and skills deficits have been shown to have a direct negative relationship on the effectiveness of comprehensive physical and physiological assessment, the use of early warning scoring systems to detect those at risk of deterioration, and also the usefulness of regular physiological monitoring. The NPSA (2007) provided an analysis of 1,804 serious incidents included in the national reporting learning system that had resulted in death of patients. The analysis indicated that just over half of these deaths (576) could be regarded as potentially avoidable. The majority of the 576 deaths occurred within acute and/or general hospitals. The NPSA (2007) also conducted an in-depth analysis of 107 patients' deaths reported to the agency because of concerns related to the safety of the care provided for these patients during their hospitalisation. In the majority of cases (64), health professionals either took too long to notice or did not recognise signs of deterioration which may have prevented these deaths; the remaining cases related to either a failure to recognise cardiac arrest or not instigating early interventions and calling the cardiac arrest team once the arrest had been recognised. The NPSA (2007) report also highlighted the existence of good practice in the NHS, but importantly the report made a series of recommendations (see Table i.4) designed to improve the care of patients who were considered to be at risk of deterioration or who were deteriorating; all of these issues will be considered in the context of case studies in later chapters of this book. The report also made a number of recommendations in relation to the resuscitation of the acutely ill individual. Recognising and responding to the importance of these issues, NICE (2007) developed detailed clinical guidelines (CG:50) designed to improve the recognition of and response to adults presenting with acute illnesses in hospital. The NICE (2007) guidelines will be reviewed in 2016 to determine if further updating is required. Currently, these guidelines, which are discussed in more detail in Chapter 1 and subsequent chapters in this book, continue to underpin practice in the NHS. An important feature of both the NPSA and NICE 2007 documents was the recognition of the need for training to improve skills, knowledge and understanding for all staff involved in assessing, treating and managing the acutely ill adult. It is also clear that, although the documents outlined above focused primarily on caring for acutely ill patients in hospital, the skills required to systematically assess the acutely ill adult are transferable to the majority of settings where patients present seeking assistance from health professionals, including primary care settings such as hospital at home and rapid response teams, outreach services, walk-in centres and polyclinics.

Table i.4   Key recommendations to improve the care of patients who were considered to be at risk of deterioration or who were deteriorating

There needs to be	*Rationale*
Better recognition of patients who are at risk of, or who have experienced, deterioration Appropriate monitoring of vital signs	In the cases reviewed: Formal or visual observations, including colour, consciousness, temperature, pulse, blood pressure and oxygen saturations were either completely or partially omitted. *The most common omission was observation of the **respiratory rate**.*
Accurate interpretation of clinical findings	In the cases reviewed: Early warning scores were not calculated correctly and health professionals did not always recognise when observations gave cause for concern, which may require more intensive monitoring.
Calling for help early and ensuring that it arrives A related recommendation was made in relation to ensuring appropriate drugs and equipment were available to facilitate appropriate and early interventions	In the cases reviewed: There was a lack of communication and health professionals did not act on concerns identified during handovers or transfer of information between professional groups.
Training and skills development	In the cases reviewed: Analysis of specific incidents resulting in death suggested that medical and nursing staff did not have the depth of knowledge and skills required to recognise deterioration and call for appropriate help.

Source: Adapted from the National Patient Safety Agency (2007). Reproduced under the Open Government Licence v1.0.

There is a continuing concern to standardise the quality of care of such services across the UK and to ensure staff providing the services have a uniform level of knowledge and competency. To this end the National Outreach Forum (NORF) (2012) has developed *Operational Standards and Competencies for Critical Care Outreach Services* (NORF, 2012). These complement those developed by the Department of Health in 2009. Despite the valuable developments in recognition of the need to improve the coordination of acute services and the knowledge and skills of staff working in these settings, there have been continuing reports drawing attention to shortfalls in systems designed to ensure patient safety, most notably the Francis Report into the Mid Staffordshire NHS Foundation Trust (Francis, 2013) and *Improving the Safety of Patients in England* (2013), commonly referred to as the Berwick Report). A key recommendation of the Berwick Report (National Advisory Group on the Safety of Patients in England, 2013: 5) was that 'mastery of quality and patient safety sciences and practices should be part of initial preparation and lifelong education of all health care professionals, including managers and executives'. We endorse this recommendation and seek to contribute to the preparation of nurses to develop this mastery.

Developments in Recording Vital Signs: The Role of Technology

A key part of ensuring patient safety in acute and critical care situations is in recognising and responding effectively to the often rapid deterioration in patients' condition. Track and trigger systems, including in the UK the National Early Warning Scoring system (NEWS) (RCP, 2012; Centre for Reviews and Dissemination (CRD), 2014) are now a central part of this process. However, it is important to recognise that these systems alone will not be sufficient to drive up the standard of care required to recognise and prevent deterioration which can rapidly lead to unnecessary deaths (Massey, 2010; Clifton et al., 2015; Odell, 2015). Factors influencing compliance with protocols for accurate recording of vital signs and for initiating reports of change and deterioration also need to be considered if these systems are to contribute to real and sustained improvements in patient care (NCEPOD, 2012; Hands, 2013). There have been rapid developments in the technology available to support vital signs recording. These include electronic charting systems which utilise tablet or smartphone technology and incorporate algorithms which enable the automatic detection and reporting of deterioration in vital signs (CRD, 2014; Cooper et al., 2015). These systems 'automate' the collection and recording of the data used in track and trigger systems such as NEWS (RCP, 2012) and allow for staff in outreach or acute care teams to review vital signs of at-risk patients remotely. Case-based examples of their use are reported in Cooper et al. (2015) by Leicester and Nottingham NHS Trusts, and at NHS England's Nursing Technology Fund pages. These systems, whether electronic or paper based, do not guarantee accuracy in reporting and so must be part of a larger culture of ensuring patient safety and must be effectively monitored and managed if the benefits claimed are to be realised (CRD, 2014; Clifton et al., 2015).

Collaboration in Acute and Critical Care Provision

Whilst collaboration, that is, working together, is a common-sense expectation for health professionals faced with providing care for patients with increasingly complex needs, there is a large volume of research evidence which identifies that collaboration cannot be taken for granted (for examples see: Allen, 2001; Snelgrove and Hughes, 2002; Annandale et al., 2004). It is beyond the scope of this text to explore the reasons why relations between nursing and medicine in acute and other settings have been often been problematic. Some common factors have been repeatedly highlighted; these include differences in professional socialisation, medical dominance and the influence of gender as well as differences in professional role expectation and opportunities to work together (see, for example, Mackay, 1993; Davies, 1995; Hudson, 2002; Leathard, 2003; Nelson et al., 2008). Despite these well-documented problems there is increasing acceptance by policy makers and health professionals that collaborative multidisciplinary working not only makes good sense but it also results in improved patient outcomes, including reductions in morbidity and mortality (Stroke Unit Trialists' Collaboration, 2013; NICE, 2007; Massey et al., 2008). Multidisciplinary teams also include allied health professionals and an important contribution is being made by assistant critical care practitioners, healthcare assistants and other support workers. In most healthcare settings there are overlapping areas of clinical work but in acute and critical care settings in particular there is a high degree of interdependence between nursing and medical work and that of other professionals (see Figure i.1).

This interdependence is in part based on the traditional roles occupied by nurses and physicians. With few exceptions, nurses spend more time

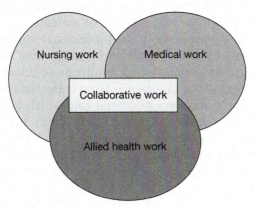

Figure i.1   Overlapping areas of work in acute and critical care

in direct contact with patients than almost all other health professional groups. As a result nurses are more likely to observe subtle changes in a patient's condition even if the signs which alert the nurse to a change are not always objective and may be based on an intuitive grasp that the patient needs close observation (Benner et al., 1996; Cioffi, 2002; Odell et al., 2009). However, whilst nurses are normally responsible for comprehensive assessment of patient need and monitor vital signs and response to treatment, determining the need for investigations and making a diagnosis remains (with exception of some advanced practice roles) a medical responsibility. However, it is not difficult to comprehend how important nursing assessment and reporting of patient data is in terms of making an early diagnosis and introducing appropriate interventions for acute and critically ill patients in a timely manner; increasingly this requires collaborative decision making. In order for there to be effective collaboration, the communication between multidisciplinary team members has to be frequent and requires use of a common, often technical language (Andrews and Waterman, 2005; Clarke, 2010). This impacts in turn on the education preparation of health professionals in pre-registration and continuing education programmes as it is within multidisciplinary or inter-professional programmes where shared understanding of roles, practice in joint problem solving and understanding and use of a common language are most likely to flourish (Young et al., 2003; Kilminster et al., 2004; Bandali et al., 2008).

The Organisation of this Book

This introduction has sought to establish the necessity for nurses to develop knowledge, understanding and competence in assessment, early recognition and appropriate management of patients in acute and critical care settings. This is based on both the professional imperative to develop the core skill of nursing assessment and the recognition that the evidence suggests that unless nurses and other health professionals develop these competencies, patients who experience acute deterioration and/or cardiac arrest will continue to receive suboptimal care which can lead to deaths which are largely preventable (NCEPOD, 2009, 2012). Early recognition of acute deterioration is dependent on skilled assessment but it also requires understanding of normal anatomy and physiology and the ways in which pathophysiology and disease result in changes and disruption in normal physiological processes. Throughout the book a series of case studies will be presented; the purpose of these is to help the reader to develop an understanding of the important interrelationship between presenting signs and symptoms, recognition of the underlying pathophysiology and the required nursing and medical assessment, and investigations and interventions required in acute and critical illness. The case scenarios will pose a series of questions to provoke the reader to reflect and think critically about their current knowledge, experience and understanding. Answers to the questions posed and further explanation will be provided in the subsequent text.

Chapter 1 of this book provides a detailed examination of the purpose and conduct of systematic history taking, physical assessment, including application of the ABCDE approach, the purpose of monitoring of vital signs, and using track and trigger systems; the chapter will establish the principles underpinning interpretation of clinical data. The information contained in Chapter 1 is designed to apply to all clinical settings where acutely ill adults are seen. Chapter 2 focuses on the key problem of shock and draws on common acute care scenarios to explain the nature and causation of shock. This chapter will also introduce key principles related to disturbances in acid–base balance and will outline the place of oxygen therapy in supporting acutely ill adults. These two chapters focus on essential aspects of assessment which will be applied and developed in each of the subsequent chapters of the book. In the remaining chapters the authors present case studies which illustrate commonly encountered problems related to a range of acute illness situations. New chapters in this edition include those focusing on caring for patients with sepsis and following stroke. The authors of each chapter identify key learning and action points and links to important resources (both online and paper based), and because no single text can cover all of the information which may be useful in acute and critical care, each chapter will also include suggestions for further reading. We believe this approach will ensure this book provides more than most narrowly focused anatomy and physiology or nursing care texts can, and will capture the interest of readers keen to develop their understanding of priorities in assessing and managing the acutely ill adult.

Note

All the case studies used in this book represent composites drawn from the common presenting signs and symptoms seen in acute and critical care patients; the names chosen for case study patients are fictitious.

Further Reading: Key Resources for Assessment and Management of Acute and Critical Illness

Clinical Guideline 50: *Acutely Ill Patients in Hospital: Recognition of and Response to Acute Illness in Adults in Hospital.* Prepared by the National Institute for Health and Clinical Excellence (NICE) (2007). Available from: http://guidance.nice.org.uk/CG50

'Resources and Good Practice Examples', in *Safer Care for the Acutely Ill Patient: Learning from Serious Incidents.* Fifth Report from the Patient Safety Observatory, pp. 26–36. (London: NHS National Patient Safety Agency, 2007). Available from: www.npsa. nhs.uk/nrls/alerts-and-directives/directives-guidance/acutely-ill-patient/

Resuscitation Council Guidelines (2015) Available from: www.resus.org.uk/resuscitation-guidelines/ Note: The 2015 guidelines do not include any significant changes to core interventions or processes.

Patient Safety First is a 'hub' for a number of patient safety improvement programmes and resources, and sits within the Patient Safety Domain Team of NHS England. The resources can be accessed via: www.patientsafetyfirst.nhs.uk/Content.aspx?path=/About-the-campaign/

References

Allen, D. *The Changing Shape of Nursing Practice* (London: Routledge, 2001).

Andrews, T. and H. Waterman. 'Packaging: A Grounded Theory of How to Report Physiological Deterioration Effectively', *Journal of Advanced Nursing* **52**(5) (2005), 473– 81.

Annandale, E, M. A. Elson, L. Prior (eds). *Medical Work, Medical Knowledge and Health Care* (Oxford: Blackwell Publishing, 2004).

Armitage, M., J. Eddlestone and T. Stokes. 'Recognising and responding to acute illness in adults in hospital: summary of NICE guidance'. *British Medical Journal*, **335** (2007), 258–9.

Bandali, K., K. Parker, M. Mummery and M. Preece. 'Skills Integration in a Simulated and Interprofessional Environment: An Innovative Undergraduate Applied Health Curriculum', *Journal of Interprofessional Care*, **22**(2) (2008), 179–89.

Bellomo, R., D. Goldsmith, S. Uchino, J. Buckmaster, G. Hart, H. Opdam, W. Silvester, L. Doolan and G. Gutteridge. 'Prospective Controlled Trial of the Effect of the Emergency Team on Morbidity and Mortality Rates', *Critical Care Medicine* **32**(4) (2004), 916–21.

Benner, P., C. A. Tanner and C. A. Chesla. *Expertise in Nursing Practice: Caring Clinical Judgment and Ethics* (New York: Springer, 1996).

Centre for Reviews and Dissemination (CRD). *Impact of Early Warning Systems on Patient Outcomes. Effectiveness Matters* (Centre for Reviews and Dissemination, University of York, 2014).

Cioffi, J. 'What are Clinical Judgements?', in C. Thompson and D. Dowding (eds), *Clinical Decision Making and Judgement in Nursing* (Edinburgh: Churchill Livingstone, 2002).

Clarke, D. J. 'Achieving Teamwork in Stroke Units: The Contribution of Opportunistic Dialogue', *Journal of Interprofessional Care*, **24**(3) (2010), 285–97.

Clifton, D. A, Lei Clifton, D. M. Sandhu et al.. 'Errors and Omissions in Paper-Based Early Warning Scores: The Association with Changes in Vital Signs – a Database Analysis', *BMJ Open* (2015), 5e:007376.

Cooper, A., J. Gorman and M. Wilson. 'Improving Observation with New Technology', *Nursing Times*, **111**(15) (2015), 12–24.

Critical Care Stakeholder Forum (CCSF). *Quality Critical Care: Beyond Comprehensive Critical Care*. A Report by the Critical Care Stakeholder Forum. (London: Critical Care Stakeholder Forum, 2005).

Davies, C. *Gender and the Professional Predicament in Nursing* (Buckingham: Open University Press, 1995).

Department of Health (DH). *Making a Difference: Strengthening the Nursing, Midwifery and Health Visiting Contribution to Health and Healthcare* (London: Department of Health, 1999).

Department of Health (DH). *Comprehensive Critical Care* (London: Department of Health, 2000a).

Department of Health (DH). *The NHS Plan: A Plan for Investment, a Plan for Reform* (London: Department of Health, 2000b).

Department of Health Modernisation Agency. *Critical Care Outreach: Progress in Developing Services* (London: Department of Health, 2003).

Eraut, M. *Developing Professional Knowledge and Competence* (London: Falmer, 1994).

Francis, R. 'Report of the Mid Staffordshire NHS Foundation Trust Public Inquiry. HC 947'. (London: The Stationery Office, 2013).

Goldhill, D. and A. McNarry. 'Physiological Abnormalities in Early Warning Scores are Related to Mortality in Adult Inpatients', *British Journal of Anaesthesia*, **92**(6) (2004), 882–4.

Hands, C., E. Reid, P. Meredith et al.. 'Patterns in the Recording of Vital Signs and Early Warning Scores: Compliance with an Escalation Protocol', *BMJ Quality and Safety*, **22** (2013), 719–26.

Hudson, B. (2002). 'Interprofessionality in Health and Social Care: The Achilles' Heel of Partnership?', *Journal of Interprofessional Care* **16**(1) (2002), 7–17.

Jevon, P. and B. Ewens. *Monitoring the Critically Ill Patient*, 3rd edn (Chichester: Wiley-Blackwell, 2012).

Kilminster, S., C. A. Hale, M. A. Lascelles, P. Morris, T. Roberts, P. Stark, J. R. Sowter and J. Thistlethwaite. 'Learning for Real Life: Patient-Focused Interprofessional Workshops Offer Added Value', *Medical Education*, **38**(7) (2004), 717–26.

Leathard, A. (ed.) *Interprofessional Collaboration: From Policy to Practice in Health and Social Care* (Hove: Brunner-Routledge, 2003).

Mackay, L. *Conflicts in Care: Medicine and Nursing* (London, Chapman Hall, 1993).

Manley, K. and S. Hardy. *Improving Services to Patients Through Ongoing Development of Critical Care Teams*. A Report Commissioned by the Department of Health (England). (London: Department of Health: 2006).

Massey, D., L. M. Aitken and C. Wendy (2008) 'What Factors Influence Suboptimal Ward Care in the Acutely Ill Ward Patient?', *Australian Critical Care*, **21**(3) (2008), 127–40.

Massey, D., L. M. Aitken and W. Chaboyer. 'Literature Review: Do Rapid Response Systems Reduce the Incidence of Major Adverse Events in the Deteriorating Ward Patient?', *Journal of Clinical Nursing*, **19** (2010), 3260–73.

McQuillan, P., S. Pilkington, A. Allan, B. Taylor, A. Short, G. Morgan, M. Nielsen, G. Barrett, and G. Smith. 'Confidential Inquiry into Quality of Care Before Admission to Intensive Care', *British Medical Journal*, **316** (1998), 1853–8.

Morgan, R. J. M., F. Williams, M. M. Wright. 'An Early Warning Scoring System for Detecting Developing Critical Illness. *Clinical Intensive Care*, **8** (1997), 100.

National Advisory Group on the Safety of Patients in England. *Improving the Safety of Patients in England* (London: Crown Publishers, 2013).

National Confidential Enquiry into Patient Outcome and Death (NCEOPD). *An Acute Problem: A Report of the National Confidential Enquiry into Patient Outcome and Death (NCEPOD)* (London: NCEPOD, 2005).

National Confidential Enquiry into Patient Outcome and Death (NCEPOD). *Deaths in Acute Hospitals: Caring to the End?* (London: NCEPOD, 2009).

National Confidential Enquiry into Patient Outcome and Death (NCEPOD). *Cardiac Arrest Procedures: Time to Intervene?* (London: NCEPOD, 2012).

National Institute for Health and Clinical Excellence (NICE). *Acutely Ill Patients in Hospital: Recognition of and Response to Acute Illness in Adults in Hospital. NICE Clinical Guideline 50* (London: National Institute for Health and Clinical Excellence, 2007).

National Outreach Forum (NORF). *Operational Standards and Competencies for Critical Care Outreach Services* [Online, 2012]. Available from: www.norf.org.uk/Resources/Documents/NOrF%20CCCO%20and%20standards/NOrF%20Operational%20Standards%20and%20Competencies%201%20August%202012.pdf (accessed 1 June 2015).

National Patient Safety Agency (NPSA). *Safer Care for the Acutely Ill Patient: Learning From Serious Incidents*. Fifth Report from the Patient Safety Observatory (London: NHS National Patient Safety Agency, 2007).

Nelson, G. A., M. L. King and S. Brodine. 'Nurse–Physician Collaboration on Medical–Surgical Units', *Medical–Surgical Nursing*, **17**(1) (2008), 35–40.

NHS England. *Patient Safety First 2015* (Leeds: NHS England, 2015).

Nightingale, F. 'Training of Nurses', in M. A. Nutting and L. Dock (eds), *History of Nursing: The Evolution of Nursing Systems from the Earliest Times to the Foundation of the first English and American Training Schools for Nurses*, Volume 2 (New York: Putman & Sons, 1907).

Odell, M. 'Detection and Management of the Deteriorating Ward Patient: An Evaluation of Nursing Practice', *Journal of Clinical Nursing* **24**(1–2) (2015), 173–82.

Odell, M., C. Victor and D. Oliver (2009). 'Nurses' role in detecting deterioration in ward patients: systematic literature review', *Journal of Advanced Nursing* **65** (2009), 1992–2006. doi: 10.1111/j.1365-2648.2009.05109.x

Priestley, G., W. Watson, A. Rashidian, C. Mozeley, D. Russell, J. Wilson, J. Cope, D. Hart, D. Kay, K. Cowley and J Pateraki. 'Introducing Critical Care Outreach: A Ward-Randomised Trial of Phased Introduction in a General Hospital', *Intensive Care Medicine* **30**(7) (2004), 1398–1404.

Royal College of Physicians (RCP). 'National Early Warning Score (NEWS) – Standardising the Assessment of Acute-illness Severity in the NHS' (2012) www.rcplondon.ac.uk/resources/national-early-warning-score-news (accessed 30 November 2015).

Seward, E., E. Greig, S. Preston, R. A. Harris, Z. Borrill, T. D. Wardle, R. Burnham, P. Driscoll, B. D. W. Harrison, D. C. Lowe and M. G. Pearson. 'A Confidential Study of Deaths after Emergency Medical Admission: Issues Relating to Quality of Care', *Clinical Medicine* **3**(5) (2003), 425–34(10).

Snelgrove, S. and D. Hughes. 'Perceptions of Teamwork in Acute Medical Wards', in D. Allen and D. Hughes (eds), *Nursing and the Division of Labour in Healthcare*. (Basingstoke, Palgrave Macmillan, 2002), 53–74.

Stroke Unit Trialists' Collaboration. 'Organised Inpatient (Stroke Unit) Care for Stroke', *Cochrane Database of Systematic Reviews*, **9** (2013), Art. No.: CD000197. DOI: 10.1002/14651858.CD000197.pub3.

Young, M. P., V. J. Gooder, K. McBride, B. James and E. S. Fisher. 'Inpatient Transfers to the Intensive Care Unit: Delays Are Associated with Increased Mortality and Morbidity', *Journal of General Internal Medicine*, **18**(2) (2003), 77–83.

1

Principles of Assessment

Julie Jackson

Introduction

The assessment and management of the acutely ill adult is an essential part of the role of the nurse. In the Introduction it was established that a consistent body of evidence shows that patients may be at risk of acute deterioration in clinical condition due to delayed recognition, the institution of inappropriate therapy, poor communication between clinical staff and a lack of escalation within medical teams (Goldhill et al., 1999; NCEPOD, 2005 and 2012; NPSA, 2007). For example, most cardio-respiratory arrests are predictable; in approximately 80 per cent of cases there is deterioration in clinical signs prior to an event. These patients often experience physiological deterioration that is unnoticed by staff or poorly treated, leading to suboptimal clinical outcome (Resuscitation Council UK, 2011). NICE guideline CG:50 *Acutely Ill Patients in Hospital: Recognition of and Response to Acute Illness in Adults in Hospital* (NICE, 2007) and the Department of Health's (2009) *Competencies for Recognising and Responding to Acutely Ill Patients in Hospital* were developed in direct response to concerns about the care of the acutely ill adult. These guidelines, which remain current, recognise that staff caring for acutely ill adults should have competencies in monitoring, measurement, interpretation and prompt response appropriate to the level of care they are providing; this chapter focuses on these important issues. Assessment is essentially a practical activity but knowledge application is vital for systematic, prioritised assessment. The Francis Report (The Mid Staffordshire NHS Foundation Trust Public Inquiry) (Francis, 2013) has had further impact at an organisational and practice level in reinforcing the importance of having an adequate number of highly skilled nurses in order to prevent adverse patient outcome. The theoretical and practical knowledge discussed in this chapter is applicable to primary, secondary and tertiary care in equal measures. A patient may present with acute illness

17

in any care setting and optimal clinical outcome is dependent upon early detection and management of deterioration.

Aim and Learning Outcomes

The Aim

The aim of this chapter is to explore the priorities in early assessment and management of the individual presenting with an acute event or a deteriorating clinical condition.

Learning Outcomes

At the end of this chapter the reader will be able to:

1. Discuss prioritisation of assessment and intervention.
2. Assess and monitor an acutely ill patient.
3. State the normal values of key physiological markers.
4. Identify a prioritised management plan appropriate to their own role.
5. Recognise the importance of multidisciplinary teamworking in acute care.

Assessment: Skills and Definitions

All patients in acute hospital settings should have a full assessment recorded at the time of admission (NICE, 2007). The preliminary assessment includes simultaneous measurement of the patient's vital signs, collection of essential biographical data, a brief accurate history of presenting signs and symptoms and specific investigation in order that life-saving intervention and symptom relief can be administered immediately. The secondary assessment includes a full clinical examination and provides more detailed information on past medical history, family, social and drug history, further diagnostic investigation and bio-psychosocial aspects of activities of daily living. The focus of this chapter is on the preliminary assessment for the acutely ill adult.

The aim of the preliminary assessment is threefold:

1. To collect a series of clues required to translate a provisional diagnosis into a definitive one that will inform prompt, appropriate and effective management.
2. To provide a baseline against which future measures can be compared to enable the early detection of improvement or deterioration in symptoms.
3. To determine current physiological status and inform the frequency and manner of ongoing assessment and investigation.

Table 1.1 Prerequisite skills for assessment

- Observation skills
- Application of knowledge and understanding of normal and abnormal physiological parameters
- Interpretation skills
- Critical thinking and decision-making skills
- Prioritisation of patient needs
- Communication skills and collaboration with the multidisciplinary team

---

Source: Adapted from Dougherty and Lister (2015) and Alfaro-LeFevre (2006).

Nursing assessment involves gathering and synthesising clinical data, recording this information and recognising and communicating abnormalities. It is an ongoing dynamic process that requires a range of prerequisite skills (Table 1.1). Monitoring of vital signs is a fundamental aspect of care that may be considered a basic, routine activity that simply requires a practical awareness of how to perform and record the physical assessment. However, accurate and meaningful assessment is more than the ability to operate an electronic device or count pulsation at the radial artery: it is important to contextualise the data collected. Therefore a high degree of knowledge application is required if results are to be correctly synthesised, reported and responded to. Knowledge of normal physiological parameters is essential but taken in isolation can be of limited value. It is of greater importance to know what is 'normal' for a particular patient, or, if previous observations are not available, what could be considered normal with a particular clinical presentation. There is, however, a danger that accepting recordings that are believed to be 'the patient's normal' may obscure evidence of deterioration and it is useful to remember that grossly abnormal observations are rarely 'normal'. Two or more deteriorating observations can be an ominous sign of imminent severe clinical deterioration, and to appreciate this and other issues fully, application of knowledge to practice is vital. Furthermore, competent observation, measurement, accurate recording and application of knowledge and understanding to interpretation of data, are essential prerequisites for informed decision making. Observations should therefore be recorded and acted upon by clinical staff with appropriate training and knowledge. Student nurses are often responsible for the monitoring and documentation of vital signs but they should only perform this clinical activity if they have been observed and assessed by experienced nurses and are competent to do so. Lastly, communication to and collaboration with a team of staff from varying backgrounds possessing a range of skills is essential for effective clinical intervention (DH, 2009).

The structure of an assessment will depend upon the clinical presentation, the care setting and clinical need. An acutely ill patient may be encountered in primary, secondary and tertiary care and optimal clinical outcome is dependent upon early recognition and management of a potentially life-threatening problem. The health professional requires good acute assessment skills in all care settings, particularly as rapid response and outreach or other acute services are now being provided in primary care. The UK Guidelines for Resuscitation were updated in late 2015; these guidelines underpin much of the practice of nurses, physicians and allied health professionals working with the acutely ill adult. The focus of this chapter is the theoretical and practical aspects of assessment of the acutely ill adult using the ABCDE approach (Airway, Breathing, Circulation, Disability and Exposure) (Resuscitation Council UK, 2015a) in a hospital setting.

Assessing the Acutely Ill Adult

The ABCDE approach provides a systematic method of clinical assessment that can be used and understood by all members of the healthcare team. It ensures that the most vital signs for life are assessed and managed in a logical manner. However, a theoretical knowledge and understanding of normal and abnormal physiological parameters is essential if data is to be appropriately interpreted and acted upon. The ABCDE assessment should then form the basis for a more detailed preliminary and secondary assessment.

Underlying Principles

- Complete an initial assessment following the ABCDE approach.
- Treat life-threatening problems when encountered, before moving on to the next part of the assessment.
- Reassess regularly. (How frequently will depend on the problem and the clinical status of the patient. But once ABCDE is completed, it will need to be repeated at intervals specified by medical or senior nursing staff.)
- Assess the effects of treatment and interventions.
- Recognise when additional help is required – for example, from other members of the multidisciplinary team – and call for help early.
  (Adapted from Resuscitation Council UK, 2015b)

Always think about personal safety before any assessment begins. Look for danger in the environment; this may be from a tripping hazard, traffic, a noxious substance, electricity or any other number of potential hazards.

The Systematic ABCDE Approach

A: Airway

Airway is assessed in order to recognise any signs of obstruction. If a patient is able to talk the airway is patent. Causes of airway obstruction include central nervous system depression causing loss of patency and protective reflexes, vomit, a foreign body, epiglottitis, infection, allergy, laryngeal spasm or bronchial secretions and bronchospasm (Resuscitation Council UK, 2011). If there is a reason to suspect that the airway may be compromised, the look, listen and feel approach will provide confirmation and potentially identify the cause (Table 1.2).

Look:

- In the mouth for any physical obstruction.
- At chest movement and breathing pattern for symmetrical movement. See-saw breathing (paradoxical abdominal and chest movement) whereby the abdomen and chest move alternately is a sign of obstruction as the air in the lungs cannot exit via the airway.

Listen:

- To the sound of breathing. Normal breathing is not noisy and so loud gurgling, snoring, wheezing or croaking is abnormal and requires intervention.

Feel:

- For breath against the hand or cheek to establish if there is evidence of air movement.
- The chest for signs of fluid. Obstruction from secretions is suspected if gurgling is heard and can sometimes be felt by placing a hand on the upper chest.

Table 1.2 Signs of compromised airway

- Difficulty talking or unable to talk
- Choking
- Shortness of breath or difficulty breathing, use of accessory muscles
- Noisy breathing: stridor, wheeze or gurgling
- See-saw respiratory pattern

Source: Adapted from Resuscitation Council UK (2011).

Airway obstruction is a medical emergency and requires urgent intervention to prevent hypoxic organ damage and death. If suspected, get expert help immediately (Resuscitation Council UK, 2015a).

TREATMENT OF AIRWAY OBSTRUCTION

Airway obstruction is a stressful clinical situation and speed is required to prevent rapid deterioration. However, relatively simple interventions can improve outcome (Table 1.3). Repositioning a patient on their side (lateral position) unless contraindicated and insertion of simple airway adjuncts – for example, a nasal or oropharyngeal airway and suctioning – can be successful in a patient with a partially obstructed airway caused by secretions (Resuscitation Council UK, 2015a). This is a common cause of airway obstruction in the clinical environment and physiotherapists are often skilled at assisting with removal of excess secretions.

OXYGEN THERAPY

If a patient is critically ill or in a peri-arrest situation then 15 L/minute of oxygen therapy should be delivered via a non-rebreathe bag and reservoir mask. Once the patient has stabilised the oxygen can be reduced to maintain a normal oxygen saturation (SpO_2) of 94 to 98 per cent. Patients with chronic obstructive pulmonary disease (COPD) and other risk factors for hypercapnia (high carbon dioxide) who develop critical illness should have the same target saturations of 94 to 98 per cent as other critically ill patients, until the results of blood gas analysis are available and there is a clinical indication to reduce the target saturation and therefore the oxygen concentration (British Thoracic Society, 2016).

B: Breathing

Breathing is often the first vital sign to alter in a patient with a deteriorating condition and respiratory dysfunction can be predictive of an adverse clinical event (NICE, 2007; NPSA, 2007). Respiration is a complex process that incorporates four distinct events. Pulmonary ventilation (breathing) promotes air

Table 1.3 Treatment of airway obstruction

- Get expert help immediately (Ring 2222 in hospital, 999 out of hospital)
- Airway opening, i.e. head tilt, chin lift or jaw thrust
- Simple airway adjuncts
- Advanced techniques, i.e. intubation or emergency tracheostomy
- Provide oxygen

Source: Adapted from Resuscitation Council UK (2011).

movement in and out of the lungs. External respiration is gas exchange at the alveoli and pulmonary capillary interface (oxygen loading and carbon dioxide unloading). Respiratory gas transport requires oxygen and carbon dioxide to be transported to and from the lungs and cells of the body via the bloodstream. Internal respiration is gas exchange at the interface between systemic capillaries and tissue cells (Marieb, 2015). All four processes must be fully functioning for effective respiration. Respiration may not only be affected by disease or injury of the respiratory system (bronchi, alveoli, chest wall etc.) but many other disorders (cerebral, neurological, cardiac, sepsis or anaphylaxis etc.) may initially present with tachypnoea (Table 1.4). Assessment of breathing should include look, listen and feel.

Look for:

- difficulty in breathing;
- sweating;
- tachypnoea (respiratory rate > 20 breaths per minute);
- accessory muscle use (use of the sternocleidomastoid and the scalene muscles, not seen in normal respiration);
- skin colour – central cyanosis is notable as a blue tinge to the lips and tongue;
- abnormal physiology, i.e. deviated trachea or uneven chest movement;
- altered consciousness level;
- a measure of SpO_2 (normal range 94 to 98 per cent);
- an increase in amount/colour/consistency of sputum.

Listen for:

- noisy breathing – wheeze, gurgling, stridor, cough;
- breath sounds (by auscultation) for bilateral air entry.

Table 1.4 Common causes of respiratory compromise

- Airway obstruction
- Underlying respiratory illness: chronic obstructive pulmonary disease (COPD), asthma
- Lung pathology: pulmonary oedema, pneumothorax, carcinoma, infection such as TB or pneumonia, pulmonary embolus, pulmonary hypertension
- Drugs: opiates, sedatives
- Central nervous system depression: disease or injury
- Shock: sepsis, cardiogenic, anaphylaxis
- Cardiac: left ventricular failure
- Chest trauma: flail chest

Feel for:

- lung expansion (this can be felt if both hands are placed on the chest wall: on inspiration hands should move apart evenly);
- presence of secretions;
- surgical emphysema (presence of gas or air in the subcutaneous tissue);
- chest percussion (an airway clearance technique to loosen secretions. It involves clapping with cupped hands on the back and chest).
  (Adapted from Resuscitation Council UK, 2015a)

RESPIRATORY RATE

Respiratory rate is measured over one minute and each count includes the rise and fall of the chest which equates to one breath (Jevon and Ewens, 2012). Opinion on normal values varies slightly but 12 to 20 breaths per minute is generally accepted as normal (Resuscitation Council UK, 2015a). Tachypnoea is an early sign of respiratory distress and a deteriorating clinical condition (Table 1.5). Respiratory depth, pattern and sound such as wheezing, stridor, obstruction or coughing should also be documented (Woodrow, 2012). Cheyne–Stokes respiration describes an irregular breathing pattern interrupted by periods of apnoea and is associated with brain stem ischaemia and end of life (Kennedy, 2007). Deep, rapid respirations or Kussmaul breathing (air hunger) is associated with metabolic acidosis (Jevon and Ewens, 2012) caused by sepsis, uraemia or diabetic ketoacidosis. A period of tachypnoea followed by a slower rate of less than 12 breaths per minute may be a sign of impending respiratory arrest that could be misconstrued as an improvement when in fact the reverse could be true. Normal breathing should be effortless whereas the use of accessory muscles, seen in

Table 1.5 Glossary of respiratory terms

- Tachypnoea: a respiratory rate above 20
- Bradypnoea: a respiratory rate below 12
- Apnoea: an absence of respiration
- Cyanosis: a bluish discolouration of the skin and mucous membranes caused by lack of oxygen in the blood
- Hypoxia: inadequate oxygen supply is available to the tissues
- Dyspnoea: laboured difficult breathing
- Hypoxaemia: reduced arterial blood oxygen ($PaO_2 < 8$ kPa). Can be with or without increased arterial carbon dioxide
- Hypercapnia: increased arterial carbon dioxide ($PaCO_2 > 6$ kPa)

Source: Adapted from Marieb (2015).

the shoulders and neck, will give the appearance of difficult and laboured breathing (dyspnoea). A bluish tinge to the skin and mucous membranes combined with clammy skin may indicate hypoxia. It is important to check the central position of the trachea in the suprasternal notch as deviation to one side suggests mediastinal shift and requires urgent intervention (Resuscitation Council UK, 2015a). A chest X-ray will provide detailed anatomical information such as the presence of a pneumothorax, pleural fluid, pulmonary oedema, infection or lung fibrosis.

OXYGEN SATURATION

During respiration oxygen crosses the alveolar capillary interface of the lungs and enters the circulation. Up to four oxygen atoms can attach to the haemoglobin of each red blood cell, forming oxyhaemoglobin which is then transported to the tissues in the bloodstream. The percentage of haemoglobin saturated with oxygen is known as the oxygen saturation (SaO_2) (Booker, 2008). Arterial blood gas saturations (SaO_2) are very similar to peripheral (capillary) saturation (SpO_2) and so differences are considered insignificant for practice (Woodrow, 2012). Pulse oximetry is an inexpensive and non-invasive method of continuous measurement of arterial oxygen saturation (Jevon and Ewens, 2012). A pulse oximeter consists of a peripheral probe, attached to a patient's finger, and a processing unit, which measures SpO_2 by calculating the amount of haemoglobin saturated with oxygen (Cooper et al., 2006). The relationship between SaO_2 and the partial pressure of oxygen in the arterial system (PaO_2) is shown by the S-shaped haemoglobin oxygen dissociation curve (Figure 1.1).

Figure 1.1 The oxygen dissociation curve

Table 1.6   Treatment of breathing problems

- Open airway
- Position patient appropriately
- Administer oxygen (BTS 2016 Guidelines)
- Get expert help
- Treat underlying cause
- Support breathing if inadequate i.e. pocket mask ventilation or bag-valve and mask

---

Source: Adapted from Resuscitation Council UK (2011).

A saturation of 93 per cent equates approximately to a PaO_2 of 8 kPa. Figure 1.1 demonstrates that as the saturation falls below 90 per cent the PaO_2 falls rapidly below 8 kPa following the steep decline of the S-shaped curve. The body at this point would become critically short of oxygen with severe hypoxaemia. Conversely, at normal levels of PaO_2 (11 to 13 kPa) the SaO_2 will be above 95 per cent. As the curve flattens an increase in SaO_2 has very little effect upon PaO_2. National guidelines suggest aiming for an SpO_2 of 94 to 98 per cent or 88 to 92 per cent in patients with type 2 respiratory failure (see Chapter 7) until blood gas results are available (British Thoracic Society, 2016). Pulse oximetry is extremely useful but care must be taken to ensure an accurate reading. A regular waveform trace should correspond to pulse rate to ensure accuracy (Jevon and Ewens, 2012). The probe should be positioned in an area that is warm and well perfused with blood (fingers and earlobes are common sites), and it should be repositioned regularly to avoid pressure ulcer development. Dark nail polish may interfere with the signal, causing inaccuracy (Booker, 2008) and anaemia can lead to an underestimate of oxygen saturation. A haemoglobin level of 8.0 g/dL (normal range 11.5–18.0 g/dL) can underestimate SaO_2 by 10 to 15 per cent (Cooper et al., 2006) and pulse oximetry is not reliable if carbon monoxide poisoning is suspected (Woodrow, 2012). A pulse oximeter is not a replacement for observation of the patient and should be interpreted alongside other vital signs and clinical signs and symptoms. It is very important to be aware that SpO_2 is only a measure of oxygenation and not ventilation (Jevon and Ewens, 2012). It provides no information regarding arterial carbon dioxide tensions ($PaCO_2$) or abnormalities such as carbon dioxide retention or blood pH; arterial blood gas (ABG) analysis provides more detailed information. The blood pH must be maintained between 7.35 and 7.45 for the cells of the body to function effectively (Marieb, 2015). A rise in arterial carbon dioxide levels above the normal range (4.6 to 6.0 kPa) will cause the blood pH to fall below 7.35, causing a respiratory acidosis in the absence of metabolic compensation (Resuscitation Council 2015a) (see Chapters 2 and 7 for further detail on ABG analysis).

PATIENT POSITIONING

Patient positioning will depend upon the clinical presentation. If a patient is conscious and struggling to breathe, sitting upright is the optimal position for lung expansion. If, however, they have an altered consciousness level and are unable to maintain an open airway, a supine position is required to facilitate airway management and breathing support. The patient can be managed in the lateral position when stabilised. Expert help will be required during the assessment of breathing to establish the underlying cause of compromise, and life-threatening conditions must be diagnosed and treated immediately: for example, acute severe asthma, tension pneumothorax and pulmonary oedema (Resuscitation Council UK, 2015a). The table 1.6 lists the key principles of treatment.

C: Circulation

Circulatory assessment includes a general observation of the patient while recording a number of vital signs. Table 1.7 lists some of the common causes of cardiovascular compromise; however, almost all pathophysiological organ dysfunction will manifest in changes to circulatory status. The look, listen and feel approach can also be used.

- Look at the patient – peripheries may be pale or cyanosed.
- Feel the pulse for rate, rhythm and depth.
- Visually assess peripheral perfusion – capillary refill time (see description below).
- Assess the state of the veins – collapsed could be a sign of hypovolaemia.
- Measure blood pressure.
- Assess organ perfusion – measure urine output (kidney perfusion), ask if there is chest pain (heart perfusion), assess level of consciousness (AVPU) (brain perfusion) (see D (disability) below for details of AVPU).
- Perform an electrocardiogram (ECG).
- Look for haemorrhage or fluid loss.
  (Adapted from Resuscitation Council UK, 2015b)

HEART RATE

The expansion and recoil of an artery that occurs with each beat of the left ventricle creates a wave of pressure that travels through the arterial system. This pressure wave can be palpated when an artery passes over a bone as the

Table 1.7 Common causes of cardiovascular compromise

- Acute coronary syndromes
- Heart failure
- Cardiac arrhythmias
- Shock (hypovolaemic, septic, cardiogenic, neurogenic, anaphylactic)
- Pulmonary embolism

Table 1.8 Glossary of cardiovascular terms

- Tachycardia: An excessive heart rate above 100 beats per minute
- Bradycardia: A slow heart beat below 60 beats per minute
- Normotensive: a blood pressure that is within a normal range 100/60–140/90 mmHg
- Hypotension: generally considered to be a systolic blood pressure below 100 mmHg (potential causes are physiological shock, acute coronary syndromes, heart failure)
- Hypertension: a condition of sustained elevated arterial pressure of 140/90 mmHg or higher

Source: Adapted from Marieb (2015).

pulse. In a healthy individual heart rate will equate to pulse rate (Marieb, 2015). The normal range is generally regarded to be 60 to 100 beats per minute, though the average heart rate is slightly faster in adult females (72 to 80 beats per minute) than in males (64 to 72 beats per minute) (Marieb, 2015). Common causes of abnormal heart rate are listed in Table 1.9.

Table 1.9 Common causes of abnormal heart rate

Increased rate	*Decreased rate*
<ul><li>Exercise</li><li>Pain, anxiety</li><li>Pyrexia</li><li>Cardiac arrhythmia</li><li>Compensatory response to low BP, e.g. myocardial infarction, left ventricular failure, hypovolaemia</li><li>Chronotropic drugs, e.g. atropine®, isoprenaline®</li><li>Inotropic drugs, e.g. dobutamine®</li></ul>	<ul><li>Increased vagal activity, e.g. carotid sinus massage</li><li>Athletic heart</li><li>Cardiac conduction defects</li><li>Raised intracranial pressure</li><li>Drugs: beta blockers, e.g. atenolol®; calcium channel blockers, e.g. verapamil®</li></ul>

When assessing the pulse it is also important to assess rhythm and amplitude (Dougherty and Lister, 2015). The pause between pulsations provides information about the heart rhythm, which should be smooth and regular. An irregular heart rate could have many causes such as ectopic (extra) beats, atrial fibrillation or conduction defects, and should be reported immediately. Application of a sound knowledge base to practice is an essential part of assessment if relevant clinical signs and symptoms are to be synthesised and communicated. The amplitude reflects the pulse strength and elasticity of the arterial wall. A pulse may be 'weak', 'strong', 'faint' or 'bounding' (Dougherty and Lister, 2015); however, assessment of amplitude is by its nature reliant upon a degree of subjectivity and therefore tends to be reported by more experienced nurses or physicians. Both peripheral and central pulses should be assessed for rate, rhythm and amplitude. Central pulses are located at the carotid artery (neck) and femoral artery (groin); commonly palpated peripheral pulses are radial artery (wrist) and brachial pulse (elbow). A bounding pulse may indicate sepsis and a barely palpable central pulse can be caused by low cardiac output (Resuscitation Council UK, 2015b). Amplitude and rhythm are rarely detected by any electronic monitoring device, so a pulse must be palpated manually for accurate assessment, usually using the radial artery for convenience and counted over one minute. The sole reliance in some clinical areas upon electronic monitoring devices may be detrimental to the assessment process and lead to some inaccuracies or incomplete data collection, and could also deskill healthcare professionals.

SYSTOLIC BLOOD PRESSURE

Blood pressure (BP) is the pressure exerted by the blood against the inner walls of arteries and is responsible for maintaining blood circulation between heartbeats. It is directly related to cardiac output (CO) (amount of blood ejected from the left ventricle in one minute) and systemic vascular resistance (SVR) (the diameter of the vessel) (Marieb, 2015):

$$BP = CO \times SVR$$

Arterial BP has two measurements. Systolic pressure is the pressure in the arteries at the peak of left ventricular (LV) contraction and diastolic pressure is the pressure exerted when the ventricles relax. Blood pressure is usually expressed in terms of millimetres of mercury (mmHg). In a normal adult at rest systolic blood pressure varies between 110 and 140 mmHg but blood pressure varies with age, weight, race, mood and physical activity (Marieb, 2015). In track and trigger systems (see page 37), a comparable numerical figure is required, which is usually the systolic pressure as it is regarded as a more reliable marker of health status than diastolic pressure.

Diastolic pressure usually varies in a normal adult at rest between 60 and 90 mmHg. BP may initially be recorded within normal limits despite underlying pathophysiological abnormality as it is maintained by stimulation of a number of compensatory mechanisms and increased peripheral resistance in response to an initial fall in BP (see Chapter 2). However, the pulse pressure may be narrowed (the difference between systolic and diastolic pressure, normally 35 to 45 mmHg). Other signs of poor cardiac output, such as altered consciousness level and oliguria (urine volume less than 0.5 mL/kg/hr), should also be noted (Resuscitation Council UK, 2015b). An increase in BP may be associated with anxiety or pain associated with the situation or may indicate underlying hypertension. The cause of essential (primary) hypertension is multifactorial, often associated with lifestyle characteristics such as obesity, physical inactivity, high salt intake and stress; it can also be hereditary. Secondary hypertension is associated with anatomical or pathophysiological disorders: for example, raised intracranial pressure (ICP) and renal, adrenal or aortic disease. Many conditions may cause low BP, such as myocardial dysfunction, low ICP, antihypertensive medication or hypovolaemia. Low BP caused by haemorrhage is not always immediately obvious. External bleeding may be visible from wounds and drains, but internal haemorrhage is less visible and is often characterised by localised pain and swelling. There are manual, electronic and invasive methods of recording BP but the most reliable and accurate method is often regarded as the manual technique, so this is an essential skill for all healthcare professionals assessing acutely ill patients.

MEAN ARTERIAL PRESSURE

In the critical care environment mean arterial pressure is often used as a marker of clinical status but this is more difficult to calculate as it requires an intra-arterial catheter or a mathematical calculation (Dougherty and Lister, 2015):

Mean arterial pressure = 1/3 systolic pressure + 2/3 diastolic pressure

CAPILLARY REFILL TIME

Peripheries are often pale and cool in cardiovascular compromise and capillary refill time (CRT) can be prolonged. CRT can be measured by applying pressure to a fingertip held at heart level for five seconds to cause blanching (loss of colour). CRT is measured as the time it takes to return to normal colour. A CRT greater than two seconds is considered abnormal although older age and low environmental temperature can have the same effect (Resuscitation Council UK, 2015b). CRT may also be misleading in pyrexial septic patients due to an inflammatory response causing peripheral vasodilation, characterised by very warm peripheries. Pale, cool peripheries can be due to poor perfusion caused by arterial vasoconstriction, suggestive of hypovolaemic shock or cardiac failure.

In almost all medical and surgical emergencies, until proven otherwise, hypovolaemia should be considered as the primary cause of shock. Unless a cardiac problem is suspected intravenous fluids should be given to any patients with cool peripheries and tachycardia (Table 1.10). Important additional evaluation of haematological, biochemical, coagulation and microbiological investigations and cross matching should aid diagnosis if haemorrhage is suspected. A fluid challenge of 500 mL of warmed intravenous crystalloid for a normotensive patient, or 1 litre if the patient is hypotensive, can be prescribed by a suitably qualified health professional (Resuscitation Council UK, 2015b). Some clinicians may prefer to give colloid (see Chapter 2). The heart rate and BP should be checked every five minutes during the acute stage of intervention to prevent fluid overload and cardiac failure (Resuscitation Council UK, 2015b). A raised jugular venous pressure (JVP) or central venous pressure (CVP) (right atrial pressure, measurable if a central line is present) could indicate fluid overload and inotropes or vasopressors may be prescribed (see Chapter 2).

D: Disability

Assessment to establish the cause of an altered state of consciousness is imperative.

LEVEL OF CONSCIOUSNESS

A reduced consciousness level is associated with potentially life-threatening complications, including airway obstruction, hypoxaemia and aspiration (Cooper et al., 2006) and so is a very important element of the assessment process. AVPU is a rapid method of neurological assessment and is particularly useful in an emergency situation where speed is required (Resuscitation Council UK, 2011).

Table 1.10 Treatment of circulatory problems

- Seek expert help
- Treat cause if known (cardiac tamponade, haemorrhage, shock)
- IV access – take bloods
- Give fluid challenge
- Reassess and monitor
- Treat acute coronary syndromes (see Chapter 6)

AVPU stands for **a**lert, **v**oice, **p**ain, **u**nresponsive:

- Alert;
- Responsive to verbal stimuli;
- Responsive to painful stimuli;
- Unresponsive.

A normal level of consciousness would include an alert patient and one who could respond to verbal stimuli from a state of sleep. A patient who requires painful stimuli to achieve a response (see Chapter 4) or who is unresponsive would be classed as having an altered level of consciousness (Table 1.11). If greater depth of neurological assessment is required, the Glasgow Coma Scale (GCS) (Teasdale, 2014a; Teasdale et al., 2014b) provides a numerical score and so a more quantifiable and comparable figure (see Chapter 4). If a patient is alert then their airway will be patent but if they present with an altered level of consciousness then their airway may be compromised and so it is essential that assessment returns to ABC to establish if the situation is a medical emergency.

Examine and assess:

- assess consciousness using AVPU and/or GCS (and check pupil, size, equality and reaction to light);
- check drug chart (Naloxone® can be given for opioid toxicity);
- measure blood glucose (exclude hypoglycaemia: if less than 3 mmol, give 50 mL of 10 per cent glucose IV) or hyperglycaemia in diabetic ketoacidosis (see Chapter 10);
- nurse unconscious patients in the lateral position if possible.
  (Resuscitation Council UK, 2015b)

Table 1.11   Common causes of neurological compromise

- Hypoxia
- Poor cerebral perfusion
- Cerebral pathology (disease or injury)
- Drugs (opiates, sedatives) and alcohol
- Hypercapnia
- Hypoglycaemia or hyperglycaemia
- Uraemia
- Hypovolaemia
- Cardiac arrhythmia
- Peri/post-cardiac arrest

E: Exposure

Full exposure of the patient's body may be required to gain a complete clinical picture, maintaining privacy and dignity and preventing heat loss. An initial examination can exclude any obvious external haemorrhage and note any skin rash, redness or oedema.

- Take a full clinical history.
- Review the case notes and charts (look for significant clinical history and abnormality).
- Note vital sign trends.
- Give prescribed medications.
- Review the results of investigations (laboratory and radiological).
- Consider the level of care required by the patient (i.e. ward, high dependency unit (HDU) or intensive care unit (ICU)).
- Record in the patient notes details of assessment, treatment and response to therapy.
(Adapted from Resuscitation Council UK, 2015b)

TEMPERATURE

In a healthy individual core body temperature is relatively constant, with a normal range of 35 to 37 °C (Woodrow, 2012), though opinion varies and 37.5 °C is accepted by some physicians as the upper end of the normal range. Higgins (2008) defines pyrexia as a temperature above 37.5 °C and hypothermia as a temperature below 35.0 °C (Table 1.12). A temperature above 41°C (hyperpyrexia) is dangerous and may cause convulsions and be fatal (Table 1.13). A temperature below 32 °C is similarly dangerous and can cause cardiac arrhythmias (Woodrow, 2012). Through autonomic nervous system pathways the hypothalamus regulates body temperature. In a pyrexial illness macrophages, white blood cells and injured tissue cells release pyrogens that act directly on the hypothalamus, altering the internal thermostat to a higher temperature. The body initiates heat-conserving mechanisms, vasoconstriction redirects blood away from the skin surface preventing heat loss from radiation and convection, and shivering creates heat (Marieb, 2015).

A patient who is pale, shivering and complaining of the cold may well have a high temperature. Once the thermostat is reset due to the administration of medication or an improvement in the clinical condition, the patient will begin to sweat and the skin may appear flushed. A fever can actually speed up the healing process and inhibit bacterial growth by increasing the metabolic rate; however, if the thermostat is set too high body proteins may be denatured and permanent brain damage can occur (Marieb, 2015).

When devising a management plan for a pyrexial patient it is important to consider the comfort of the patient, the dangers associated with an elevated temperature and the protective nature of fever.

Body temperature can be recorded orally, per axilla, rectally, via the ear canal (tympanic) or via a skin probe. There are a wide range of thermometers available and the choice will depend upon the availability of the equipment and the condition of the patient, though oral and tympanic thermometers are commonly used. If a patient is to have an oral reading taken they must not have had a hot or cold drink or smoked in the 15 minutes prior to assessment in order to ascertain accurate data (Dougherty and Lister, 2015). As with any equipment, training and competency will be required before use and with any multi-use equipment it should be clean in line with infection control policies.

Oxygen consumption will be elevated in a pyrexial patient so SpO_2 will often decrease as temperature rises. A pyrexia will shift the oxygen dissociation curve to the right (Figure 1.1) so the affinity of haemoglobin for oxygen decreases, causing unloading of oxygen at the tissues and increased tissue oxygenation. Conversely, hypothermia shifts the curve to the left and the haemoglobin affinity for oxygen increases (Woodrow, 2012). An increase in body temperature will have a marked effect upon

Table 1.12   Glossary of temperature terms

Pyrexia	Temperature above 37.5 °C
Febrile	Temperature above 37.5 °C
Apyrexial	Temperature between 36–37.5 °C
Afebrile	Temperature between 36–37.5 °C
Hypothermia	Temperature below 35 °C

Source: Adapted from Marieb (2015).

Table 1.13   Causes of hypothermia and hyperthermia

Causes of hypothermia	*Causes of hyperthermia (pyrexia)*
• Exposure	• Infection (commonly)
• Metabolic derangement	• Central nervous system problem
• Medication	• Systemic inflammatory response
• Alcohol	syndrome (Sirs)
• Septic shock	• Medication

Source: Adapted from Higgins (2008).

other vital signs. Heart rate and respiratory rate will rise as the metabolic rate increases, so as with all vital sign interpretation assessment must be comprehensive to be accurate.

Additional Assessment Data

In addition to the physiological observations required NICE (2007) suggests monitoring:

- biochemistry (Table 1.14);
- haematology (Table 1.15);
- ABGs (see Chapter 2, Table 2.5);
- microbiology if infection is suspected;
- liver function tests (LFT) (see Chapter 11, Table 11.3);
- hourly urine output;
- pain.

Nurses are often responsible for accepting blood and urine results so it is essential to have a good working knowledge of 'normal values'.

Hourly Urine Output

A fluid balance chart collated over a 24-hour period will provide valuable information regarding a patient's fluid status. In health, intake will largely

Table 1.14   Blood biochemistry normal values (mmol/L)

Urea and electrolytes (U&E)	
Sodium (Na⁺)	135–145
Potassium (K⁺)	3.5–5.0
Chloride (Cl)	95–105
Urea	2.2–7.7
Creatinine	50–120 (µmol/L)
Bicarbonate (HCO₃)	22–32
Glucose	3.0–5.0
Calcium	2.1–2.6
Magnesium	0.7–1
Cholesterol	3.0–5.0
Triglyceride	0.0–2.3

Note: Normal values differ between men and women and local laboratory test procedures.

Table 1.15 Haematology normal values

Full blood count (FBC)	
Haemaglobin (Hb)	11.5–16 g/dL
Mean cell volume (MCV)	70–100 fL
Red blood cells (RBC)	$3.7–5.5 \times 10^{12}/L$
White blood cells (WBC)	$4–11 \times 10^9/L$
Platelets	$130–400 \times 10^9/L$
Clotting	
Prothrombin time (PT)	12–16 seconds
International normalised ratio (INR)	1
Fibrinogen	1.5–4.0 g/L

Note: Normal values differ between men and women and local laboratory test procedures.

equal output, with a degree of insensible loss. The amount of urine produced will depend upon intake but a healthy individual can be expected to produce 1 mL/kg/hr (Scales and Pilsworth, 2008). A urine output of less than 30 mL/hr in an adult patient suggests the kidneys are underperfused and requires further investigation and intervention (see Chapter 8). Fluid resuscitation for hypovolaemia should result in a positive fluid balance over 24 hours, whereas diuretic or renal therapy should culminate in a negative balance.

Pain

Pain assessment and control is required to ensure patient comfort and a variety of pain assessment tools exist to aid this process. The choice of tool will depend upon patient presentation. There are also important physiological reasons for good pain control as the effects of severe pain include:

- tachycardia, hypertension and increased myocardial oxygen demand;
- nausea and vomiting;
- inadequate lung expansion and inability to cough – basal atelectasis and chest infections;
- urinary retention;
- thromboembolism due to inactivity;
- pressure sores due to immobility.
  (Adapted from Cooper et al., 2006)

Physiological Track and Trigger Systems

Physiological track and trigger systems should be used to monitor all patients in acute care environmenets (NCEPOD, 2005; NICE, 2007). Track and trigger systems are also known as early warning scoring systems (EWSS). They emerged from the review of adult critical care services (DH, 2000) and were designed to recognise early signs of deterioration in level 0 and 1 patients (Oakey and Slade, 2006). There are a wide variety of systems that all rely on observation of selected basic physiological signs (tracking) with predetermined calling criteria (triggers) for requesting the attendance of staff who have competencies in the management of acute illness (NICE, 2007). NCEPOD (2012) found that 98.9 per cent of hospitals studied were using an EWSS. The National Early Warning Score (NEWS) was launched in 2012 by the Royal College of Physicians (RCP, 2012). It is a standardised system devised by doctors and nurses and is now in use throughout much of the NHS. Figure 1.2 shows the NEWS scoring system and Figure 1.4 NEWS thresholds and triggers for action. The National Early Warning Score aims to help both nursing and medical staff to identify patients who are acutely ill or at risk of deterioration. The tracking signs are respiratory rate, oxygen saturations, any supplemental oxygen, temperature, systolic BP, heart rate and level of consciousness relating to AVPU. Each tracking sign receives a score depending upon patient presentation and scores are added together to provide a final score. The final National Early Warning Score triggers a response, shown in Figure 1.5. A low National Early Warning

PHYSIOLOGICAL PARAMETERS	3	2	1	0	1	2	3
Respiration Rate	≤8		9 – 11	12 – 20		21 – 24	≥25
Oxygen Saturations	≤91	92 – 93	94 – 95	≥96			
Any Supplemental Oxygen		Yes		No			
Temperature	≤35.0		35.1 – 36.0	36.1 – 38.0	38.1 – 39.0	≥39.1	
Systolic BP	≤90	91 – 100	101 – 110	111 – 219			≥220
Heart Rate	≤40		41 – 50	51 – 90	91 – 110	111 – 130	≥131
Level of Consciousness				A			V, P, or U

Figure 1.2 National Early Warning Score (NEWS)

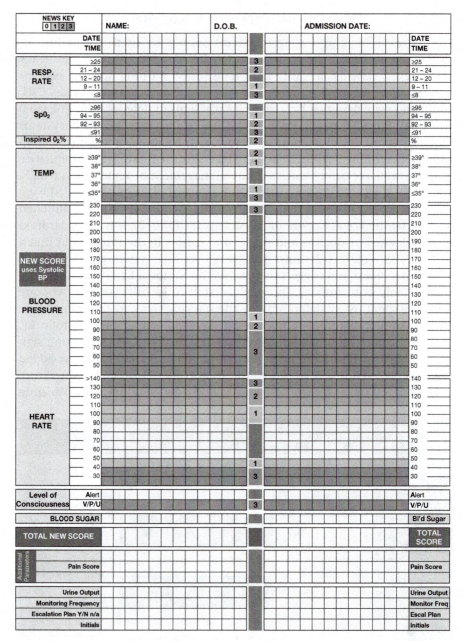

Figure 1.3 NEWS observation chart

NEW scores	Clinical risk
0	Low
Aggregate 1–4	
RED score* (Individual parameter scoring 3)	Medium
Aggregate 5–6	
Aggregate 7 or more	High

Figure 1.4   NEWS thresholds and triggers
Copyright © 2012 Royal College of Physicians. Reproduced with permission.

Score (0 to 1) suggests the patient is stable and at low risk of deterioration, which is reflected by the trigger response for 12-hourly observations in line with NICE guidelines (NICE, 2007). The NEWS observation chart for ongoing monitoring of acutely ill adults is shown in Figure 1.3. It can be seen that an elevated National Early Warning Score triggers an increased intervention in terms of monitoring and clinical response; a score of 7 or more requires continuous monitoring of vital signs, specialist registrar review, critical care assessment and potential transfer to a level 2 or 3 facility (see Figure 1.5).

The NICE (2007) guideline suggests that the frequency of monitoring should increase if abnormal physiology is detected. Track and trigger systems are objective and provide direct guidance to clinical staff when faced with an acutely ill patient, and anecdotal evidence suggests they are generally regarded as useful tools. There is, however, limited good quality research evidence supporting their use (McGaughey et al., 2009; McNeill and Bryden, 2013). A number of hospitals are now using electronic devices such as smartphones and tablets to complete track and trigger scores; an example of such an approach was discussed in the Introduction. One benefit of this is the automation of the trigger for referral to outreach or medical/nursing staff with the specialist skills required to escalate care if required. However, this is clearly dependent on accurate and complete scoring; automated recording of vital signs does not remove the need for nurses' experience and clinical judgement.

Julie Jackson

NEWS SCORE	FREQUENCY OF MONITORING	CLINICAL RESPONSE
0	Minimum 12 hourly	• Continue routine NEWS monitoring with every set of observations
Total: 1–4	Minimum 4–6 hourly	• Inform registered nurse who must assess the patient; • Registered nurse to decide if increased frequency of monitoring and / or escalation of clinical care is required;
Total: 5 or more or 3 in one parameter	Increased frequency to a minimum of 1 hourly	• Registered nurse to urgently inform the medical team caring for the patient; • Urgent assessment by a clinician with core competencies to assess acutely ill patients; • Clinical care in an environment with monitoring facilities;
Total: 7 or more	Continuous monitoring of vital signs	• Registered nurse to **immediately** inform the medical team caring for the patient–this should be at least at Specialist Registrar level; • Emergency assessment by a clinical team with critical care competencies, which also includes a practitioner/s with advanced airway skills; • Consider transfer of Clinical care to a level 2 or 3 care facility, i.e. higher dependency or ITU;

Figure 1.5   Outline clinical response to NEWS triggers

Assessment, Communication and SBAR

Good communication skills are essential to high quality nursing care and nurses are required to develop their use of appropriate communication and interpersonal skills in order to achieve therapeutic relationships with patients (NMC, 2015). Some nurses, however, find communicating with other health professionals more difficult than communicating with patients. This can have a negative effect on the assessment process. The use of ABCDE and track and trigger systems relies upon communication with team members who have specific expertise. There is recent evidence to suggest that acutely ill patients are not receiving appropriate medical review and that a lack of escalation is leading to suboptimal clinical outcome (NCEPOD, 2012); focused communication is essential to address this issue. SBAR – Situation–Background–Assessment–Recommendation – is a tool that can be used to frame critical conversations between members of the team (Figure 1.6). It provides standardised prompt questions ensuring staff provide the information needed by colleagues, it encourages assessment skills and it enables staff to communicate effectively (NHS Institute for Innovation and Improvement, 2010).

Situation
- Identify yourself and the site where you are
- Identify the patient by name and the reason for the call
- Describe your concern

Background
- Give the reason for admission
- Explain significant medical history
- Provide relevant diagnostic results

Assessment
- Vital signs
- Clinical impressions concerns

Recommendations
- Explain what you need – be specific about time frame
- Make suggestions
- Clarify expectations

Figure 1.6 Assessment and communication: SBAR
Reproduced with permission from NHS IQ (NHS England Sustainable Improvement).

Summary

Inadequate monitoring of basic vital signs and an inability to act upon documented abnormal results are, it seems, not uncommon in clinical practice (NPSA, 2007). Hypoxaemia with increased respiratory rate and hypotension leading to hypoperfusion, metabolic acidosis and tissue hypoxia are the most common abnormalities prior to cardiac arrest (Cooper et al., 2006). If undetected and untreated a patient will rapidly and often irretrievably deteriorate. In order to prevent this it is crucial for front-line nursing staff in all clinical settings to have good assessment skills, the ability to accurately record, interpret and document vital signs and to prioritise assessment, intervention and care. Knowledge and understanding of normal and abnormal physiology is essential for prompt recognition and interpretation of data collected. A structured, systematic approach based on Airway, Breathing, Circulation, Disability and Exposure (ABCDE), as recommended by the Resuscitation Council UK (2015a), will ensure that assessment is prioritised and any abnormalities are responded to before moving on to the next stage, and track and trigger systems can provide guidance and direction for less experienced healthcare staff. Lastly, effective communication and collaborative teamworking are more likely to result in successful clinical outcomes.

References

Alfaro-LeFevre, R. *Applying Nursing Process: A Tool for Critical Thinking* (Lippincott Williams & Wilkins, 2006).

Booker, R. 'Pulse Oximetry', *Nursing Standard*, **22**(30) (2008), 39–41.

British Thoracic Society (BTS). *Guideline for Emergency Oxygen Use in Adult Patients*, 2nd edn (London: British Thoracic Society, 2016). Available from: www.brit-thoracic.org.uk (accessed 31 March 2016).

Cooper, N., K. Forrest and P. Cramp. *Essential Guide to Acute Care*, 2nd edn (Oxford: Blackwell, 2006).

Department of Health (DH). *Comprehensive Critical Care: A Review of Adult Critical Care Services* (London: The Stationery Office, 2000).

Department of Health (DH). *Competencies for Recognising and Responding to Acutely Ill Patients in Hospital* (London: The Stationery Office, 2009). Available from http://webarchive.nationalarchives.gov.uk/20130107105354/http://www.dh.gov.uk/en/Publicationsandstatistics/Publications/PublicationsPolicyAndGuidance/DH_096989 (accessed 10 January 2016).

Dougherty, L. and S. Lister. *The Royal Marsden Manual of Clinical Nursing Procedures*, 9th edn (Oxford: Wiley-Blackwell, 2015).

Francis, R. 'Report of the Mid Staffordshire NHS Foundation Trust Public Inquiry. HC 947'. (London: The Stationery Office, 2013). Available from: www.midstaffspublicinquiry.com (accessed 13 April 2015).

Goldhill, D. R., L. Worthington, A. Mulcahy, M. Tarling and A. Sumner. 'The Patient at Risk Team: Identifying and Managing Seriously Ill Patients', *Anaesthesia*, **54** (1999), 853–60.

Higgins, D. 'Patient Assessment: Part 2 – Measuring Oral Temperature', *Nursing Times*, **104**(8) (2008). Available from: www.nursingtimes.net/nursing-practice/

clinical-zones/assessment-skills/patient-assessment-part-2-measuring-oral-temperature/808198.article (accessed 13 April 2015).

Jevon, P. and B. Ewens. *Monitoring the Critically Ill Patient*, 3rd edn (Chichester: Wiley-Blackwell, 2012).

Kennedy, S. 'Detecting Changes in the Respiratory Status of Ward Patients', *Nursing Standard*, 21(49) (2007), 42–6.

Marieb, E. N. *Essentials of Human Anatomy and Physiology*, 11th edn (San Francisco: Pearson Benjamin Cummings, 2015).

McGaughey, J., F. Alderdice, R. Fowler, A. Kapila, A. Mayhew and M. Moutray. *The Cochrane Database of Systematic Reviews. Outreach and Early Warning Systems (EWS) for the Prevention of Intensive Care Admission and Death of Critically Ill Adult Patients on General Hospital Wards* (2009). Available from: www.update-software.com/pdf/CD005529.pdf (accessed 9 April 2015).

McNeill, G. and D. Bryden. 'Do Either Early Warning Scoring Systems or Emergency Response Teams Improve Hospital Patient Survival? A Systematic Review'. *Resuscitation* 84(12) (2013), 1652–67.

National Confidential Enquiry into Patient Outcome and Death (NCEPOD). *An Acute Problem?* (London: National Confidential Enquiry into Patient Outcome and Death, 2005).

National Confidential Enquiry into Patient Outcome and Death (NCEPOD). 'Time to Intervene? A Review of Patients who Underwent Cardiopulmonary Resuscitation as a Result of an In-hospital Cardiorespiratory Arrest' (2012). Available from: www.ncepod.org.uk/2012report1/downloads/CAP_summary.pdf (accessed 13 April 2015).

National Institute for Health and Clinical Excellence (NICE). *Acutely Ill Patients in Hospital: Recognition of and Response to Acute Illness in Adults in Hospital. Clinical Guideline 50* (London: NICE, 2007).

National Patient Safety Agency (NPSA). *Safer Care for the Acutely Ill Patient: Learning from Serious Incidents* (London: NPSA, 2007).

NHS Improving Quality. NHS England Sustainable Improvement Team. Online. Available at: www.nhsiq.nhs.uk (accessed 10 January 2016).

NHS Institute for Innovation and Improvement. 'SBAR – Situation–Background–Assessment–Recommendation' (2010). Available from: www.institute.nhs.uk/quality_and_service_improvement_tools/quality_and_service_improvement_tools/sbar_-_situation_-_background_-_assessment_-_recommendation.html (accessed 8 April 2015).

Nursing Midwifery Council (NMC). *The Code: Professional Standards of Practice and Behaviour for Nurses and Midwives* (London: Nursing Midwifery Council, 2015).

Oakey, R, J. and V. Slade. 'Physiological Observation Track and Trigger System', *Nursing Standard*, 20(27) (2006), 48–54.

Resuscitation Council (UK). *Advanced Life Support*, 6th edn (London: Resuscitation Council, 2011).

Resuscitation Council (UK). 'A Systematic Approach to the Acutely Ill Patient (ABCDE Approach)' (2015a). Available from: www.resus.org.uk/resuscitation-guidelines/abcde-approach/ (accessed 20 October 2015).

Resuscitation Council (UK) 'Resuscitation Guidelines 2015' (2015b). Available from: www.resus.org.uk/resuscitation-guidelines/ (accessed 20 October 2015).

Royal College of Physicians (RCP). 'National Early Warning Score (NEWS) – Standardising the Assessment of Acute-illness Severity in the NHS' (2012) www.rcplondon.ac.uk/resources/national-early-warning-score-news (accessed 9 April 2015).

Scales, K. and J. Pilsworth. 'The Importance of Fluid Balance in Clinical Practice', *Nursing Standard*, **22**(47) (2008), 50–7.

Teasdale, G. 'The Glasgow Structured Approach to Assessment of the Glasgow Coma Scale' (2014a). Available from: www.glasgowcomascale.org (accessed 9 April 2015).

Teasdale, G., D. Allen, P. Brennan, E. McElhinney, L. Mackinnon. 'The Glasgow Coma Scale: An Update after 40 Years'. *Nursing Times*, **110** (2014b), 12–16.

Woodrow, P. *Intensive Care Nursing*, 3rd edn (Abingdon: Routledge, 2012).

2

Shock Presentation

Ian Goulden

Introduction

Shock is never a primary diagnosis but is a physiological consequence of a range of pathophysiological problems. It can be broadly classified into cardiogenic, neurogenic, anaphylactic, septic or hypovolaemic shock. Regardless of the underlying cause of shock, without prompt assessment and intervention it will almost certainly lead to death. Yet shock is a common presentation and it is therefore crucial that nurses understand the causes, physiological responses, assessment strategies and management priorities in order to provide optimum care for the patient.

Aim and Learning Outcomes

The Aim

The aim of this chapter is to outline the various classifications of shock and to explore by use of a case study the priorities of early accurate assessment and management of the individual presenting with hypovolaemic shock.

Learning Outcomes

At the end of this chapter the reader will be able to:

1. Describe the main causes of shock.
2. Identify and explain the pathophysiological basis of the presenting signs and symptoms observed in the patient with shock.
3. Prioritise the immediate assessment, specific monitoring and key investigations required to enable an accurate and timely diagnosis.

4. Outline the main aspects in the management of the patient with shock.
5. Recognise indicators of patient deterioration.

The Definition of Shock

Fundamental Physiological Concepts

Body cells require an adequate supply of oxygen to enable them to produce energy from food fuels and to function correctly. This is known as aerobic metabolism. The cardiovascular and respiratory systems work together to transport oxygen from the environment to the cells. Inspired oxygen in the lungs is transported into the bloodstream at the alveolar capillary membrane, where it binds to haemoglobin for circulation around the body to the tissues. On arrival at the cells haemoglobin releases the oxygen, which enters the cells by a process of diffusion, i.e. from an area of high concentration to an area of lower concentration. Adequate perfusion of body cells is therefore dependent upon:

1. Efficient respiration – inspiration of oxygen (O_2) and expiration of carbon dioxide (CO_2).
2. An efficient cardiac pump to maintain cardiac output (CO) (Table 2.1).
3. Adequate blood pressure (BP) (Table 2.2).
4. A vascular system that transports oxygenated blood from the left heart via arteries to the tissues, permits release of O_2 from capillaries to cells and returns deoxygenated blood via veins to the right heart and lungs.
5. Sufficient blood volume to fill the vascular system.
6. Cells that are able to use and extract O_2 from the blood.

Table 2.1 Determinants of cardiac output (CO)

- Cardiac output = heart rate × stroke volume (normal range 4–8 L/min)
- Average CO at rest = 75 × 70 ml = 5.25 L/min
- Heart rate (Hr) is influenced by the autonomic nervous system:
  - Sympathetic nervous stimulation = increased heart rate, atrioventricular (AV) conduction and myocardial contractility
  - Parasympathetic nervous stimulation = decreased heart rate and atrioventricular conduction (no effect upon myocardial contractility)
- Stoke volume (SV) is influenced by:
  - Preload = the volume of blood in the ventricle at the end of diastole (filling)
  - Afterload = the resistance against which the ventricle must eject blood volume (equates to blood pressure)
  - Contractility = myocardial contractile strength to enable complete ventricular emptying
  - Distensibility = myocardial relaxation to enable complete ventricular filling

Table 2.2 Determinants of systemic blood pressure (BP)

- Blood pressure is defined as the force which the blood exerts on the walls of the vessels in which it is contained. It is composed of systole and diastole. Systolic pressure reflects the force of ventricular contraction, degree of systemic vascular resistance and compliance of the arteries. Diastolic pressure reflects the velocity of run-off of blood from the aorta, the elasticity of the arterial walls and the degree of vasoconstriction.
- Blood pressure (BP) = cardiac output (CO) × systemic vascular resistance (SVR).
- Blood pressure is determined by:
  o cardiac output
  o circulating blood volume
  o systemic vascular resistance
  o venous return
  o elasticity of arterial walls
  o blood viscosity.

When one or more of these factors is compromised there may be *inadequate oxygen delivery to the cells*. When oxygen delivery to the cells is reduced, they use a less effective energy production process known as anaerobic metabolism. Anaerobic metabolism does not rely upon oxygen for energy production but does result in a severe reduction in the level of energy produced within the cells and the formation of lactic acid as a metabolic waste product. An increase in cellular lactic acid leads to a fall in blood pH. This is potentially harmful to the cells and is known as metabolic acidosis.

Metabolic acidosis has a detrimental effect upon intracellular and cell membrane function. As cell function deteriorates, the cell membrane becomes more permeable and allows abnormal leakage of electrolytes and fluids in and out of the cells. If this process is not rapidly reversed, cell structures are damaged and cell necrosis will ensue, leading to potential organ failure. Failure of organ systems increases the likelihood of death (Jevon and Ewens, 2012).

The Classification of Shock

Shock is the term used to describe a 'clinical syndrome characterised by inadequate tissue perfusion that results in impaired cellular metabolism' (McKinley, 2005: 249). Shock is an unstable and dynamic state of great complexity. It is *never* a primary diagnosis, but is always a physiological adaptation to a potentially life-threatening situation. The most consistent clinical

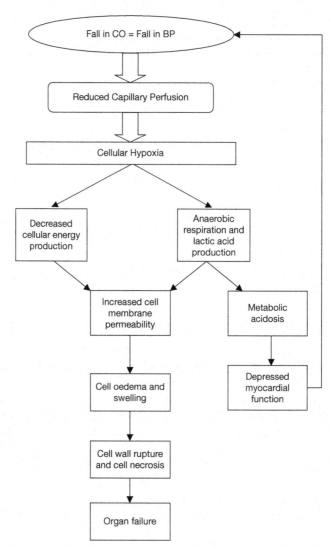

Figure 2.1   The hypoxic sequence in shock

features in all forms of shock are a reduced BP, diminished capillary blood flow (hypoperfusion), widespread tissue hypoxia and abnormalities in cell metabolism (Figure 2.1).

The primary goal of resuscitation is to restore adequate tissue oxygen delivery, to treat the underlying pathology and to prevent further deterioration.

Although sharing much of the underlying physiology, shock has traditionally been classified according to its cause or to reflect the failing organ.

Cardiogenic Shock

Cardiogenic shock occurs when the heart's ability to pump effectively is impaired, causing CO and BP to fall. It may be caused by open heart surgery or trauma to the heart, but it is seen most commonly after a large myocardial infarction (MI). The prognosis for patients with cardiogenic shock is poor and it is the most common cause of death in patients hospitalised with an acute MI (Topalian et al., 2008). Treatment includes restoration of blood supply to the damaged myocardium and the use of drugs to support the damaged heart and circulation. New techniques to revascularise or restore blood flow to the heart muscle may improve survival rates (see Chapter 6).

Neurogenic Shock

The autonomic nervous system controls involuntary muscles within blood vessel walls that maintain the squeeze (vascular tone) so that the volume within the vessels stays constant even if the body changes position against gravity. Neurogenic shock results from a loss of vasomotor tone. It can occur following anaesthesia (both general and spinal), in patients with spinal cord injury, at times of profound emotional distress and in those with severe pain. Impulses from the sympathetic autonomic nervous system are lost, allowing unopposed parasympathetic activity. Massive vasodilatation results and the patient's blood pressure falls. This situation looks like hypovolaemic shock, although there is no absolute loss of blood volume. As a consequence of the unopposed parasympathetic activity, in contrast to other types of shock the heart rate may be slower than normal. Management includes treating the cause, fluid resuscitation and occasionally the use of drugs such as adrenaline (Epinephrine®) to increase vascular tone.

Anaphylactic Shock

This represents an exaggerated, violent and systemic allergic response to a drug or other substance. Common triggers include bee and wasp stings, nuts, shellfish, eggs, latex and certain drugs such as penicillin. There is sudden profound vasodilatation, pooling of blood in the peripheries and increased capillary permeability. This is again a type of hypovolaemic shock, but in this case the loss of blood volume is real. An urticarial rash is common and there may be obvious oedema in the face. Bronchospasm may result in a pronounced wheeze and laryngeal oedema can obstruct the upper airway. Untreated severe anaphylaxis may be life threatening. Treatment is by airway management, fluid resuscitation and drugs such as adrenaline (Epinephrine®), antihistamines and steroids (for example, hydrocortisone).

Septic Shock

Septic shock results from an overwhelming infection commonly caused by gram-negative organisms such as *Escherichia coli*, *Proteus*, *Klebsiella* and *Pseudomonas*, although gram-positive organisms and fungi are also implicated. There is widespread peripheral vasodilatation and increased capillary wall permeability. As with anaphylactic shock this is a subset of hypovolaemic shock and again the loss of blood volume is real. Septic shock is further compounded by sepsis-related depression of the myocardium and by a range of life-threatening complications such as disseminated intravascular coagulation (DIC) and multiple organ dysfunction syndrome. Septic shock is fatal in nearly 50 per cent of cases and warrants admission to an intensive care unit. Treatment is based on support of organ perfusion with fluids and vasoactive agents while attempts are made to interrupt the septic cascade. Septic shock is a major cause of death in the UK; septic shock is discussed in more detail in Chapter 3.

Since the observed pathophysiology seen in neurogenic, anaphylactic and septic shock states relates to abnormal fluid distribution they are often referred to by the collective term distributive shock (Jevon and Ewens, 2012).

Hypovolaemic Shock

In health, fluid intake and urine output are the most important mechanisms for regulating blood volume. Table 2.3 lists the pathological conditions that promote or reflect fluid loss and may lead to hypovolaemic shock. Hypovolaemic shock is the most common type of shock seen in practice.

It is characterised by diminished circulating volume such that there is inadequate filling of the blood vessels and the body's metabolic needs cannot be met. This loss can be either visible (external) or invisible (internal) and can result from actual blood loss due to haemorrhage or from the excessive loss of plasma or water (Table 2.3).

The degree of shock is determined not only by the volume of fluid lost, but also by the rate of loss. A loss of 10 per cent of normal blood volume can

Table 2.3　Pathological causes of fluid loss

- Haemorrahage: loss of whole blood, e.g. fractured femur, trauma injury
- Dehydration: fluid, e.g. excessive diaphoresis (sweating)
- Severe vomiting and diarrhoea
- Excessive urine output, e.g. diabetes mellitus, diabetes insipidus, diuretic overdose
- Burns injury: loss of plasma
- Sepsis

be tolerated without any significant effects if the rate of loss is controlled, such as in blood donation. Rapid loss of a lesser volume may not result in significant symptoms and as haemorrhage may not always be immediately evident; the amount of blood loss after blunt trauma is often underestimated. A simple rib fracture can account for up to 125 mL, a closed fracture of the femur can result in loss of up to 2 litres of blood (40 per cent of circulating volume) and a pelvic fracture may cause the loss of 3 to 4 litres (60 to 80 per cent) of circulating blood volume. The abdominal cavity may contain a large amount of blood or fluid without any obvious distension. All causes of shock including hypovolaemia can lead to cardiac arrest and death, and therefore early accurate assessment, monitoring and diagnosis is imperative if appropriate management is to be instigated and death avoided. The acute assessment and management of hypovolaemic shock is the focus of the remainder of this chapter.

The Case Scenario: The Presenting Complaint

Billy is a 34-year-old, previously fit and well man who is brought to the accident and emergency department after feeling unwell while playing rugby. He is complaining of left-sided upper quadrant abdominal pain and feels lightheaded. Billy is communicating with members of the healthcare team but he appears to be restless and a little confused. He is complaining of nausea, but has not vomited. His initial observations are:

Temperature: 36.5°C
Heart rate: 105 beats per minute
BP: 110/70 mmHg
Respiratory rate: 16 breaths per minute

Billy's skin is cool to touch and clammy, and he looks pale.

Blood is taken for full blood count, urea and electrolytes, lactate, glucose, blood group cross match and save. A 12-lead ECG is performed. Billy has a 14 gauge cannula inserted and is commenced on a 0.9 per cent sodium chloride IV infusion. Oxygen is administered at 40 per cent via face mask.

A provisional diagnosis of ruptured spleen is made. Doctors decide to manage the condition conservatively.

Consider the following:

1. With reference to his current observations, what might be your first impression?
2. What pathophysiological mechanisms might account for the vital signs recorded so far?
3. What would be your immediate assessment priorities?

The Compensatory Stage of Shock

Shock represents a severe disturbance in homeostasis and no matter what the cause the body will initially respond with the same compensatory mechanisms. In hypovolaemic shock, compensatory mechanisms come into play when the loss of circulating volume reaches 10 to 15 per cent (loss of about 750 mL). A reduction in blood volume causes a fall in venous return (preload), leading to a fall in stroke volume (SV), cardiac output (CO) and blood pressure (BP) (Tables 2.1 and 2.2):

$$\downarrow SV \times HR = \downarrow CO. \text{ This in turn leads to } \downarrow CO \times SVR = \downarrow BP$$

Compensatory mechanisms are induced in an effort to increase SV and CO and so restore BP. In the elderly and in those with chronic disease compensatory mechanisms may be less effective, and in cardiogenic shock, as a consequence of damage to the myocardium, compensatory mechanisms are counterproductive and progression through the stages of shock is much more rapid.

The Compensatory Mechanisms

$$HR \times SV = CO$$

There is a direct relationship between heart rate (HR), SV and CO whereby an increase in either HR or SV will result in an increase in CO and conversely a decrease in either of the factors will result in a fall in CO. In the event of a sudden fall in SV, a compensatory increase in HR will normally occur in an effort to maintain CO. The increase in Billy's heart rate to 105 beats per minute may be evidence of this mechanism.

Sympathetic Nervous Activation

A fall in BP caused by fluid loss will be detected by sensory receptors to stretch, known as baroreceptors, located in the aortic arch and carotid sinus. The detection of a fall in sensory stretch will be transmitted to the medulla oblongata in the brain, which houses the cardiac vasomotor (acceleratory and inhibitory) centre. In response to the fall in BP the acceleratory centre will increase sympathetic nervous stimulation with the following consequences:

1. Noradrenaline (Norepinephrine®) release at the beta 1 (β_1) receptors located at the sinus node will stimulate a further increase in heart rate.
2. Noradrenaline release at the beta 1 (β_1) receptors located at the atrioventricular (AV) node will increase electrical impulse conduction from atria to ventricles.

3. Noradrenaline release at the beta 1 (β_1) receptors located within the myocardium will enhance the force of contraction.
4. Noradrenaline release at the beta 1 (β_1) receptors located within the arterial walls will cause arterial vasoconstriction and lead to an increase in BP.
5. Adrenaline (Epinephrine®) and noradrenaline (Norepinephrine®) release will cause selective vasoconstriction and a redistribution of blood flow. Blood is diverted away from less vital centres such as the gut, skin and kidneys to vital centres such as the brain, heart and lungs. This may explain why Billy looks pale and his skin is cool and clammy to touch. Reduced peripheral perfusion will increase capillary refill time beyond the normal two-second period and diversion of blood flow away from the gut may explain Billy's feeling of nausea. Increased levels of circulating adrenaline are associated with a feeling of impending doom and this should be seen as a significant sign in patients expressing such thoughts (Sheppard and Wright, 2006). Catecholamines stimulate the liver's conversion of glycogen to glucose, resulting in hyperglycaemia.

Renin–Angiotensin–Aldosterone Activation

A fall in BP and subsequent selective vasoconstriction may reduce renal artery perfusion and glomerular filtration rate (GFR) to approximately 25 per cent of the normal rate, causing a fall in diuresis. The kidneys are

Figure 2.2   Renin–angiotensin–aldosterone release

highly sensitive to a fall in renal perfusion pressure and will activate the renin–angiotensin–aldosterone compensatory mechanism (Figure 2.2).

Vasoconstriction and increased circulating volume may initially maintain Billy's BP within the normal range. A satisfactory BP may be maintained with as much as 1500 mL of blood loss (Sheppard and Wright, 2006) and clinicians may well not recognise the signs of shock until there is a dramatic fall in BP (Tippins, 2005; Jevon and Ewens, 2012). Therefore monitoring of BP alone in this early or compensatory stage may not be a good indicator of the patient's actual condition. Observations of heart rate, skin temperature, skin colour and capillary refill time are all essential additions to the monitoring regime. Billy may experience a small increase in respiratory rate as the body tries to increase the amount of oxygen in the blood and any reduction in blood flow to the brain may manifest as mild confusion.

The Case Scenario: Assessment and Diagnosis

Since admission two hours previously Billy appears to be becoming increasingly difficult to arouse and is less responsive to commands. A more recent set of observations reveals:

Temperature: 36.2°C
Heart rate: 132 beats per minute
BP: 80/55 mmHg
Respiratory rate: 28 breaths per minute
SpO_2: 95 per cent
Billy has not passed urine since admission.
He is receiving oxygen 40 per cent via a face mask.
Arterial blood gas (ABG) results are as follows:

- pH: 7.25
- PaO_2: 12.5 kPa
- $PaCO_2$: 4.8 kPa
- HCO_3: 20 mmol/L
- SaO_2: 96 per cent
- BE: –2

Immediate Assessment
1. What are the immediate assessment priorities in Billy's case and what is the rationale for each measure?
2. Identify the common characteristics that help to distinguish the different causes of shock.
3. What is the most likely cause of Billy's sudden deterioration?

The Progressive Stage of Shock

Once 30 to 40 per cent of the circulating blood volume has been lost the ability to compensate diminishes, leading to the progressive stage of shock. The BP will fall, tissues become hypoxic and continued cellular anaerobic metabolism leads to a worsening metabolic acidosis. Metabolic acidosis leads to depression of myocardial function and then to vasodilatation and pooling of blood in the peripheries, which will in turn lead to a further fall in BP. The heart rate and respiratory rate will increase in an attempt to increase the delivery of oxygen to the tissues, but any sustained period of cellular hypoxia will compromise the function of vital organs. The brain is affected, leading to altered consciousness, and decreased kidney function results in low urine output (less than 30 mL/hour). If interventions are unsuccessful the patient will enter a decompensation (or refractory) phase.

Assessment and Reaching a Diagnosis

In practice, a full systematic preliminary assessment should have commenced on admission. However, in order to demonstrate the importance of early, accurate recognition of potential signs of deterioration and to highlight the potential to miss important clues if the practitioner lacks sufficient knowledge and awareness, the detailed assessment will be discussed here. Assessment must include simultaneous measurement of the patient's vital signs, a brief accurate history of presenting signs and symptoms and specific investigations in order that life-saving intervention and symptom relief can be administered immediately. For the sake of narrative fluency each aspect will be discussed separately; however, in practice it is the integration of assessment information that is essential for an accurate and prompt definitive diagnosis. Table 2.4 identifies the key signs and symptoms to be aware of.

The Preliminary Assessment

Airway

Initially Billy was conscious and talking so his airway was clearly patent, but constant observation and assessment of his airway is imperative (see Chapter 1). The sequence of shock events can cause rapid deterioration and loss of consciousness, which can lead to airway problems requiring prompt intervention. This may require the use of adjuncts, such as an oral airway, or in the seriously ill patient endotracheal intubation and mechanical ventilation may be required.

Table 2.4   Signs and symptoms of shock

Compensatory stage	*Progressive stage*
• Tachycardia	• Increasing tachycardia
• Possible weak thready pulse	• Weak, rapid, thready pulse
• Blood pressure may be normal	• Hypotension
• Increased respiratory rate: tachypnoea	• Tachypnoea with shallow respirations
• Cool, pale skin	• Cold and cyanotic skin
• Reduced urine output/concentrated urine	• Further reduction in urine output
• Confusion/anxiety	• Further deterioration in level of consciousness
• Nausea	
• Sweating	• Signs of hypoxaemia
• Increased blood sugar	• Hyperkalaemia

Note: This typical picture may show some variation. For example, in the early stages of septic shock the skin may be warm and dry and the pulse bounding, and in neurogenic shock the heart rate may be low.

Breathing

On admission Billy's respiratory rate is slightly elevated; however, there was no other information about the effectiveness of his respiratory system. It is imperative that Billy's respiratory rate, depth and pattern should be monitored and documented at least every 30 minutes to reveal a trend and draw attention to any potential changes. A chest X-ray may be requested. A pulse oximeter should be applied to measure Billy's peripheral oxygen saturation (SpO_2). Peripheral vasoconstriction can cause problems with the quality of the signal and therefore SpO_2 may not provide a completely accurate picture. Since a pulse oximeter assesses the amount of haemoglobin (Hb) saturated with oxygen, if large amounts of blood have been lost the value of SpO_2 displayed may be inappropriately high (Casey, 2001). An ABG analysis will provide a more accurate measure of Billy's respiratory status.

Initially Billy was showing signs of the compensatory stage of shock and was prescribed supplemental oxygen. The amount of oxygen prescribed would depend upon his respiratory rate, SpO_2, skin colour, ABG results and co-morbid history. Although unlikely in Billy's case, should there be a history of chronic obstructive pulmonary disease (COPD) he would need to be given oxygen with caution, with close monitoring for any reduction in his respiratory rate (see Chapter 7). The second set of observations reveals an elevated respiratory rate. Low oxygen and rising carbon dioxide levels in the blood will stimulate the respiratory centre to increase the rate of oxygen inspiration and expiration to 'blow off' excess carbon dioxide. At this stage Billy requires continued monitoring and unless contraindicated he should receive 100 per cent oxygen via a non-rebreathe mask at 10 to 15 litres per minute (British Thoracic Society, 2008). Humidification is recommended to minimise the risk of sputum retention and chest infection, which are associated with the drying effect of the oxygen (Pilkington, 2004; Ricard and Boyer, 2009). If Billy's BP will allow he should be nursed with a degree of head elevation to aid his breathing. Supine positioning (lying flat on his back) increases the risk of respiratory infection and should be avoided whenever possible. ABG measurement will guide the management of Billy's respiratory system and involves the use of a needle and syringe to withdraw a small amount of arterial blood. The radial artery in the wrist is the most common site, but other arteries such as the femoral artery in the groin can be used. Billy's blood sample is tested and results compared with normal values (Table 2.5).

Billy's low pH indicates that his blood is more acidotic than normal. The pH of arterial blood can fall for a number of reasons: for example, retention of respiratory acid carbon dioxide (see Chapter 7), retention of normal metabolic acids as a consequence of acute kidney injury (see Chapter 8) or the over-production of metabolic acids in diabetic ketoacidosis (see Chapter 10). In Billy's case the fall in arterial pH is a consequence of excess production of lactic acid associated with impaired tissue perfusion (anaerobic metabolism). Base excess (BE) provides a numerical value of the degree of acid–base imbalance. The level of bicarbonate, an alkali (or base), has fallen as the body attempts to buffer the rising level of acid with a base. The level of arterial carbon dioxide ($PaCO_2$) has fallen to the low side of normal as a consequence of Billy's increased respiratory rate. The amount of oxygen in the blood (PaO_2) and the oxygen saturation are initially maintained; however, the normal limits shown are for a patient breathing atmospheric air

Table 2.5 ABG: normal range and Billy's results

	Normal range of ABG values on air	*Billy's ABG results 2 hours after admission on 40% oxygen*
pH	7.35–7.45	7.25
PaO_2	11–13.3	12.5
$PaCO_2$ (kPa)	4.8–6.0	4.8
HCO_3 (mmol/L)	21–28	20
BE	–2 to +2	–2
SaO_2 (%)	95–100	96

Note: Normal values differ between men and women and local laboratory test procedures (oxygen content 21 per cent). Billy is receiving supplemental oxygen so the measured values must be seen with some caution and continued monitoring of respiratory parameters is vital.

Circulation

On admission Billy's BP was within the normal range and the changes to his peripheral circulation (cool and pale skin) and the increase in his heart rate suggested that compensatory mechanisms had been activated to counteract an earlier reduction in BP. At this stage frequent monitoring of his pulse and blood pressure should occur and if available three- or five-lead cardiac monitoring should have been commenced. Billy's radial pulse should be manually palpated at least every 30 minutes to gain an indication of the volume and strength. In hypovolaemic states the pulse is likely to be fast but to lack volume and strength and may even be described as 'weak and thready'. In severe cases it may be necessary to palpate a more central artery such as the carotid pulse, although in practice this is not always easy to locate. Electronic monitoring of Billy's BP every 30 minutes may initially suffice as a means of recording and documenting a trend over time. However, as the BP begins to fall below a systolic pressure of 90 mmHg electronic monitoring may become inaccurate and necessitate manual BP recording at 10 to 15 minute intervals in the first instance. Patients who are nursed in high dependency or critical care environments may have an arterial catheter inserted, which permits a continuous display of arterial blood pressure. A 20 mmHg fall in blood pressure when moving a patient from lying to standing indicates at least a 20 per cent loss in circulating blood volume, and hypotension in the supine patient is indicative of a loss of approximately 40 per cent (Marini and Wheeler, 2010). Pulse pressure is the difference between the diastolic and systolic blood pressure and in hypovolaemia the pulse pressure is often narrow (Table 2.6). Billy's fall in skin temperature reflects poor peripheral perfusion and lack of urine output indicates low renal perfusion.

A large-bore (14 to 16 gauge) intravenous cannula was inserted on admission but as Billy's condition has deteriorated he will require a second

Table 2.6 Billy's blood and pulse pressures

	On admission	After 2 hours
Blood pressure (mmHg)	110/70	80/55
Pulse pressure (mmHg)	40	25

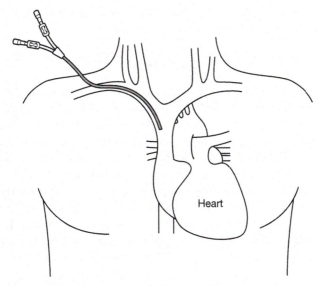

Figure 2.3   Placement of a central venous catheter

intravenous cannula for continued fluid resuscitation. To allow closer monitoring of his central venous pressure, Billy may have a central venous line
inserted into either the subclavian or internal jugular vein and advanced
along the vein until its tip is close to the right atrium (Figure 2.3).

Central venous pressure (CVP) is the pressure within the right atrium of
the heart. It normally reflects the volume of blood being returned to the
right side of the heart, which is referred to as the venous return or preload.
The normal CVP is in the range 5 to 12 cmH$_2$O (3 to 10 mmHg), although
there is considerable variation as to what is considered the norm. A fall
in CVP is often associated with hypovolaemia. A single reading of CVP is
less important than the monitoring of trends over time and the measurement of its change following fluid replacement therapy. If Billy's CVP does
not change after a fluid challenge with 500 mL of crystalloid fluid such as
0.9 per cent sodium chloride given over 30 minutes, then he is still volume
depleted and will require more fluid. If the CVP rises slightly, but falls after
10 minutes, again he will require additional fluid. If, however, following
a fluid challenge Billy's CVP rises above 10 cmH$_2$O and does not fall then
he has been adequately resuscitated. It is important to remember, however,
that monitoring of CVP alone is not a reliable measure of fluid balance, but
when used in conjunction with continuous measurement and documentation of BP, pulse, cardiac rhythm, urine output and level of consciousness
will give a more complete picture of Billy's physiological status. Central

venous catheters are not ideal for rapid fluid volume resuscitation as a consequence of their length and narrow diameter.

Disability

Although initially awake and communicating Billy was a little confused, which may be indicative of reduced blood flow to the brain. Billy's confusional state and level of consciousness should be monitored at least hourly using the AVPU system (see Chapter 1) and if there is further cause for concern, or should his condition deteriorate, the Glasgow Coma Scale (GCS) will provide a more detailed evaluation of Billy's neurological status (see Chapter 4). Billy reported abdominal pain, which can lead to further physiological as well as psychological complications (Woodrow, 2012) and he will therefore need a thorough assessment of the site, character and intensity of his pain and administration of analgesia as prescribed. Billy describes his pain as being in the upper left part of his abdomen with radiation to the left shoulder when he lies down. Referred pain such as this is common in many situations, but coupled with his left-sided abdominal pain, the history of trauma and the signs of hypovolaemia tends to support the diagnosis of ruptured spleen. Opioids such as IV morphine remain at the forefront of acute pain management and will be prescribed according to Billy's age, body mass and pain response.

Exposure

As the body redirects blood flow to the vital centres it reduces blood flow to the kidneys. When the kidneys have reduced perfusion their function is impaired and urine output declines. An accurate measure of urine output can provide further evidence of the function of the cardiovascular system. Normal urine output is 0.5 mL/kg/hr or approximately 30 mL/hour for a patient weighing 65 kg. Reduced urine output (oliguria) is a key sign of a shocked presentation. On admission it would not be appropriate to insert a self-retaining urinary catheter to monitor Billy's urine output, but as his condition deteriorated this option would be considered to ensure accuracy of measurement. As a consequence of the reduced renal perfusion and the renal retention of water any urine passed will be dark and concentrated and have a higher than normal specific gravity. Billy will be kept nil by mouth until the potential for emergency surgery is excluded. Gastric distension may increase pressure on the spleen and so a nasogastric tube will be passed to enable gastric decompression.

Billy is now tachycardic, hypotensive, cool, pale and clammy and these and the lack of diuresis are all indications that he is in the progressive stage of hypovolaemic shock. However, although Billy's condition may be as a result of internal blood loss following a ruptured spleen, there are many causes of a shocked presentation and assessment of signs and symptoms and further investigations are necessary to determine the primary cause.

Specific Investigations

Full blood count (FBC), urea and electrolytes (U and E), serum lactate, blood group, save and cross matching for potential blood transfusion, coagulation studies, blood glucose, liver function tests and a 12 lead ECG will be adequate to determine the type of shock. For example, blood loss may be reflected in a low Hb and haematocrit but if the blood test was taken after aggressive fluid resuscitation, haemodilution may have occurred, so the results must be reviewed with some caution. Early stage sepsis should be suspected if there is a raised temperature, warm, dry skin, a bounding pulse, a raised white cell count and a raised C-reactive protein (CRP), and should be confirmed with positive blood cultures. As a consequence of the stress, response patients with shock often present with a raised blood glucose level and elevated serum lactate confirms the presence of anaerobic metabolism. Chest pain, palpitations, changes on a 12-lead ECG and raised troponin may indicate an underlying MI or arrhythmia induced cardiogenic shock. A detailed history of current events may reveal sources of anaphylaxis or spinal cord injury. A rash and signs of peripheral oedema are more common with anaphylaxis. Billy describes receiving a blow to his abdomen during a rugby match, which would be classed as a blunt trauma injury, and is complaining of abdominal pain, so imaging including plain X-rays, abdominal ultrasound and an abdominal computerised tomography (CT) scan may be indicated.

Medical Management Strategies

Management strategies must focus upon:

- restoring circulating blood volume;
- control of fluid loss/treatment of cause;
- restoration of the oxygen carrying capacity of the blood.

Fluid Resuscitation

The average adult requires a fluid intake of about 3 litres a day to maintain homeostasis; however, in illness this may change dramatically in terms of both the volume and the composition of the fluid required. For example, when a patient has a high temperature they will require an additional

The Case Scenario: Management and Care Issues

Billy's condition has not yet shown any signs of recovery. He remains increasingly difficult to arouse and is less responsive to commands. He has been commenced on 500 mL of IV Gelofusine® to infuse over 20 minutes via a wide-bore peripheral cannula and has a CVP line inserted into the subclavian vein attached to 1 litre of IV 0.9 per cent sodium chloride solution. He has had IV morphine 5 mg for pain relief with some effect. A more recent set of observations reveals:

AVPU: V
GCS: 12 (E3, V4, M5)
Temperature: 36.0°C
Heart rate: 130 beats per minute
BP: 80/55 mmHg
CVP: 2 cmH$_2$O
Respiratory rate: 28 breaths per minute
SpO$_2$: 98 per cent
Billy has a urinary catheter in situ and has passed a total of 35 mL of dark coloured urine in the past two hours.
He is receiving oxygen 100 per cent via a face mask.
Arterial blood gas (ABG) results are as follows:

- pH 7.15
- PaO$_2$ 14.5 kPa
- PaCO$_2$ 5.2 kPa
- HCO$_3$ 18 mol/L
- SaO$_2$ 98 per cent
- BE –2

Billy's Hb level is reported as 9.5 g/dL with a PCV (haematocrit) of 25 per cent.

Consider the following:

1. What are Billy's management priorities now?
2. Describe the rationale for the treatment interventions given.
3. What are Billy's main care issues?

500 mL of maintenance fluid for every degree above 37°C. To fully appreciate the importance of fluid replacement therapy it is necessary to understand about body fluid compartments. About 60 per cent of the total body weight of an adult is fluid (almost entirely water). This fluid is distributed either within the cells (intracellular fluid) or outside of the cells (extracellular fluid) in a ratio of about two-thirds to one-third (Figure 2.4). When considering fluid volume replacement the key components of the extracellular

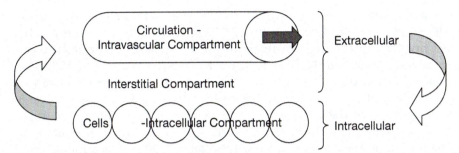

Figure 2.4 Body fluid compartments

fluid are the fluid contained within the blood vessels (the intravascular compartment) and the fluid contained in the spaces between the blood capillaries (the interstitium or interstitial compartment) and the cells. Fluid is constantly moving between the compartments and loss should largely equal gain. The interstitial compartment gains a small amount of fluid and this is drained away as lymph.

Circulating blood volume is approximately 5 litres and at any given time about 65 per cent of this volume is contained within the intravascular compartment. When fluid moves out of or is lost from the intravascular compartment, blood pressure will fall and tissue perfusion will be compromised. To compensate for this, fluid is drawn out of the cells and the interstitium. The rapid loss of about 1 litre of blood will be compensated within about 10 minutes by the movement of approximately 600 mL of fluid from the cells and the interstitium into the vascular compartment. This has been referred to as an 'internal transfusion' (Noble et al., 2010). When fluid shifts out of the intracellular compartment, cells can become dehydrated and cellular processes become less efficient. Depletion of the interstitial compartment is not in itself life threatening.

The importance of fluid volume replacement is proven but the type, amount and speed of infusion remains a focus of debate (Perel et al., 2013). The National Institute for Health and Care Excellence (NICE) produced guidelines on intravenous fluid therapy in adults in hospital (NICE:CG174, 2013). It is important to note, however, that NICE states that these guidelines do not apply to patients needing inotropes (see below) and those on intensive monitoring; as a result the guidelines are less relevant to intensive care settings. Crystalloids such as 0.9 per cent sodium chloride solution and Hartmann's solution and colloids such as Haemaccel® and Gelofusine® are capable of restoring blood volume, but each has a different impact upon physiological systems. Crystal fluids temporarily replace fluid lost in the circulatory volume but the majority of the fluid is absorbed from the circulation into the extracellular fluid and then into the cells. In the case of 0.9 per cent sodium chloride solution, 750 mL of each litre given is rapidly lost from the vascular compartment to the extracellular and cellular compartments (Jordan, 2000). It will therefore replace not only the fluid lost from the bloodstream, but also that lost from the cells. The Resuscitation Council UK (2015) recommends that a 1 litre fluid challenge is given over 5 to 10 minutes for the management of hypotension, as in Billy's case. Alternatively, though less commonly adopted in the UK, 1 to 2 litres of Hartmann's solution may be given for shock-related fluid resuscitation because when metabolised in the liver and kidneys bicarbonate is produced, which will act to buffer the lactic acid produced from anaerobic metabolism (Evans and Tippins, 2007). In addition, the increased chloride load associated with the infusion of large volumes of 0.9 per cent sodium chloride solution may produce a hyperchloraemic acidosis, which will result in renal vasoconstriction and reduced GFR. For this reason Powell-Tuck et al. (2009) recommend that Ringer's lactate or Hartmann's solution should replace 0.9 per cent sodium chloride solution.

Colloids are much larger molecules that do not readily cross capillary membranes like crystalloids and therefore provide a more sustained expansion of circulating blood volume. They are, however, associated with an increased risk of complications such as cellular dehydration, and so large volumes of colloid for resuscitation and volume expansion should be used with caution, though small volumes are still used in practice (Perel et al., 2013). Bunn and Trivaldi (2012) also suggested that no colloid has any advantage over another. The rapid infusion of small amounts of colloid will provide for a more sustained improvement in blood volume and will increase the amount of oxygen available to the cells. Billy was commenced a fluid challenge of 500 mL of Gelofusine® over 10 to 20 minutes at the first sign of fluid volume depletion. Because of the way crystal fluid moves out of the vascular compartment, much greater volumes of crystalloid than colloid will be needed. Two to four litres of crystal fluid will provide the same level of vascular expansion as one litre of colloid. The use of such large volumes of crystal fluid is not without complications and patients must be observed for the development of pulmonary oedema and adult respiratory distress syndrome. The Cochrane Review (Perel et al., 2013) concluded that there was no evidence that colloids were superior to crystalloids when used as a treatment for intravascular volume resuscitation in critically ill patients and stated that given the higher cost of colloids, their ongoing use was unjustified.

Crystal and colloid fluids increase the volume but not the oxygen carrying capacity of the blood and when blood loss is suspected or proved a blood transfusion may be required. There is no advantage in using blood for fluid volume resuscitation when blood has not been lost (Marini and Wheeler, 2010). Whole blood contains red and white cells, platelets, plasma and electrolytes and provides for the best volume expansion in the haemorrhaging hypovolaemic patient. Packed red cells contain the same volume of red blood cells, but have a smaller volume of plasma and as such produce less volume expansion (Kneale, 2003). Although the normal Hb is in the range 12 to 18 g/dL the optimal Hb value following blood transfusion is patient- and circumstance-dependent. A balance needs to be drawn between the value of Hb required to ensure adequate oxygen carrying capacity and a lower Hb, which will decrease blood viscosity and promote organ perfusion (Woodrow, 2012). A consequence of the 'internal transfusion' described earlier is haemodilution and a fall in haematocrit. Sheppard and Wright (2006) suggest that a blood transfusion should be given if the measured haematocrit or packed cell volume (PCV) is less than 30 per cent or if the Hb is less than 10 g/dL. As Billy's Hb was 9.5 g/dL and his PCV was 25 per cent the need for a blood transfusion became more evident. The amount of blood transfused will depend upon repeat haematological results. If large volumes of blood are required it is common also to give regular transfusions of platelets and fresh frozen plasma to minimise the risk of blood clotting problems. The infusion of mismatched blood or blood products can lead to a potentially life-threatening transfusion reaction and vigilance and checking are required to ensure that the patient receives the correct blood. Once a transfusion is in progress frequent observations of temperature, pulse, respirations and BP plus observation of the skin for flushing or the development of a rash will enable early detection of a transfusion anaphylaxis. Complications can occur during any form of fluid resuscitation and it is important to continue monitoring of pulse, BP, CVP, respirations and temperature. In addition the patient's jugular veins can be assessed, as fluid overload may result in jugular vein distension. The infusion of large volumes of fluid at room temperature, or much cooler if blood (usually about 4°C), can cause a rapid reduction in the patient's body temperature and the use of fluid warming devices is recommended. When treating haemorrhage a rapid increase in BP is contraindicated due to the risk of dislodging any clot formation and producing a worsening of the blood loss. Therapy to aim for a systolic blood pressure of 90 mmHg is recommended (Evans and Tippins, 2007).

Oxygen Therapy

It is essential to increase the arterial oxygen concentration and as such the amount of oxygen delivered to the tissues. All shocked patients should receive high flow oxygen via a non-rebreathe face mask. Billy's PaO_2 and $PaCO_2$ are within normal parameters, but he will continue to receive

100 per cent oxygen via the non-rebreathe mask until his overall condition improves. Where the required level of tissue oxygenation is not achieved, non-invasive respiratory support (see Chapter 7) or intubation and mechanical ventilation is indicated.

Vasoactive and Inotropic Drugs

Pharmacological support is rarely needed in hypovolaemic shock except when it is severe or when surgical intervention is delayed (McLukie, 2009). If, however, after volume loading the BP is still too low, drugs such as positive inotropes (Dobutamine® or vasopressors (adrenaline/Epinephrine®, noradrenaline/Norepinephrine®) might be considered to optimise cardiac output and to increase BP. Positive inotropes will act to increase myocardial contractility, whereas drugs with vasopressor properties act upon the tone of blood vessels and tend to increase venous return (preload). Patients with septic or cardiogenic shock are most likely to need vasoactive or inotropic drugs, but in all cases patients needing these drugs should be transferred to a high dependency or intensive care environment.

Electrolyte Management

When a patient has a major haemorrhage there is a total loss of electrolyte volume relative to each other and before the body's compensatory mechanisms begin, blood biochemistry would appear largely unchanged (O'Shea, 2005). However, the developing altered physiology, renal impairment and fluid replacement therapy will all disrupt Billy's normal electrolyte balance, requiring regular monitoring of serum electrolytes (see Chapter 1, Table 1.14). Abnormalities in the levels of sodium, potassium, calcium and magnesium affect myocardial and smooth muscle contractility and elevated potassium (hyperkalaemia) or a low level of calcium (hypocalcaemia) is a frequent cause of cardiac dysrhythmias. Elevated levels of chloride (hyperchloraemia) and sodium (hypernatraemia) may occur following the infusion of large quantities of 0.9 per cent sodium chloride solution and this may cause or worsen a metabolic acidosis (Marini and Wheeler, 2010). Monitoring of acid–base balance via ABG analysis is essential.

Acid–Base Balance

The body is very intolerant of an arterial blood pH outside of the normal range (7.35 to 7.45). All causes of shock lead to a metabolic acidosis, which if untreated will lead to cardiac dysrhythmias, impaired cardiac conduction, a further decline in CO and BP and depression of the central nervous system.

A pH of 7.0 or below may lead to disorientation and coma, and a pH of less than 6.8 is usually incompatible with life. In Billy's case the cause of his metabolic acidosis is the increased production of lactic acid from cellular anaerobic metabolism. The treatment aimed at improving cell perfusion will in many cases result in the normalisation of acid–base balance. Should this not occur then small amounts of sodium bicarbonate may be given intravenously. Metabolic acidosis related to acute kidney injury will require renal replacement therapy (see Chapter 8).

Surgical Intervention

If conservative management is unsuccessful in managing Billy's underlying cause of a ruptured spleen, he will be transferred to the operating theatre for surgery once he is haemodynamically stable. If the damage is limited it may be possible to repair the spleen; however, a splenectomy to remove the entire spleen is more likely. The spleen plays a major role in filtering foreign organisms from the blood and in the production of protective antibodies, so when it is removed the body's ability to fight infection is impaired. Billy should be made aware of the need to take extra care to protect himself against infection and he should be vaccinated against pneumococcal infection. Annual vaccination against influenza is recommended and some people take prophylactic antibiotics to try to prevent infections.

Ongoing Care Issues and the Role of the Nurse

In addition to care in support of the management strategies, patients in shock require a broad range of nursing care interventions. Close observation, frequent monitoring and location within the ward should be considered and transfer to a high dependency or intensive care unit may be required. There is a direct relationship between the stress response and the manifestation of anxiety, and expressions of fear and anxiety are common in shock. Information giving, psychosocial support, communication and the development of trusting, supportive relationships with Billy and his close family and friends are essential aspects of shock management (Bench, 2004; Jevon and Ewens, 2012). An impaired level of consciousness will impact upon Billy's ability to meet his own personal hygiene needs. This, coupled with fluid loss, a restricted oral intake and ongoing oxygen therapy, makes assistance with oral hygiene of vital importance. Failure to meet Billy's oral hygiene needs will increase discomfort and the incidence of oral and systemic infection (Woodrow, 2012). Skin integrity may also be compromised by reduced tissue perfusion and immobility, and regular position changes coupled with frequent assessment and the use of pressure-relieving aids or mattresses is indicated.

The Refractory Stage of Shock: What if the Interventions Don't Work?

When 40 per cent (2 litres) or more of the circulating blood volume is lost the body is no longer able to compensate and death is assured with blood loss of 50 per cent (Evans and Tippins, 2007). In this decompensated stage there is a persistent tachycardia and severe hypotension. Poor coronary artery blood flow results in reduced myocardial contraction, a predisposition to arrhythmias and an increased risk of MI. Ischaemia of alveolar cells leads to rapidly worsening respiratory function, with hypoxaemia, CO_2 retention and rapid irregular respirations. Acute respiratory distress syndrome with severe hypoxaemia and bilateral pulmonary infiltrates may supervene. As brain cell ischaemia progresses the patient will become unconscious, and the pupils dilate and become slow to react to light. A prolonged reduction in renal blood flow will lead to renal failure and liver failure will lead to jaundice and the accumulation of waste products in the blood. Poor perfusion of the gastrointestinal tract may promote gastric ulceration, haemorrhage and the movement (translocation) of bacteria from the gut into the bloodstream, leading to sepsis. A multiple organ dysfunction syndrome (MODS) will exist, reflecting irreversible dysfunction of more than one organ system. Organ systems commonly associated with MODS are cardiovascular, respiratory, hepatic, renal and gastrointestinal, although there are no universal criteria. Mortality is in the region of 50 per cent and this worsens as more organ systems become involved. Treatment is largely organ-specific and supportive, and may include mechanical ventilation, optimised fluid resuscitation, renal replacement therapy and pharmacological interventions to support the failing heart.

Summary

Shock is a life-threatening presentation that arises from the body's inability to maintain its own internal homeostasis. Inadequate treatment or delay in the recognition and treatment of shock can lead to an increase in morbidity and mortality. Assessment and monitoring of the patient in shock are crucial and nurses must ensure that they have the necessary knowledge and skills. Treatment of the underlying cause and management of the pathophysiological sequelae of hypovolaemic shock with appropriate, timely fluid and electrolyte resuscitation can reverse the shock pattern and lead to a successful outcome.

Further Reading

Higgins, C. *Understanding Laboratory Investigations: For Nurses and Health Professionals*, 2nd edn (Oxford: Blackwell, 2007).

Jevon, P. and B. Ewens. *Monitoring the Critically Ill Patient*, 3rd Edn (Chichester: Wiley-Blackwell, 2012).

Scott, W. *Fluids and Electrolytes Made Incredibly Easy!* (London: Lippincott, Williams and Wilkins, 2010).

References

Bench, S. 'Clinical Skills: Assessing and Treating Shock. A Nursing Perspective', *British Journal of Nursing*, **13**(12) (2004), 715–21.

British Thoracic Society. 'BTS Guideline for Emergency Oxygen Use in Adult Patients', *Thorax*, **63** (suppl. VI) (2008), 1–68.

Bunn F. and D. Trivedi. *Colloid Solutions for Fluid Resuscitation* (John Wiley & Sons, Ltd, 2012). Cochrane Database Syst. Rev. [Internet] Available from: http://onlinelibrary.wiley.com/doi/10.1002/14651858.CD001319.pub5/abstract (accessed August 2015).

Casey, G. 'Oxygen Transport and the Use of the Pulse Oximeter', *Nursing Standard*, **15**(47) (2001), 46–53.

Evans, C. and E. Tippins. *The Foundations of Emergency Care* (Maidenhead: Open University Press, 2007).

Jevon, P. and B. Ewens. *Monitoring the Critically Ill Patient*, 3rd Edn (Chichester: Wiley-Blackwell, 2012).

Jordan, K. S. 'Fluid Resuscitation in Acutely Injured Patients', *Journal of Intravenous Nursing*, **23**(2) (2000), 81–7.

Kneale, J. 'Understanding Hypovolaemic Shock', *Journal of Orthopaedic Nursing*, **7** (2003), 207–13.

Marini, J. J. and A. P. Wheeler. *Critical Care Medicine: The Essentials*, 4th edn (Philadelphia: Lippincott, Williams and Wilkins, 2010).

McKinley, M. G. 'Shock and Sepsis', in M. L. Sole, D. G. Klein and M. J. Moseley (eds), *Introduction to Critical Care Nursing* 4th edn (St Louis: Elsevier Saunders, 2005).

McLukie, A. 'Shock: An Overview', in A. D. Bernsten, N. Soni (eds), *Oh's Intensive Care Manual*, 6th edn (Philadelphia: Butterworth Heinemann, 2009).

NICE. 2013. *Intravenous Fluid Therapy in Adults*. (CG:174) (London: NICE, 2014) [Online]. Available from: www.nice.org.uk/Guidance/CG174 (accessed 26 February 2016).

Noble, A., R. Johnson, A. Thomas and P. Bass. *The Cardiovascular System. Basic Science and Clinical Conditions* (Edinburgh: Churchill-Livingstone Elsevier, 2010).

O'Shea, A. *Principles and Practice of Trauma Nursing* (Edinburgh: Churchill Livingstone, 2005).

Perel, P., I. Roberts and K. Ker. 'Colloids Versus Crystalloids for Fluid Resuscitation in Critically Ill Patients', *Cochrane Database of Systematic Reviews*, **2** (2013). Art. No.: CD000567. DOI: 10.1002/14651858.CD000567.pub6.

Pilkington, P. 'Humidification for Oxygen Therapy in Non-ventilated Patients', *British Journal of Nursing*, **13** (2004), 111–15.

Powell-Tuck, J., P. Gosling, D. Lobo, S. Allison, G. Carlson, M. Gore, A. Lewington, R. Pearse and M. Mythen. 'Summary of the British Consensus Guidelines on Intravenous Fluid Therapy for Adult Surgical Patients (GIFTASUP)', *Journal of the Intensive Care Society*, **10**(1) (2009), 13–15.

Resuscitation Council UK. *A Systematic Approach to the Acutely Ill Patient (ABCDE approach)* (London: Resuscitation Council UK, 2015). Available from: www.resus.org.uk/resuscitation-guidelines/abcde-approach/ (accessed 20 October 2015).

Ricard, J. D., A. Boyer, 'Humidification During Oxygen Therapy and Non-invasive Ventilation: Do We Need Some and How Much?', *Intensive Care Medicine*. **35**(6) (2009), 963–5.

Sheppard, M. and M. Wright. *Principles and Practice of High Dependency Nursing*, 2nd edn (London: Bailliere Tindall, 2006).

Tippins E. 'How Emergency Department Nurses Identify and Respond to Critical Illness', *Emergency Nurse*, **13**(3) (2005), 24–33.

Topalian, S., F. Ginsberg and J. E. Parrillo. 'Cardiogenic Shock', *Critical Care Medicine*, **36**(1) (2008), S66–S74.

Woodrow, P. *Intensive Care Nursing: A Framework for Practice*, 3rd edn (London: Routledge, 2012).

3

Understanding Sepsis

Peter O'Donnell and Catherine Waskett

Introduction

Sepsis is a serious condition and remains the primary cause of death from infection despite advances in medicine including antibiotic provision, vaccines and developments in acute and trauma care. Worldwide, millions of people die of sepsis every year; in the UK 102,000 cases of sepsis occur annually resulting in up to 37,000 deaths (UK Sepsis Trust, 2016). The incidence of sepsis has increased annually by 8–13 per cent over the last decade. Reasons for this include an ageing population, increases in high-risk medical interventions and the development of drug-resistant and more virulent varieties of microbes. Sustained campaigning from the UK Sepsis Trust led to a publication in 2013 by the Parliamentary and Health Service Ombudsman (PHSO) of *Time to Act. Severe Sepsis: Rapid Diagnosis and Treatment Saves Lives*. This report focused on the cases of ten NHS patients who died because of failure to diagnose and rapidly treat severe sepsis. A Stage Two Patient Safety Alert on sepsis care followed (NHS England, 2014). The alert aimed to heighten awareness of sepsis, cement existing progress such as the changes in clinical care driven by the Surviving Sepsis Campaign (SSC) (Dellinger et al., 2013) and signpost health professionals to a new set of resources or toolkits developed to support prompt recognition and initiation of treatment for patients suspected of having sepsis. These toolkits included the Sepsis Six care bundle (Daniels et al., 2011) which has been associated with significant numbers of lives saved and reduced hospital stays.

Sepsis is a medical emergency. As in other medical emergencies such as heart attack, stroke or major trauma, there is a narrow window of opportunity in which timely, evidence-based treatment can improve survival. It must be emphasised, however, that treatment of sepsis can only begin after appropriate assessment and diagnosis have been made. Therefore the importance of a full clinical assessment, monitoring and management of a patient presenting with suspected sepsis is the focus of this chapter.

Aim and Learning Outcomes

The Aim

In this chapter the pathophysiology of sepsis, severe sepsis and septic shock will be outlined, and by way of a case scenario the priorities of early, accurate assessment and management of patients presenting with suspected sepsis will be explored.

Learning Outcomes

At the end of this chapter the reader will be able to:

1. Discuss the major causes of sepsis.
2. Describe the sepsis continuum.
3. Identify and explain the pathophysiology of sepsis, severe sepsis and septic shock.
4. Recognise the immediate assessment, specific monitoring and key investigations required to enable accurate and timely diagnosis.
5. Understand and apply the Surviving Sepsis Campaign Guidelines and Surviving Sepsis Campaign care bundles.
6. Discuss indicators of patient deterioration in sepsis.

Causes of Sepsis

Sepsis does not arise on its own; it stems from an infection in the lungs, urinary tract, skin, abdomen (such as appendicitis) or other parts of the body. Body systems most frequently affected by sepsis are respiratory, cardiovascular and renal (Dombrovskiy et al., 2007). Invasive medical procedures such as the insertion of vascular catheters, urinary catheters or surgical procedures can also introduce pathogens into the bloodstream leading to the development of sepsis. Sepsis can also be caused by neutropenia. Neutropenia is a decrease in the number of circulating neutrophils and is a common complication of systemic anti-cancer treatments such as chemotherapy (Moreau et al., 2009). It can result in a life-threatening episode of neutropenic sepsis, the risk of which is related to the degree of immunosuppression and the causative pathogen.

Any pathogenic microbe can cause sepsis, but bacteria, especially gram-negative organisms, are the most common. However the incidence of gram-positive sepsis such as methicillin-resistant *Staphylococcus aureus* (MRSA) has increased. Viruses or fungi, particularly *Candida*, cause one-tenth of all cases (Dombrovskiy et al., 2007).

The Continuum of Sepsis

There is evidence that early treatment for sepsis existed as far back as the early Chinese emperors but it was not until 1991 that definitions of sepsis were agreed and later published (Table 3.1) (Bone et al., 1992). These

Table 3.1 Clinical indicators of sepsis

Term	Definition
Systemic inflammatory response syndrome (SIRS)	The systemic inflammatory response to a variety of severe clinical insults. The response is manifested by two or more of the following conditions: • Temperature > 38 °C or <36 °C; Heart rate > 90 bpm • Respiratory rate > 20 breaths/min or PaCO < 32 mmHg • White blood cell count > 12,000/mm³ • < 4,000 cells/mm³, or > 10 per cent immature (band) forms.
Sepsis	The systemic response to infection, manifested by two or more of the following, as a result of infection: • Temperature > 38 °C or < 36 °C; Heart rate > 90 bpm • Respiratory rate > 20 breaths/min or PaCO < 32 mmHg • White blood cell count > 12,000 cells/mm³ • < 4,000 cells/mm³ or > 10 per cent immature (band) forms.
Severe sepsis	Associated with organ dysfunction, hypoperfusion or hypotension. Hypoperfusion and perfusion abnormalities may include, but are not limited to: • Lactic acidosis • Oliguria • Acute alteration in mental status.
Septic shock sepsis	Induced with hypotension despite adequate fluid resuscitation, along with the presence of perfusion abnormalities that may include, but are not limited to, lactic acidosis, oliguria or an acute alteration in mental status. Patients receiving inotropic or vasopressor agents may not be hypotensive at the time that perfusion abnormalities are measured.
Sepsis-induced hypotension	A systolic blood pressure < 90 mmHg or a reduction of 40 mmHg from baseline in the absence of other causes for hypotension.
Multiple organ dysfunction syndrome (MODS)	The presence of altered organ function in an acutely ill patient such that homoeostasis cannot be maintained without intervention.

Table 3.2   Signs and symptoms of serious infection

Term	Clinical Indicator
Signs of serious infection (SSI)	Temperature: < 36 °C or > 38 °C Heart rate: > 90 bpm Respiratory rate: > 20 per minute White cell count: < 4,000 or > 12,000 cells/mm^3
Sepsis	Bloodstream infection
Severe sepsis	Sepsis with evidence of organ failure
Septic shock	Sepsis with shock
SIRS	Systemic inflammatory response syndrome

underpin more recent research and guidance from leading campaign groups such as SSC (Dellinger et al., 2013) and Global Sepsis Alliance.

Sepsis can also be seen as a continuum progressing through stages identified in Table 3.1, with each stage having more severe consequences, and unless treated rapidly and effectively, ultimately will result in Multiple Organ Dysfunction Syndrome (MODS) (Fry, 2012).

In addition to the above Dellinger et al. (2013) describe clinical indicators which can lead to early diagnosis of sepsis and are recognised internationally. These terms are summarised in Table 3.2.

The Case Scenario: The Presenting Complaint

Brian Phelps, a 54-year-old man who has previously been fit and well has arrived at accident and emergency (A&E), accompanied by his wife Janet, with a two-day history of abdominal pain, initially on the left side but now widespread. His abdomen is rigid and tender when touched. Brian feels nauseous and has vomited once. He is alert but in obvious distress due to pain. He reports occasional abdominal discomfort and bouts of diarrhoea over the past six months. His initial observations are:

- Temperature: 38.2 °C
- Heart rate: 118 beats per minute
- Blood pressure (BP): 115/65 mmHg
- Respiratory rate: 22 breaths per minute.

Consider the following:

- With reference to the history and current observations what is your first impression?
- What pathophysiological mechanisms might account for these observations?
- What signs of serious infection are present?
- What actions should follow immediately?

Sepsis is diagnosed when patients show two or more of these signs of serious infection (SSI) and there is evidence of a new infection. In this way early treatment can be initiated before microbiological evidence of a bloodstream infection is available.

The Pathophysiology of Sepsis

The homeostatic response to infection is an inflammatory defence against the pathogen which should result in recovery. If the defensive response is unable to overcome the infection then the patient may die; also if the inflammatory response is excessive, death may result. Inflammatory responses trigger the release of mediators promoting vasodilation and capillary permeability. Excessive release of these mediators is termed SIRS. It is important to note that although sepsis is a common cause of systemic inflammatory response syndrome (SIRS) there are non-infective triggers also such as trauma or burns. If there is excessive mediator release, shock will result. If sepsis is the causative mechanism then it is termed septic shock.

Once sepsis occurs an abnormal inflammatory response is likely. The presence of pathogens in the bloodstream triggers mediator release from epithelial cells lining blood vessels (Angus and van der Poll, 2013). These mediators include tumour necrosis factor (TNF), interleukins, nitric oxide and platelet activating factors. The result is increased capillary permeability, activation of the clotting cascade and vasodilation. Neutrophils, a type of white blood cell, are mobilised. In the case of a localised infection this process supports homeostasis but in sepsis the systemic response results in hypotension. Severe infection increases oxygen consumption and releases radical oxide compounds which have a dampening effect on cardiac output (Kumar et al., 2015). This combination of events has profound effects. Reduced cardiac output and systemic vasodilation combine to induce severe hypotension resulting in poor tissue perfusion. Triggering of the clotting cascade may lead to disseminated intravascular coagulation (DIC); a syndrome characterised by widespread coagulation and thrombus formation in small blood vessels (Wada et al., 2013). The culmination of all of these effects, if not interrupted, is the failure of organs.

MODS is defined as the failure of more than one organ system. Table 3.3 lists indicators of organ dysfunction. In sepsis the respiratory system frequently fails first and it is this respiratory failure which often prompts admission to intensive care units (ICU).

As a result of the above sequelae cardiac dysfunction is compounded by the reduced cardiac output associated with sepsis. Systemic hypotension

Table 3.3 Signs of acute organ failure

Cardiovascular system	Pulse > 100 beats per minute Dysrhythmias Systolic blood pressure 90 mmHg or 40 point drop from baseline Mean arterial pressure < 65 mmHg
Respiratory system	Respiratory rate > 24 breaths per minute O_2 saturation < 90 per cent with new/more oxygen
Renal system	Creatinine > 177 µmol/L or urinary output < 0.5 mL/ kg/hr for 2 hr
Coagulation	International normalised ratio > 1.5 or partial thromboplastin time > 60 seconds
Gastrointestinal system	Ileus
Hepatic system	Bilirubin >34 µmol/L
Central nervous system	Altered level of consciousness Confusion Psychosis
Hypoperfusion	Lactate > 2 mmol/L

inevitably reduces renal perfusion and acute kidney injury (AKI) results if this is left uncorrected (see Chapter 8). Cellular injury in the affected organs releases more inflammatory mediators resulting in sustained development of septic shock.

Medical Management Strategies

International guidelines exist for the management of sepsis (Dellinger et al., 2013). There are also nursing considerations to complement the guidelines (Aitken et al., 2011). A care bundle is a group of interventions which, if taken together, have been shown to improve patient outcomes. The Surviving Sepsis Campaign Guidelines recommend a resuscitation bundle for severe sepsis and septic shock. This care bundle should be delivered in the first six hours after recognition of sepsis. When two or more SSIs are detected the steps outlined in Table 3.4 should occur within the set timescale. The bundle contains simple tasks as well as the more complex tasks listed. All acute NHS trusts in the UK are required to have protocols in place which meet these guidelines.

Table 3.4 Sepsis Six care bundle

To be completed within three hours	• Give oxygen • Measure lactate level • Obtain blood culture sample before administering antibiotics • Administer broad-spectrum antibiotics • Administer 30 mL/kg crystalloid for hypotension or if lactate ≥ 4 mmol/L • Monitor hourly urine output • Referral for critical care advice/transfer
To be completed within six hours	• Administer vasopressors if hypotension does not respond to fluid resuscitation. Attempt to raise mean arterial pressure (MAP) ≥ 65 mmHg • Measure central venous pressure (CVP) if hypotension is persistent or if lactate ≥ 4 mmol/L (target 8 mmHg) • Measure central venous oxygen saturation if hypotension is persistent or if lactate ≥ 4 mmol/L (target 70 per cent) • Repeat lactate measurement if initial lactate is raised

The initial three-hour bundle, referred to as the 'Sepsis Six' (BMJ, 2015), should be initiated as soon as possible within the immediate clinical environment. Oxygen can be administered and the patient should have a urinary catheter inserted. Continuous cardiac monitoring, if available, is advisable. Nursing care in the initial stages involves advocating for and implementing these interventions.

Implementation of the Sepsis Six bundle has also been promoted by the use of mnemonics such as **BUFALO** (Blood cultures, Urine output, Fluids, Antibiotics, Lactate and Hb, Oxygen) or **O2 FLUID** (Oxygen, Fluids IV, Lactate measurement, Urine output measurement (catheterisation), Infection screening, Drugs – antibiotics as appropriate).

The steps outlined to be completed within six hours will usually require admission to a critical care unit. The patient will need repeated arterial blood sampling which can be made less uncomfortable if an arterial cannula is inserted; this will also allow constant and accurate blood pressure measurement. Central venous pressure and oxygen saturation measurement requires the insertion of a central venous catheter (CVC). Vasopressors are medications which act on the cardiovascular system to raise blood pressure and/or increase cardiac output. In sepsis noradrenaline is most commonly used; sometimes adrenaline and vasopressin are added. These drugs are usually administered using a CVC and all patients receiving them should have arterial blood pressure monitoring. Transfer to a critical care unit is usually indicated and therefore referral to the critical care unit is also indicated as an initial step.

Assessment and Reaching a Diagnosis

In practice a full systematic, preliminary assessment should have commenced on admission. However, in order to demonstrate the importance of early, accurate recognition of potential signs of deterioration and to highlight the potential to miss important clues if the practitioner lacks sufficient knowledge and awareness, the detailed assessment will be discussed here. Assessment must include simultaneous measurement of the patient's vital signs, an accurate history of presenting signs and symptoms, and specific investigations in order that life-saving interventions can be commenced immediately. In this chapter each aspect will be discussed separately; however, in practice several aspects are conducted simultaneously to facilitate an accurate, prompt diagnosis, a factor that in sepsis has already been highlighted as a major contributor to reducing mortality rates. Please also see Table 2.4 in Chapter 2 for key signs and symptoms to be aware of.

The Case Scenario: Assessment and Diagnosis

After an abdominal X-ray revealed free gas under the diaphragm Brian was consented for a laparotomy and informed that he would be admitted to HDU post operatively. IV fluid resuscitation is commenced according the Sepsis Six and BUFALO (Dellinger et al., 2013) guidelines for acutely ill adults.

Intra-operative findings were a perforated large bowel secondary to diverticular disease. There was extensive faecal soiling of the peritoneal cavity. A bowel resection and formation of colostomy was performed. A peritoneal lavage to remove the faecal soiling was performed. Brian was commenced on broad-spectrum antibiotic therapy via the central venous catheter (CVC) that was inserted in theatre.

It is the morning following Brian's surgery. He is difficult to rouse and appears confused. His most recent observations are:

- Temperature: 38.9 °C
- Heart rate: 125 beats per minute
- BP: 90/50 mmHg

The Case Scenario *continued*

- Respiratory rate: 26 breaths per minute
- Urine output 30 mL over the prior two hours
- Pulse oximeter not reading from finger probe, 94 per cent when attached to ear lobe
- Oxygen via venturi mask 28 per cent
- CVP 6 mmHg
- His skin is warm and flushed

His latest arterial blood gas analysis (ABG), which was taken three hours ago shows:

- pH: 7.32
- lactate: 5.0 mmol
- paO_2: 10.5 kPa
- HCO_3: 17.8
- $paCO_2$: 3.9 kPa
- BE: -4

1. With reference to the history and current observations what is your first impression?
2. What pathophysiological mechanisms might account for these observations?
3. What signs of serious infection are present?
4. What actions should follow immediately?

The Preliminary Assessment

Airway

Initially Brian was conscious and talking so his airway was patent, but constant observation and assessment of his airway is vital (see Chapter 1). Sepsis can cause rapid deterioration resulting in reduced conscious levels leading to airway patency problems. These problems will need immediate action and may require the use of an airway adjunct or, in the seriously ill patient, endotracheal intubation and mechanical intervention.

Breathing

Brian's observations reveal an elevated respiratory rate at 26 bpm. His arterial blood gases (ABGs) had been taken two hours previously (Table 3.5) revealing low oxygen and high carbon dioxide levels. Low oxygen and high

Table 3.5 Arterial blood gases

	Normal range of ABG values on air	Brian's ABG results eight hours after his return from theatre on 28 per cent oxygen
pH	7.35–7.45	7.32
PaO_2 (kPa)	11–13.3	10.5
$PaCO_2$ (kPa)	4.8–6.0	3.9
HCO_3 (mmol/L)	21–28	17.8
BE	–2 to +2	–4
SaO_2 (%)	95–100	94
Lactate (mmol/L)	0.5 to 2.2	5.0

carbon dioxide levels in the blood will stimulate the respiratory centre to increase the rate of breathing to 'blow off' excess carbon dioxide. At this stage Brian's respiratory rate, depth and pattern should be monitored and documented at least every 15 minutes to detect any trends or deterioration and unless contraindicated he should receive 100 per cent oxygen via a non-rebreathe mask at 10 to 15 litres per minute (British Thoracic Society, 2016). Although unlikely in Brian's case, if there was a history of chronic obstructive pulmonary disease (COPD), oxygen would need to be given with caution, with close monitoring for any reduction in his respiratory rate (see Chapter 7).

Brian's pH indicates that his blood is acidotic. The pH of arterial blood can fall for a number of reasons and these are discussed in Chapters 2, 7, 8 and 10. In Brian's case the fall in arterial pH is a consequence of excess production of lactic acid associated with cellular hypoxia. Brian's lactate level is high at 5.0. Hyperlactaemia is typically present in patients with severe sepsis or septic shock and may be secondary to anaerobic metabolism due to hypoperfusion or other complex factors. The prognostic value of raised blood lactate levels has been well established in sepsis, particularly if the high levels persist. Obtaining a lactate level is essential to identifying tissue hypoperfusion in patients who are not yet hypotensive but who are at risk for septic shock (Focht et al., 2009).

Given the high risk for septic shock, all patients with elevated lactate >4 mmol/L enter the early goal-directed therapy portion of the six-hour septic shock bundle: (see Table 3.4) (Dellinger et al., 2013), regardless of blood pressure.

In addition, Brian's base excess (BE) has fallen as his body attempts to buffer the rising level of acid with a base. The level of carbon dioxide ($PaCO_2$) is low as a consequence of Brian's increased respiratory rate. The amount of oxygen in the blood (PaO_2) and the oxygen saturation are reduced even though Brian was receiving 28 per cent supplemental oxygen. On the sepsis continuum (Table 3.1) Brian at this point can be said to have severe sepsis.

Circulation

When Brian presented at A&E his blood pressure was within the normal range but the increase in his heart rate suggests that compensatory mechanisms had been activated to maintain blood pressure. His skin was warm, flushed and dry which may be opposite to what is seen in a typical 'shock picture' where cool and clammy skin is often observed. This is a result of the systemic vasodilation that occurs in sepsis and can confuse staff when assessing patients. It is usually seen before the onset of septic shock when the patient's condition is hyperdynamic. The skin is warm and flushed, pulse volume is increased, and pulse pressure is wide. At this stage monitoring of his pulse (including palpation to monitor volume and strength and blood pressure) are required along with cardiac monitoring if available. After return from theatre Brian's pulse has increased to 125 bpm and his blood pressure has fallen to 90/50 mmHg; his mean arterial pressure is now 46 mmHg. This is caused by the presence of bacteria in the bloodstream triggering the release of mediators resulting in systemic vasodilation and subsequent hypotension. In addition, increased capillary permeability and vascular leakage due to the abnormal inflammatory response lead to hypovolaemia. Brian's low urine output indicates low renal perfusion.

Brian has had a subclavian CVC inserted in theatre; his central venous pressure (CVP) is 4 mmHg (see Chapter 2 for CVP measurement). Ideally Brian's CVP should be maintained between 8 and 12 mmHg so he now requires fluid replacement therapy (see Chapter 2) and should be administered 30 mL/kg crystalloid to increase both his CVP and mean arterial pressure. To achieve adequate fluid resuscitation the Surviving Sepsis Campaign Guidelines recommend at least 30 mL/kg of crystalloids (1.5–3 litres) to be infused for most patients in severe sepsis or septic shock. Brian may require more and fluid should be aggressively infused for as long as he continues to improve haemodynamically. If Brian remains hypotensive after fluid resuscitation, vasopressors via his CVC should be commenced to target a mean arterial pressure of 65 mmHg. Norepinephrine should be provided as the first line vasopressor (Dellinger et al., 2013). Epinephrine is considered the next line agent after norepinephrine if Brian's mean arterial pressure is not maintained at 45 mmHgs. Vasopressin at 0.03 units/minute is appropriate to use with norepinephrine either to improve perfusion (increase mean arterial pressure) or to reduce the dose of norepinephrine (Dellinger et al., 2013).

Disability

Although awake and communicating when in A&E, three hours after he returned from theatre Brian became difficult to rouse and appeared confused. This may indicate reduced blood flow to the brain and also renal and hepatic impairment due to hypoperfusion. Brian's level of consciousness and any signs of confusion should be monitored at least hourly using the AVPU system (see Chapter 1) and if there is further cause for concern, or should he deteriorate, the Glasgow Coma Scale (GCS) will provide a more detailed evaluation of Brian's neurological status (see Chapter 4).

Brian has had occasional abdominal discomfort and bouts of diarrhoea over the past six months and his abdominal X-ray indicated that he had diverticular disease. Diverticular disease is a condition in which the mucosal layer of the colon herniates through the muscularis layer which is then termed a diverticulum (Porth, 2015). Most people with diverticular disease remain asymptomatic. The disease is often found when X-ray studies are completed for other purposes (as in Brian's case). When symptoms do occur, they are often attributed to irritable bowel syndrome or other causes. Ill-defined lower abdominal discomfort, a change in bowel habits (e.g., diarrhoea, constipation), bloating and flatulence are common and were some of the symptoms Brian had been having for a few months. Diverticulitis is a complication of diverticular disease in which there is inflammation and gross or microscopic perforation of the diverticulum. One of the most common complaints of diverticulitis is pain and tenderness in the lower left quadrant, accompanied by nausea and vomiting and a slight fever (Porth, 2015). These signs and symptoms were all present when Brian was admitted. Complications include perforation with peritonitis, haemorrhage and bowel obstruction. Brian's perforated bowel was a result of a perforated diverticulum and has resulted in leakage of intestinal content into the abdominal cavity causing peritonitis and development of severe sepsis.

Due to this infection Brian was commenced on broad-spectrum intravenous antibiotics after blood cultures were taken; this is in line with initial management indicated in the Surviving Sepsis care bundle (Society of Critical Care Medicine, 2013) (see medical management strategies section).

Post-operatively, pain management should include assessment of the wound site and intensity and character of pain, along with the use of a pain assessment tool and administration of prescribed intravenous analgesia.

Exposure

Skin condition should be assessed as its integrity can be compromised during bed rest and while in the operating theatre itself. Brian's pressure areas should therefore be observed on admission and assessment undertaken to determine whether a pressure-relieving mattress is required. In order to monitor urine output Brian had a urinary catheter inserted. As a result of the reduced renal perfusion and subsequent retention of water, any urine passed will be dark, concentrated and have a high specific gravity. Brian will also be nil by mouth and have a nasogastric tube passed to enable gastric decompression and drainage of gastric aspirate after surgery. Post-operatively Brian is now oliguric, tachycardic and hypotensive but his skin is still warm and flushed. These are all indications of severe sepsis.

Specific Investigations

The following specific investigations to detect a clinically suspected focal infection, the presence of a clinically occult focal infection, and complications of sepsis and septic shock are indicated and would have been completed both pre- and post-operatively:

- Full blood count (FBC) with differential leukocyte count
- Blood group, save and cross matching for potential blood transfusion
- Coagulation studies (prothrombin time (PT), activated partial thromboplastin time (aPTT), fibrinogen levels)
- Serum lactate
- Electrolytes (sodium, chloride, magnesium, calcium, phosphate, glucose)
- Renal and hepatic function tests (creatinine, blood urea nitrogen, bilirubin, alkaline phosphatase, alanine aminotransferase, aspartate aminotransferase, albumin, lipase)
- Blood cultures
- Urinalysis and urine cultures
- Gram stain and culture of secretions and tissue.

The following radiological studies may also be undertaken to evaluate patients with suspected severe sepsis and septic shock although in Brian's case, as he had an abdominal focus to his presenting symptoms, only a chest and abdominal X-ray was necessary:

- Chest, abdominal, or extremity radiography
- Abdominal ultrasonography
- Computed tomography (CT) of the abdomen or head.

Brian's vital signs indicate he is now at the septic shock stage of the sepsis continuum (see Tables 3.1 and 3.2); he has persistent hypotension despite adequate volume resuscitation and requires vasopressors to maintain cardiac output and tissue perfusion. Septic shock is far easier to recognise, as by this time patients are very unwell and usually present as pale, cold and clammy rather than the warm and flushed appearance that can manifest in earlier stages of sepsis. The survival rate for patients in septic shock is very low with estimates of between 40 and 60 per cent mortality rates despite critical care support (McPherson et al., 2013). Further management strategies in severe sepsis and septic shock focus upon the restoration and maintenance of adequate tissue perfusion to prevent multiple organ

---

The Case Scenario: Management and Care Issues

Following anaesthetic review Brian's oxygen was changed to 15 L via a non-rebreathe mask and a repeat ABG sample was taken:

- pH: 7.30
- PaO_2 9.8
- $PaCO_2$ 3.5
- Lactate 6.0 mmol/L
- HCO_3 16.5
- BE −10

The decision was taken to transfer Brian to ICU in order to intubate and ventilate him. 1L normal saline was administered over 30 minutes. This has not significantly altered Brian's blood pressure. Janet is present and very upset at Brian's apparent deterioration.

1. At what stage of the sepsis continuum is Brian now?
2. What are the treatment priorities now according to the sepsis care bundle? Describe the rationale for these steps.
3. What are the nursing care priorities?

dysfunction. Haemodynamic support in severe sepsis and septic shock is provided by:

- Restoring adequate circulating blood volume
- Optimising perfusion pressure and cardiac function with vasoactive and inotropic support to improve tissue oxygenation by reversing inappropriate vasodilation and improving cardiac output.

Please refer to Chapter 2 for further detail regarding fluid resuscitation and the use of vasoactive and inotropic drugs in the management of all types of shock.

Ongoing care issues and the role of the nurse

Although the Surviving Sepsis Campaign Guidelines (Dellinger et al., 2013) provide a comprehensive review of the medical management of patients with sepsis and septic shock, essential nursing care for optimal outcomes is not identified. Expert nursing knowledge and skills are required for the early recognition of SSI as well as both the identification of the patient deteriorating as a result of developing sepsis and the ongoing implementation of competent care for the known severe sepsis patient. In addition many of the sepsis bundle recommendations involve aspects of nursing care. Nurses can play an important role in promoting implementation of the guidelines. The guidelines include prevention measures addressing education, accountability, surveillance of nosocomial infection, hand hygiene and prevention of respiratory, central catheter-related, surgical site and urinary tract infections with infection management recommendations targeting both focused control of the infection source and transmission-based precautions. In addition, consideration needs to be given to the patient's family and carers. Open and frank discussions with the patient and family about treatment and possible outcomes will help them understand the severity of the condition and its expected outcome. Please also refer to Chapter 2 for further detail regarding ongoing care issues and the role of the nurse when caring for patients in shock.

Summary

Sepsis is a systematic response to overwhelming infection and is a serious condition carrying a high risk of mortality. The hallmarks of severe sepsis and septic shock are changes that occur at the microvascular and cellular level and may not be clearly manifested in recorded vital signs or on clinical examination. The nurse is often the closest to the patient and in a key position to identify any subtle changes at their earliest onset and is therefore able to advocate early intervention. Knowledge of the signs and symptoms of SSI, SIRS, sepsis and septic shock is key to this. Once sepsis is diagnosed, early and aggressive treatment in accordance with the Surviving Sepsis Campaign guidelines can begin, which greatly reduces mortality rates associated with sepsis.

Further Reading and Additional Resources

Daniels, R. and T. Nutbeam (eds), *ABC of Sepsis*. (Oxford: Wiley-Blackwell, 2010).

McClelland H. and A. Moxon. 'Early Identification and Treatment of Sepsis', *Nursing Times*; 110(4) (2014), 14–17.

Sepsis Six Saving Lives video (15 minutes of content) can be accessed at: www.youtube.com/watch?v=CrUHnYIZbpM

ICNARC Intensive care national audit and research centre. Can be accessed at:

www.icnarc.org/Our-Audit/Audits/Cmp/Our-National-Analyses/Reason-For-Admission

The UK Sepsis Trust can be accessed at: http://sepsistrust.org/

References

Aitken, L. M., G. Williams, M. Harvey et al.. (2011) 'Nursing Considerations to Complement the Surviving Sepsis Guidelines', *Critical Care Medicine* 39 (7) (2011), 1800–18.

Angus, D. and T. van der Poll. 'Severe Sepsis and Septic Shock', *N Engl J Med*, 369 (2013, 29 August), 840–51.

Bone, R. C., R. A. Balk, F. B. Cerra, R. P. Dellinger, A. M. Fein, W. A. Knaus, R. M. Schein and W. J. Sibbald. 'Definitions for Sepsis and Organ Failure and Guidelines for the Use of Innovative Therapies in Sepsis', The ACCP/SCCM Consensus Conference Committee, American College of Chest Physicians/Society of Critical Care Medicine, *Chest*, **101**(6) (1992),1644–55.

British Medical Journal (BMJ). 'Sepsis in Adults', *BMJ* Best practice monograph 245 (2015).

British Thoracic Society (BTS). *Guideline for Emergency Oxygen Use in Adult Patients*, 2nd edn (London: British Thoracic Society, 2016). Available from: www.brit-thoracic.org.uk (accessed 31 March 2016).

Daniels, R., T. Nutbeam, G. McNamara and C. Galvin. 'The Sepsis Six and the Severe Sepsis Resuscitation Bundle: A Prospective Observational Cohort Study', *Emerg Med*, **28**(6) (2011), 507–12.

Dellinger, R., M. Levy, A. Rhodes, D. Annane, H. Gerlach, S. Opal and J. Sevransky, C. Sprung, I. Douglas, et al.. 'Surviving Sepsis Campaign: International Guidelines for Management of Severe Sepsis and Septic Shock', *Critical Care Medicine*, **41**(2) (2013), 580–637.

Dombrovskiy, V. Y., A. A. Martin, J. Sunderram and H. L. Paz. 'Rapid Increase in Hospitalization and Mortality Rates for Severe Sepsis in the United States: A Trend Analysis from 1991 to 2003', *Critical Care Medicine*, 35(5) (2007), 1244–50.

Focht, A., A. E. Jones and T. J. Lowe. 'Early Goal-Directed Therapy: Improving Mortality and Morbidity of Sepsis in the Emergency Department', *Jt Comm J Qual Patient Saf*, **35** (2009), 186–91.

Fry, D. E. 'Sepsis, Systemic Inflammatory Response, and Multiple Organ Dysfunction: The Mystery Continues'. *The American Surgeon*, **78**(1) (2012), 1–8.

Kumar D., A. Kumar, S. Singh and R. Tilak. 'Candidemia-induced Pediatric Sepsis and its Association with Free Radicals, Nitric Oxide, and Cytokine Level in Host', *Journal of Critical Care*, **30**(2) (2015), 296–303.

McPherson, D., C. Griffiths, M. Williams et al.. (2013) 'Sepsis-Associated Mortality in England: An Analysis of Multiple Cause of Death Data from 2001 to 2010', *BMJ Open*, **3**(8) (2013), 3:e002586. doi:10.1136/bmjopen-2013- 002586.

Moreau, M., J. Kiastersky, A. Schwarzbold et al.. 'A General Chemotherapy Myelotoxicity Score to Predict Febrile Neutropenia in Haematological Malignancies', *Annals of Oncology*, **20**(3) (2009), 513–19.

NHS England. *Stage Two: Resources to Support the Prompt Recognition of Sepsis and the Rapid Initiation of Treatment* (2014). Available from: http://tinyurl.com/k5lenqt (accessed 25 January 2016).

Parliamentary and Health Service Ombudsman. *Time to Act. Severe Sepsis: Rapid Diagnosis and Treatment Saves Lives* (2013). Available from: http://tinyurl.com/q31oc4u (accessed 25 January 2016).

Porth, C. *Essentials of Pathophysiology: Concepts of Altered Health States*, 4th edn (Philadelphia: Wolters Kluwer, 2015).

Society of Critical Care Medicine. *Surviving Sepsis Campaign – Sepsis Care Bundles* (London, 2013).

The UK Sepsis Trust Professional Resources (2016). Available from: http://sepsistrust. org/professional/professional-resources/ (accessed 25 January 2016).

Wada, H., J. Thachil, M. Di Nisio, P. Mathew, S. Kurosawa, S. Gando, H. K. Kim, J. D. Nielsen et al.. 'Guidance for Diagnosis and Treatment of Disseminated Intravascular Coagulation from Harmonization of the Recommendations From Three Guidelines'. *J Thromb Haemost*, **11** (2013), 761–7.

4

Traumatic Brain Injury

Ian Goulden and David Clarke

Introduction

Head injury is a broad term that can refer to any injury of the scalp, the skull or the brain and may be associated with widely varying levels of morbidity and mortality. Head injury is the commonest cause of death and disability in people aged 1–40 years in the UK. In those under 45, traumatic brain injury (TBI) is the leading cause of death and severe lifelong disability worldwide (Werner and Engelhard, 2007). In the UK, 1.4 million people attend accident and emergency departments every year following a head injury and between 33 per cent and 50 per cent of these are under 16 years of age (National Institute for Clinical Health and Excellence (NICE), 2014). Although only 10 per cent of head injuries are classed as moderate (Glasgow Coma Score (GCS) 9–12) or severe (GCS 3–8), approximately 5,000 people die in the UK each year as a result of head injury. In excess of 30 per cent of those that survive severe TBI will be left with a long-term disability (Bader and Arbour, 2005). Management of the patient with an acute severe head injury is complex and challenging. Damage at the time of injury (primary damage) is largely irreversible; however, the effects of secondary damage can be reduced by rapid accurate assessment and intervention. Guidelines for the assessment and management of head injured patients were published by NICE in 2014 (revised), and the Scottish Intercollegiate Guidelines Network (SIGN) in 2009.

Aim and Learning Outcomes

The Aim

The aim of this chapter is to explore the priorities of early accurate assessment and management of the individual presenting with elevated intracranial pressure (ICP) following a head injury that has resulted in traumatic

brain injury. A case scenario will be used to provide the template for application of evidence-based decision making to clinical practice.

Learning Outcomes

At the end of this chapter the reader will be able to:

1. Describe the main causes of altered consciousness.
2. Describe the main mechanisms of TBI.
3. Identify and explain the pathophysiological basis of a range of presenting neurological signs and symptoms.
4. Consider the immediate assessment, specific monitoring and key investigations required to enable an accurate and timely diagnosis in the
   patient with neurological dysfunction.
5. Outline the priorities in the management of the patient with raised ICP.
6. Appreciate the potential long-term impact of TBI.

The Case Scenario: The Presenting Complaint

Louise is a previously fit and well 28 year old. She is brought to the accident and
emergency (A&E) department complaining of headache and nausea. She appears
somewhat restless and confused. Louise's husband tells you that she fell down a
flight of stairs yesterday while out shopping, but that she had refused to attend
A&E as 'she was alright'. Her initial observations are:

Temperature: 36.7 °C
Heart rate: 90 beats per minute
Blood pressure (BP): 130/70 mmHg
Respiratory rate: 14 breaths per minute
She is moving all limbs equally
AVPU score is A
SpO_2: 97 per cent (on air)
A bruise is noted to the right side of her forehead

Consider the following:

1. With reference to the underlying pathophysiology explain Louise's signs and
   symptoms.
2. What do the initial observations reveal?
3. How might the head injury affect Louise's behaviour?

Fundamental Physiological Concepts

'The human brain is by far the most complex structure in the known universe' (Thompson, 1993, in Sheppard and Wright, 2006: 159) and it is beyond the scope of this chapter to discuss complex brain function. However, a basic understanding of brain structure (Figure 4.1), function (Table 4.1) and a number of fundamental physiological principles is an essential prerequisite for accurate assessment and management of TBI.

There are multiple potential diseases and disorders (Table 4.2) that will affect the structure and function of one or more parts of the brain. The manifestation of common clinical signs and symptoms will be dependent upon the type of disease or disorder and the affected part of the brain. Louise may have suffered cerebral trauma as a result of her fall and the associated changes in pressure within the brain may give rise to a number of specific clinical signs and symptoms.

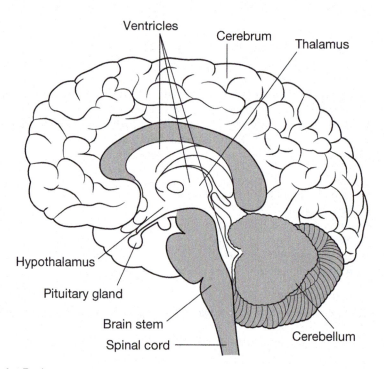

Figure 4.1 Brain structure

Table 4.1 Brain structure and function

Cerebrum	Consists of the two cerebral hemispheres. Multiple roles including the direction of conscious movement, sensory processing, speech and language, learning and memory and the sense of smell.
Cerebellum	Processing centre for coordination of muscular movement and balance.
Ventricles	Four connected ventricles contain cerebrospinal fluid (CSF). The main function of CSF is to cushion the brain from injury.
Hypothalamus	Responsible for autonomic regulation via the sympathetic and parasympathetic nervous system.
Thalamus	Relay and processing centre for all sensory information other than smell.
Pituitary Gland	Complex two-lobed endocrine gland secreting multiple hormones, including thyroid stimulating hormone, growth hormone and antidiuretic hormone.
Brain Stem	Connection between the brain and spinal cord. Contains cardiac, respiratory and vasomotor centres and the reflex centres of coughing, swallowing, vomiting and sneezing. Contains the reticular activating system. Site of origin of 10 of the 12 pairs of cranial nerves.
Meninges	The meninges cover the brain and spinal cord. There are three layers. The outer dura mater lines the inside of the skull. The middle arachnoid mater loosely encloses the brain and the inner pia mater covers the entire surface of the brain.

The Monro–Kellie Doctrine

The Monro–Kellie doctrine (Figure 4.2) describes the relationship between the intracranial contents and the pressure within the skull, termed the ICP. The intracranial contents are brain and intracellular water (80 to 85 per cent), cerebral blood volume (3 to 7 per cent) and cerebrospinal fluid (5 to 12 per cent). These are contained within a structure (the skull) the volume of which is for all practical purposes fixed. As pressure is related to volume, any increase in the volume of one of the compartments will have to be buffered by a decrease in the volume of the others. Should such compensation not occur or be inadequate the ICP will become elevated.

Table 4.2 Diseases and disorders of the brain

Problem	Examples
Trauma	Concussion, contusion, extra-/sub-dural haematoma, subarachnoid haemorrhage
Vascular	Transient ischaemic attack (TIA), stroke due to cerebral bleed or infarction (thrombus)
Infection	Meningitis: bacterial, e.g. meningococcal, tuberculosis (TB) Encephalitis: viral, e.g. herpes simplex
Neoplasm	Primary benign or malignant tumour Secondary metastases
Endocrine	Pituitary problems
Auto-immune	Systemic lupus erythematosus
Congenital	Cerebral palsy, hydrocephalus
Degenerative	Alzheimer's disease
Metabolic	Glycogen storage disorder
Iatrogenic	Drug toxicity
Idiopathic	No known cause
Psychological	Psychological, e.g. anxiety, depression Psychiatric, e.g. schizophrenia, bipolar disorder

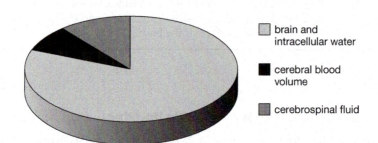

Figure 4.2 The Monro–Kellie doctrine

Intracranial Pressure

ICP is a normal phenomenon that can be measured and is a reflection of the total intracranial volume against the rigid skull. The normal value is less than 15 mmHg. A number of homeostatic mechanisms work to maintain the ICP within its normal range. The most important of these is cerebrospinal fluid (CSF) displacement. This represents a process by which CSF volume is reduced by increased reabsorption, decreased production or increased displacement into the subarachnoid space. The large cerebral veins are readily compressed and will expel some of their blood into the extracranial veins; however, this option is limited by available volume and by adequate venous drainage pathways and is therefore not a major player. Brain volume displacement refers to displacement of the brain tissue itself, e.g. by brain tumour, but this can only occur to a very slight degree. If the tumour increases above this displaceable volume then the ICP will begin to rise. Normal fluctuations in ICP occur with respect to respiration and blood pressure and transient rises are associated with activities such as coughing, straining at stool and sneezing. However, a persistent increase in ICP will give rise to symptoms such as headache and nausea and may be detected as changes in consciousness level, heart rate, blood pressure (BP) and respiratory status, though this is not yet evident in Louise's case.

Cerebral Perfusion Pressure (CPP)

CPP is the pressure required to maintain an adequate cerebral blood flow. It is the difference between mean cerebral arterial and cerebral venous blood flow and as such reflects the blood pressure gradient across the brain. Cerebral perfusion pressure can be calculated as:

$$CPP = \text{mean arterial pressure} - ICP$$

An acceptable CPP is above 60 mmHg. A CPP below 30 mmHg may lead to cessation of the cerebral blood flow.

Cerebral Blood Flow

The brain is only 2 per cent of the total body mass, yet it requires 750 mL of oxygenated blood each minute, which equates to 15 per cent of the cardiac output. Cerebral blood flow is essential for the supply of oxygen and nutrients to the cerebral tissues. A critical relationship exists between cerebral blood flow and ICP. Cerebral blood flow is disadvantaged in the presence of elevated ICP. The automatic adjustment of blood vessel diameter is an important factor involved in maintaining a constant cerebral blood flow. Homeostatic processes can maintain cerebral blood flow within normal limits using mechanisms of vasodilatation and vasoconstriction (Marieb, 2015). However this mechanism is impaired by ischaemia, hypoxia or hypercapnia and begins to fail when the CPP is below 60 mmHg or above 160 mmHg.

Traumatic Brain Injury

At a basic level the brain can be traumatically injured by one or more of the four following mechanisms:

1. Stretching of nerve fibres
2. Shearing, which is damage caused by the movement of nerve fibres over each other
3. Contusion, which is bruising of brain tissue
4. Haemorrhage

When the brain is injured by deceleration, such as from a fall, in Louise's case, or following a road traffic accident, a concept called coup/contrecoup must be considered (Figure 4.3). The brain strikes the inside of the skull at one point and if the force of impact is great enough the brain tissue will rebound and strike the skull again at the opposite point. As such the brain may receive two distinct points of damage.

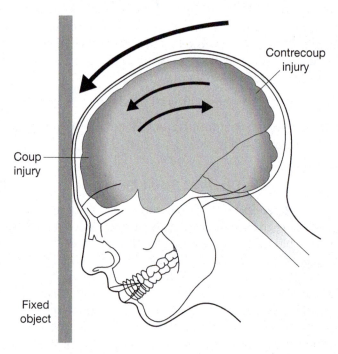

Figure 4.3 Contrecoup injury

The Case Scenario: The Immediate Assessment Priorities

Louise appears to be becoming increasingly drowsy and though she makes some attempt to answer questions when prompted she is not always clear or coherent. A further set of observations reveals:

Temperature: 36.7 °C
Heart rate: 80 beats per minute
BP: 140/75 mmHg
Respiratory rate: 12 breaths per minute
SpO_2: 95 per cent (on air)
She is moving all limbs equally
AVPU score is A
GCS is 12/15 (E3, V4, M5)
PERLA (pupils equal, reacting to light and accommodation)

Consider the following:

1. What are the immediate assessment priorities for Louise and what is the rationale for each measure?
2. What do the observations indicate in Louise's case?
3. How would a definitive cause and diagnosis be established in Louise's case?

Assessment and Reaching a Diagnosis

As per NICE (2014) guidelines for the management of head injured patients Louise should be seen by a doctor or nurse within 15 minutes of her arrival in A&E and the ABCDE approach to assessment should be used. Louise has a clear airway and is breathing adequately. Her vital signs are within the normal range and she is graded A on the AVPU system. In the initial assessment of consciousness, the AVPU scale (see Chapter 1) together with examination of the pupils, which is discussed in more detail later, is useful (Jevon, 2007). However, the nature of Louise's injury and her altered level of consciousness require a more focused assessment of her neurological condition. Neurological assessment should include measurement of vital signs, an assessment of the level of consciousness, evaluation of motor function and assessment of pupillary signs (Table 4.3). Consciousness is defined as a general awareness of oneself and the surrounding environment (Hickey, 2013). When conscious, individuals are capable of responding to sensory stimuli, whereas a state of unconsciousness represents an inability to respond to sensory stimuli. Alterations in consciousness level may be slow and progressive or may be acute; loss of consciousness may be brief or prolonged. Assessment

Table 4.3 Neurological assessment

Vital signs: T, P, R, BP and SpO$_2$
Level of consciousness: Glasgow Coma Score
Motor function: limb assessment
Pupillary function

Source: Adapted from NICE guideline CG:176 (2014)

of consciousness is difficult because it cannot be measured directly, it can only be assessed by observing a person's behaviour in response to different stimuli (Hickey, 2013). There are two aspects to consciousness:

1. Arousal or wakefulness is a function of the reticular activating system (RAS) located in the brain stem.
2. Awareness or cognition is a function of the cerebral hemispheres.

Consciousness is dependent upon the cerebral hemispheres being intact and interacting with the ascending RAS. It is maintained by a constant stream of impulses that are sent from the brain stem upwards into the two cerebral hemispheres. Changes in the level of consciousness therefore reflect two general mechanisms, which are cerebral hemisphere malfunction and brain stem malfunction. The Monro–Kellie doctrine demonstrates that the brain stem is at particular risk from elevated ICP and many causes of brain stem malfunction are secondary to cerebral hemisphere dysfunction. Louise's drowsiness and altered consciousness level suggests some brain stem malfunction, which may be indicative of raised ICP. Some potential causes of altered consciousness are given in Table 4.4.

Table 4.4 Potential causes of altered consciousness

Cerebral hemisphere malfunction	*Brain stem malfunction*
Drug and alcohol intoxication	Direct damage:
Hypoxic brain injury	Brain stem infarct
Stroke	
Metabolic disorders such as hypoglycaemia	Indirect damage:
Infection	Cerebral mass (clot, tumour,
Post seizure	abscess)
	Cerebral oedema (infarct,
	hypoxia, infection, injury)

Accurate assessment of consciousness level is one of the most important roles of the healthcare practitioner. Assessment of the patient following head injury should only be performed by professionals competent in the assessment of brain injury (NICE, 2014).

The Glasgow Coma Scale

The Glasgow Coma Scale (GCS) (Table 4.5) was introduced in 1974 (Teasdale and Jennett, 1974) as a tool for grading the severity of traumatic head injury and is the most widely used scoring system for quantifying consciousness. It assesses the two aspects of consciousness, arousal and awareness and permits standardisation of assessment. The GCS consists of three aspects of behavioural response, each of which is evaluated independently:

- eye opening;
- best verbal response;
- best motor response.

The GCS was updated in 2014 to take account of a range of concerns which have been expressed in the 40 years since this important tool was introduced (Teasdale et al., 2014). Minor changes have been made to both the content of the scale and how it is intended to be used. A new structured schema for use of the tool has been developed; its goal is to reinforce a standard approach to assessment and hence to enhance the consistency of its use (Teasdale et al., 2014). A video presentation and new 'GCS aid: "do it this way"' has been made available (www.glasgowcomascale.org); the minor changes which have been made to the tool are detailed on this site.

A derivative of the GCS is the Glasgow Coma Score. This is an artificial index obtained by adding scores from the three categories. The highest score that can be achieved is 15, the lowest 3. The total score when recorded and communicated should be stated as a fraction of 15, such as 15/15 or

Table 4.5 The Glasgow Coma Scale

	6	5	4	3	2	1
Eye opening (E)			Spontaneous	To speech	To pain	None
Best verbal response (V)		Orientated speech	Confused speech	Words only	Sounds only	None
Best motor response (M)	Obeys commands	Localises to pain	Withdraws from pain	Flexion to pain	Extension to pain	None

12/15, and monitoring and exchange of information about patients should clearly identify the score for each category, e.g. GCS 13/15, E4, V4, M5 (NICE 2014). One of the main criticisms of the GCS as an assessment tool is its subjectivity; however, further exploration of each of the assessment themes can minimise that risk.

Eye Opening

Eye opening assesses the arousal aspect of consciousness. A score of 4 is given when the patient is able to open their eyes without any active stimulation by the observer, 3 indicates that the patient will only open their eyes when spoken to and 2 is when a painful stimulus (pressure) is required. In the updated 2014 version of the GCS, eye opening to pain has been renamed eye opening to pressure (Teasdale et al., 2014). If the patient does not open their eyes even with the application of pressure a score of 1 is given. 'C' is recorded if the patient is physically unable to open their eyes due to trauma, pre-existing disease or the presence of a dressing (Jevon and Ewens, 2012). Louise scores 3 for eye opening.

Best Verbal Response

This category assesses awareness by determining whether the patient understands what has been said and can formulate and articulate a reply (Waterhouse, 2005). First, a brief assessment of hearing, language difficulties and understanding is necessary (Adam and Osborne, 2005). Scores are given as follows:

> 5 = Patient can hold a normal conversation and is orientated in time and place.
> 4 = A degree of confusion with an inability to identify time, place, month, year, as in Louise's case.
> 3 = Patient responds with single words only and conversation is absent.
> 2 = Sounds that cannot be identified as words, such as mumbling and groaning.
> 1 = No verbal response at all.

It is worth noting that patients scoring 3 and below will tend to respond to physical rather than verbal stimulation and are largely unaware of their surroundings (Dawes et al., 2007). A 'T' is recorded if the patient is unable to vocalise as a consequence of tracheal intubation (Jevon and Ewens, 2012).

Best Motor Response

This category is perhaps the most confusing as it introduces terms and patterns of movement that may only be seen in patients with severe neurological dysfunction. The GCS is an assessment of conscious level and not motor function so there is no need to record left and right differences and the best arm response should be recorded. Leg responses are not measured as these may be spinal rather than brain initiated. If the patient will obey commands such as lift up your arms, stick out your tongue or raise your eyebrows then they score 6. For patients who will not obey commands then a painful stimulus is applied and the response to stimulus observed. If the patient can localise to the source of the pain – that is, they move their hand towards it with purpose – then a 5 is given. If the patient moves their hand towards the pain but does not localise to the source this is graded with a 4. A 3 is given for flexion (a decorticate response). This is a slower response than above and is characterised by internal rotation of the shoulder with flexion of the elbow and wrist. If the patient extends their arm to pain, that is the elbows and wrists straighten and the hands tend to drift away from the body, this is a poor neurological sign (called decerebrate posture) and is scored 2. No movement at all to a painful stimulus scores 1.

Applying a Painful Stimulus

Louise scored 6 for best motor response and therefore application of a painful stimulus is not necessary. However, in some cases a full GCS assessment may require the application of a painful stimulus to illicit a purposeful and specific response to the painful stimulus (not just a response to the irritation). Only a central painful stimulus will demonstrate localisation to pain. The 'normal' expected response is the patient moving their hand upwards, ideally to at least chin level (Waterhouse, 2005; McLernon, 2014). Two techniques, either pinching of the trapezius muscle (Figure 4.4) or application of pressure to the supraorbital ridge of the eye (Figure 4.5) or are favoured (Teasdale et al., 2014). To minimise soft tissue injury no stimulus should be applied for longer than 10 seconds (Waterhouse, 2005). The application of pressure to the supraorbital ridge is considered to be the best approach as the patient's response is less likely to be misinterpreted (Fairley, 2005). However, pressure should not be applied to the supraorbital ridge if trauma to the face is identified or suspected. Application of a painful stimulus should start with light pressure and gradually increase. If the patient finds objects such as nasogastric tubes and oxygen masks irritating and localises spontaneously to such sources of irritation then the application of a painful stimulus is not necessary.

Figure 4.4   Trapezius muscle pinch

Figure 4.5   Supraorbital ridge pressure

Pupillary Signs

Reaction of the pupil to light is dependent upon the normal functioning of two cranial nerves. The optic nerve (cranial nerve II) reacts to light entering the eye, while the occulomotor nerve (cranial nerve III) causes constriction of the pupil. Any change in pupil size and response to light potentially indicates elevated ICP and compression of the optic or occulomotor nerves. Louise's pupils will be assessed and monitored for their size, shape and reaction to light. The resting size of both pupils should be assessed and should be equal (average size 2 to 5 mm). The shape should be round; an oval shape could indicate intracranial hypertension (Fairley, 2005). To test pupil reaction, room lights should be dimmed and a pen torch or other source of bright light briefly directed towards each pupil. The normal response is a brisk constriction of the pupils. The direct response, which is the pupil response in the eye you are shining the light into, and the consensual reaction of the other eye should be noted. Pupils should react as a pair. The cranial nerves do not cross over so altered reaction in one pupil indicates a pressure build-up on the same side of the brain as the affected pupil (Hickey, 2013). In the early stages of elevated ICP the pupil on the affected side will begin to gradually dilate, but is still reactive to light. As ICP continues to rise the pupil becomes more dilated and ultimately becomes unreactive (fixed). Although unlikely in Louise's case, a range of drugs, both prescribed and recreational, can alter pupil responses (Fairley, 2005). Benzodiazepines such as diazepam can cause bilateral dilation of the pupils, whilst opioid drugs including morphine and its derivatives cause bilateral constriction.

Limb Assessment

Limb assessment is required to assess for focal damage such as stroke. Spontaneous movement of all four limbs should be observed. If movement is limited then a painful stimulus should be applied to the limb and the response noted. Comparison of one side of the body to the other is necessary, as symmetry is the most important consideration when identifying focal findings. Hemiparesis or hemiplegia will usually (but not always) be seen in the limbs on the opposite side to the brain lesion.

Louise had her GCS assessed at 12/15 (Table 4.6) and her pupils were equal and reacting normally. This is often recorded as PERLA – pupils equal, reacting to light and accommodation. Her temperature, pulse, blood pressure and respirations are within normal limits but she has a reduced GCS and is complaining of headache and nausea. These, coupled with her history of head injury, suggest the possibility of the early stages of elevated ICP. In TBI, ICP rises globally due to cerebral oedema. Increased ICP leads to a reduction in cerebral blood flow and to brain tissue hypoxia. Brain cells when deprived of oxygen switch to anaerobic metabolism and produce acidic by-products. The pH falls locally and this

Table 4.6 Louise's GCS on admission

Eye opening	3
Best verbal response	4
Best motor response	5
Total	12/15

promotes local vasodilatation and a further increase in the ICP. A vicious circle may develop. Brain tissue does not have pain fibres, but headache results from traction on pain sensitive structures such as the meninges and blood vessels. Headache associated with elevated ICP is generalised rather than local to one area (Lindsay and Bone, 2010). Increasing pressure on the floor of the fourth ventricle of the brain leads to nausea and vomiting, and altered consciousness may be caused by increased ICP. Further eye examination using a fundoscope to examine Louise's retina may be performed by a doctor. Increased pressure on the optic nerve results in oedema of the nerve head, which is called papilloedema. NICE (2014) guidelines state that any patient with a GCS of < 13 on initial assessment should be referred for immediate computed tomography (CT) scan; the scan should be performed and interpreted, and a provisional written radiological report provided, within one hour of the request being made. Louise will be scheduled for urgent CT scan, and vital signs monitoring and neurological assessment will continue. Other criteria for urgent CT scanning can be found at recommendation 1.4.7 of the revised NICE (2014) guidelines. If a patient has, or is found to be at risk of developing, brain injury, GCS observations should be conducted every half an hour until a GCS of 15/15 has been achieved (NICE, 2014). Once 15/15 has been achieved GCS should be recorded half hourly for a further two hours, then every hour for four hours and every two hours afterwards, providing that their GCS remains at 15/15. Should the GCS fall observations should return to half hourly. Louise will have vital signs and neurological assessment performed at least every 30 minutes and ideally would be placed on continuous cardiac monitoring.

Louise's GCS has fallen from 12 to 8 (Table 4.7). With a GCS of 8 and below Louise's airway is at risk so a doctor will insert an endotracheal tube to secure her airway. Intubation following head injury must be performed with caution until the risk of associated injury to the cervical spine has been eliminated by X-ray. Once the airway is protected a nasogastric or orogastric tube will be inserted to allow the stomach to be emptied. Elevated ICP is associated with an increased risk of vomiting. Vomiting will in

The Case Scenario: Reaching a Diagnosis

One hour later Louise is very difficult to rouse and is unresponsive to commands. A more recent set of observations reveals:

Temperature: 36.7 °C
Heart rate: 70 beats per minute
BP: 140/80 mmHg
Respiratory rate: 10 breaths per minute
SpO_2: 95 per cent on 40 per cent oxygen via a face mask
GCS: 8/15 (E2, V2, M4)
Left pupil is reacting, normally size 4 mm. Right pupil is now 7 mm with a sluggish response.

1. What are the immediate assessment priorities now?
2. What is the most likely cause of Louise's deterioration?
3. How will her management plan change?

turn further increase the ICP. If imaging studies have not excluded the risk of a skull base fracture an orogastric tube will be used due to the danger of passing a nasogastric tube into the brain. Having secured the airway Louise will be placed on a mechanical ventilator to ensure her breathing. Louise now has abnormal pupil responses, with the right pupil being dilated and slow to respond. This indicates compression of the occulomotor nerve on the right side of the brain. Her pulse and BP show her cardiovascular system to be unaffected at this time, but close monitoring would continue, as an elevated ICP may cause bradycardia and systemic hypertension. Louise would be referred to the neurosurgeons and an immediate CT scan is required to determine the cause of Louise's rapid deterioration although an intracranial bleed is highly likely. CT scanning remains the most important imaging tool for TBI as it is better able to demonstrate fresh bleeding

Table 4.7 Louise's GCS scores

	Admission	*1 Hour Post Admission*
Eye opening	3	2
Best verbal response	4	2
Best motor response	5	4
Total	12/15	8/15

and bony trauma than Magnetic Resonance Imaging (MRI). Plain X-rays of the skull are no longer recommended for the assessment of head injury (NICE, 2014).

The CT scan reveals that Louise has an extradural haematoma. Impact to the front and temporal regions of the skull can result in partial or complete rupture of the middle meningeal artery. This artery lies between the dura mater and the skull and the resultant bleeding separates the dura from the skull. The haematoma formed exerts increasing pressure within the skull (Evans and Tippins, 2007). Extradural haemorrhage is seen in approximately 10 per cent of severe head injuries and has a significant mortality. For a given severity of injury, women appear to have more brain swelling and intracranial hypertension than men (Farin et al., 2003).

Medical Management Strategies

Primary injury is damage that occurs at the time of the initial insult and cannot be avoided. Therefore the focus of attention is prevention or reduction of secondary injury. This refers to a group of physiological conditions such as hypoxia, hypotension, elevated ICP, infection and seizure activity that, if not managed, will exacerbate the primary injury and result in a poorer outcome. The principal aims of medical management are maintenance of adequate and stable cerebral perfusion, adequate oxygenation, avoidance of hyper/hypocapnia and avoidance of hyper/hypoglycaemia (Moppett, 2007).

Respiratory Interventions

Once Louise's airway is secure, through either positioning or endotracheal intubation, the aim is to maintain normal blood levels of oxygen (PaO_2) and to maintain the $PaCO_2$ towards the low side of normal (4.5 to 5.0 kPa) (Oertel et al., 2002). The cerebral arterioles are very sensitive to changes in their metabolic environment. As such cerebral blood flow 'responds' to the metabolic needs of the tissues. CO_2 is a potent vasodilator and can produce unwanted effects on both cerebral blood flow and ICP. The effect of raised levels of CO_2 is vasodilatation of the cerebral vessels, with a resultant increase in cerebral blood flow and therefore the ICP. A fall in PaO_2 produces an increase in cerebral blood flow, but only after a threshold has been reached (PaO_2 less than 6.6 kPa). In a state of hypoxaemia at or around these levels, ICP will be elevated as a direct result of an increase in cerebral blood flow. Blood flow through the brain is increased to compensate for the reduction in available oxygen. Oxygen therapy will be given as required or the patient will be mechanically ventilated, as in Louise's case. SpO_2 monitoring will be in place and arterial blood gas (ABG) analysis will be performed as required. Neurogenic pulmonary oedema is a reasonably common complication of elevated ICP and represents increased blood flow to the lungs and damage to the pulmonary capillaries. The aetiology is not well understood, but it may be caused by vascular changes associated with elevated ICP. Treatment is by diuretics and respiratory support, coupled with measures to reduce the ICP.

Cardiovascular Interventions and Fluid Balance

IV fluids will be prescribed to maintain normovolaemia. Infusions such as 5 per cent glucose should be avoided as they may worsen any cerebral oedema. It is essential that hypotension is avoided and drugs to support blood pressure (positive inotropes) and to control any cardiac dysrhythmias will be prescribed. Head injury results in a hypermetabolic state and enteral feeding should be commenced as soon as is possible. Early feeding has been shown to improve outcome in patients with TBI (Härtl et al., 2008). Elevated ICP can compress the pituitary gland and cause a reduction in secretion of the anti-diuretic hormone (ADH), leading to the loss of large volumes of dilute urine and potential hypovolaemia. This is known as diabetes insipidus. Louise is likely to have a urinary catheter inserted to enable accurate hourly output monitoring and early detection of excessive diuresis. This may require the use of a drug called vasopressin, which mimics the action of ADH.

Control of ICP

Following admission to a neurosurgical intensive care unit Louise's ICP can be invasively monitored by insertion of a special catheter into her brain. When elevated ICP is proven it is common practice for it to be managed with a range of interventions including analgesia, sedation, neuromuscular blockade, control of PaCO2 and diuretic therapy. Hypertonic saline is being used increasingly as a therapy to manage elevated ICP. It has been shown to produce a reduction in cerebral oedema by moving water out of the cells; the decrease in cell size reduces the intracranial volume and ICP falls (Helmy et al., 2007).

Management of Blood Glucose

Severe head injury provokes a complex sympathetic and hormonal response, with increased secretion of catecholamines such as adrenaline. This leads to hyperglycaemia with approximately 50 per cent of patients showing blood glucose levels > 11.1 mmol/L within the first 24 hours after admission. Failure to normalise blood glucose is associated with increased mortality (Laird et al., 2004), but the best approach to managing hyperglycaemia in the head injured patient is yet to be decided. Hypoglycaemia may mimic the effects of TBI (Table 4.4), but is not itself a direct result of severe head injury.

Seizure Activity

A seizure represents intermittent and abnormal neural activity within the brain. They are relatively common following TBI, with a reported incidence of between 4 and 25 per cent in the first week following injury (Moppett, 2007). They must be controlled as they increase ICP and if continuous can lead to cerebral oedema. The patient's safety must be maintained throughout the seizure and details such as type of seizure and duration should be noted. Anticonvulsants such as phenytoin or carbamazepine may be prescribed both as prophylaxis against seizure activity and to aid control should a seizure occur.

Surgical Intervention

As discussed earlier there is very little capacity for an increase in volume within the skull and a haematoma in excess of 75 mL is usually fatal (Michael-Titus et al., 2007). Surgical aspiration of the haematoma is therefore a potentially life-saving procedure.

Ongoing Care Issues and the Role of the Nurse

Following surgical intervention Louise will be nursed on a neurosurgical ICU. She will be sedated, ventilated and will require specialist care. Texts such as Adam and Osborne (2005) and Woodrow (2012) provide detailed information on caring for the ventilated patient. Continuous neurological and cardiovascular monitoring will continue until a stable trend of measurements within normal parameters is maintained. There are, however, a number of care issues more specific to the management of head trauma and these include the following. NICE (2014) recognises the importance of supporting families of those who experience traumatic brain injury. Clark et al. (2009) discuss the support that can be provided to families during management and treatment of people following TBI; they advocate drawing on the frameworks provided by family systems theory and family-centred care to help structure approaches to meet the informational and emotional support needs of families.

The Case Scenario: Ongoing Care Issues

Louise's neurological condition continued to deteriorate. The CT scan revealed a right-sided extradural haematoma and so she was transferred to the ICU where she was sedated, intubated and mechanically ventilated. A nasogastric tube, was inserted though enteral feeding, was not commenced until a surgical opinion was obtained. Continuous cardiac and SpO$_2$ monitoring was commenced to assess Louise's heart rate, BP and respiratory status, and an ICP measurement catheter was inserted and regular assessment of ABGs and capillary blood glucose maintained. An infusion of IV 0.9 per cent sodium chloride was commenced and Louise was prepared for neurosurgery to remove the haematoma and relieve the raised ICP.

Nursing Care Issues
1. Consider the appropriate post-operative monitoring required for Louise.
2. What specific care needs will Louise require?
3. What will happen if the interventions do not work?
4. What are the long-term implications of TBI?

Positioning

Correct positioning and careful movement can promote cerebral venous drainage and minimise spikes in ICP. The head of Louise's bed will be elevated 15 to 30 degrees to facilitate venous outflow and her head will be maintained in neutral alignment to prevent jugular vein compression. Hip flexion will be avoided to prevent any increase in intra-abdominal pressure, which would in turn increase intrathoracic pressure, which would impede venous drainage from her brain. Uncoordinated repositioning must be avoided and to maintain neutral head and neck alignment, Louise will be log rolled when turned.

Temperature Control

Elevated ICP impacts upon the ability of the hypothalamus to control body temperature and so Louise may become hyperthermic. This must be avoided as an elevated temperature is associated with an increased body demand for oxygen and with the production of increased levels of CO$_2$. For every 1 °C rise in body temperature, cerebral oxygen use rises by 10 per cent (Evans and Tippins, 2007). Normothermia is the goal and cooling methods such as fans, tepid sponging, ice packs and cooling blankets may be used. Anti-pyretic drugs such as paracetamol may be prescribed.

Control of Noxious Stimuli

Louise's care environment will be controlled to prevent clustering of activities and excessive stimulation. Painful and distressing procedures will be limited and unnecessary instrumental touch avoided.

What if the Interventions Don't Work?

If homeostatic compensatory mechanisms fail, a small additional change in intracranial volume results in a large increase in ICP. An ICP greater than 33 mmHg is associated with a reduction in cerebral blood flow. This causes stimulation of the vasomotor centre within the brain stem, causing a rise in systemic BP, a widening pulse pressure and bradycardia. This phenomenon of rising BP and falling heart rate is called Cushing's reflex and reflects a compensatory response that attempts to provide adequate CPP in the presence of markedly elevated ICP (Hickey, 2013). When hypertension and bradycardia are associated with an abnormal respiratory pattern such as bradypnoea this is called Cushing's triad and is a warning of imminent or actual brain stem herniation. The descent of the brain stem into the foramen magnum is the end point of malignant brain swelling. The brain stem becomes compressed and brain stem death is imminent. With ICP at this level both pupils are generally fixed and dilated. The diagnosis of brain stem death is governed by clinical guidelines and is rarely seen outside of an intensive care unit. Solid organ donation may be possible after brain stem death.

The Long-Term Impact of Traumatic Brain Injury

Nearly half of all patients admitted to hospital following TBI are left with long-term physical or psychological problems (Whitnall et al., 2006); 65 per cent of adults with moderate injury and 85 per cent of adults with severe injury are disabled at one year. Recovery often continues for two to three years, although in many cases patients never fully recover. The potential disabling effects of TBI are multiple (Table 4.8) and include: physical problems, such as difficulty with balance and coordination; emotional and behavioural problems, such as agitation, depression and apathy; and cognitive difficulties, including loss of memory, an inability to concentrate and changes in the speed of information processing (see http://www.headway.org.uk for more information).

Table 4.8 Potential long-term impact of traumatic brain injury

Physical problems	• Movement, balance and coordination
	• Loss of sensation
	• Tiredness
	• Headaches
	• Speaking and swallowing disorders
	• Bladder and bowel incontinence
	• Seizures
	• Sexual problems
Emotional and behavioural problems	• Agitation, anger and irritability
	• Lack of awareness and insight
	• Apathy and poor motivation
	• Depression
	• Anxiety
	• Inflexibility and obsessionality
	• Sexual problems
Cognitive problems	• Memory
	• Attention and concentration
	• Speed of information processing
	• Planning, organising and problem solving
	• Visio-spatial and perceptual difficulties
	• Language skills

Patients who have had sustained TBI requiring surgery must notify the DVLA and will lose their driving licence for a period of between six months and one year. In 2009 the brain injury charity Headway received Department of Health funding to establish an 'approved provider' scheme, in order to set standards for nursing homes, residential homes, transitional living units and those providing respite for someone who has sustained a brain injury.

Summary

The past 20 years have seen major progress in our understanding of the physiology of secondary brain injury. Research as to the optimum way to manage the patient with elevated ICP goes on, but there is no doubt that patient outcome is improved when secondary problems are reduced or prevented. Accurate assessment is crucial and this chapter has focused on the nurse's role in the assessment of the patient with altered consciousness.

Further Reading and Additional Resources

Adam, S. K. and S. Osborne. *Critical Care Nursing: Science and Practice*, 2nd edn (Oxford: Oxford Medical, 2005).

Jevon, P. 'How to Ensure Patient Observations Lead to Effective Management of Altered Consciousness', Nursing Times, 106(6) (2010), 17–18.

National Institute for Clinical Health and Excellence (NICE). *Head Injury: Triage, Assessment, Investigation and Early Management of Head Injury in Infants, Children and Adults, CG:176* (London: NICE, 2014).

Scottish Intercollegiate Guidelines Network (SIGN). *Early Management of Patients with a Head Injury: A National Clinical Guideline* (Edinburgh: Scottish Intercollegiate Guidelines Network, 2009).

The Glasgow structured approach to assessment of the Glasgow Coma Scale can be accessed at: www.glasgowcomascale.org

Headway, a UK-wide charity that works to improve life after brain injury, has a website which can be accessed at: www.headway.org.uk/home.aspx

References

Adam, S. K. and S. Osborne. *Critical Care Nursing: Science and Practice*, 2nd edn (Oxford: Oxford Medical, 2005).

Bader, M. K. and R. Arbour. 'Refractory Increased Intracranial Pressure in Severe Traumatic Brain Injury', *AACN Clinical Issues*, 16(4) (2005), 526–41.

Clark, C., J. Brown, C. Bailey, C., P. Hutchinson. 'Supporting Families in the Context of Adult Traumatic Brain Injury. *British Journal of Neuroscience Nursing*, 5(5): 216–221.

Dawes, E., H. Lloyd, H. L. Durham. 'Monitoring and Recording Patients' Neurological Observations. *Nursing Standard*. 22(10) (2007), 40–5.

Evans, C. and E. Tippins. *The Foundations of Emergency Care* (Maidenhead: Open University Press, 2007).

Fairley, D. 'Using a Coma Scale to Assess Patient Conscious Levels', *Nursing Times*, 101 (2005), 38–47.

Farin, A., R. Deutsch, A. Biegon and L. F. Marshall. 'Sex-related Differences in Patients with Severe Head Injury: Greater Susceptibility to Brain Swelling in Female Patients 50 Years of Age and Younger', *Journal of Neurosurgery*, 98 (2003), 32–6.

Härtl, R., L. M. Gerber, Q. Ni and J. Ghajar. 'Effects of Early Nutrition on Deaths Due to Severe Traumatic Brain Injury', *Journal of Neurosurgery*, 109 (2008), 50–6.

Helmy, A., M. Vizcaychip and A. K. Gupta. 'Traumatic Brain Injury: Intensive Care Management', *British Journal of Anaesthesia*, 99(1) (2007), 32–42.

Hickey, J. V. *The Clinical Practice of Neurological and Neurosurgical Nursing*, 7th edn. (Philadelphia: Lippincott Williams & Wilkins, 2013).

Jevon, P. *Treating the Critically Ill Patient* (Oxford: Blackwell, 2007).

Jevon, P. and B. Ewens (eds). *Monitoring the Critically Ill Patient*, 3rd edn (Chichester: Wiley-Blackwell, 2012).

Laird, A. M., P. R. Miller, P. D. Kilgo, J. W. Meredith and M. C. Chang. 'Relationship of Early Hyperglycaemia to Mortality in Trauma Patients', *Journal of Trauma: Injury, Infection and Critical Care*, 56 (2004), 1058–62.

Lindsay, K. W. and I. Bone. *Neurology and Neurosurgery Illustrated*, 5th edn. (Edinburgh: Churchill Livingstone, 2010).

Marieb, E. N., and K. N. Hoehn. *Human Anatomy and Physiology* 10th edn. (Cambridge, UK: Pearson Publishing Ltd, 2015).

McLernon, S. 'The Glasgow Coma Scale 40 Years On: A Review of its Practical Use', *British Journal of Neurological Nursing*, 10(4), 179–84.

Michael-Titus, A., P. Revest and P. Shortland. *The Nervous System: Basic Science and Clinical Conditions* (Edinburgh: Churchill Livingstone, 2007).

Moppett, I. K. 'Traumatic Brain Injury: Assessment, Resuscitation and Early Management', *British Journal of Anaesthesia*, 99(1) (2007), 18–31.

National Institute for Clinical Health and Excellence (NICE). *Head Injury: Triage, Assessment, Investigation and Early Management of Head Injury in Infants, Children and Adults, CG:176* (London: NICE, 2014).

Oertel, M., D. F. Kelly, J. H. Lee et al.. 'Efficacy of Hyperventilation, Blood Pressure Elevation, and Metabolic Suppression Therapy in Controlling Intracranial Pressure after Head Injury', *Journal of Neurosurgery*, 97 (2002), 1045–53.

Scottish Intercollegiate Guidelines Network (SIGN). *Early Management of Patients with a Head Injury: A National Clinical Guideline* (Edinburgh: Scottish Intercollegiate Guidelines Network, 2009).

Sheppard, M. and M. Wright. *Principles and Practice of High Dependency Nursing*, 2nd edn. (London: Bailliere Tindall, 2006).

Teasdale, G. and B. Jennett. 'Assessment of Coma and Impaired Consciousness, a Practical Scale', *Lancet*, 2 (1974), 81–4.

Teasdale, G., D. Allen, P. Brennan, E. McElhinney and L. Mackinnon. 'The Glasgow Coma Scale: An Update After 40 years', *Nursing Times*, 110 (2014), 12–16.

Waterhouse, C. 'The Glasgow Coma Score and Other Neurological Observations', *Nursing Standard*, 19(33) (2005), 56–64.

Werner, C. and K. Engelhard. 'Pathophysiology of Traumatic Brain Injury', *British Journal of Anaesthesia*, 99 (2007), 4–9.

Whitnall, L., T. M. McMillan, G. D. Murray and G. M. Teasdale. 'Disability in Young People and Adults after Head Injury: 5–7 Year Follow up of a Prospective Cohort Study', *Journal of Neurology, Neurosurgery and Psychiatry*, 77(5) (2006), 640–5.

Woodrow P. *Intensive Care Nursing: A Framework for Practice*, 3rd edn (London: Routledge, 2012).

5

Acute Stroke

David Clarke and Pamela Beaumont

Introduction

Stroke is the second most common cause of death worldwide, resulting in up to 7 million deaths annually (World Health Organization (WHO), 2015). In the UK stroke is the fourth most common cause of death, accounting for 11 per cent of all deaths, and represents the largest cause of adult disability (National Institute for Health and Care Excellence (NICE), 2013). The commonly accepted definition of stroke is: a rapidly developing syndrome with sudden onset, with focal neurological deficit, of presumed vascular origin and with symptoms lasting more than 24 hours or leading to death (WHO, 2015). Cerebral infarction causes about 85 per cent of strokes with the remaining 15 per cent due to primary haemorrhage (10 per cent) and subarachnoid haemorrhage (5 per cent) (Stein et al., 2015). Symptoms of stroke include numbness, weakness or paralysis, altered speech pattern, swallowing problems, visual impairment, confusion and severe headache.

It is commonly assumed that stroke results in physical impairment and disability. Whilst this is true for a significant number of stroke survivors, it is also true that stroke can have wide-ranging effects including impairment of speech and language, cognition, vision and psychological effects including anxiety and depression (Lincoln et al., 2012; Stroke Association, 2015). Some of these effects are not immediately apparent. Stroke happens to individuals but is often thought of as a family illness in that the effects of stroke can impact significantly on the lives of those who are close to stroke survivors. At one time the prevailing attitude to stroke was that little or nothing could be done but palliate and wait; however, stroke and transient ischaemic attack are now viewed as medical emergencies. In England, Wales and Northern Ireland, the National Stroke Strategy (Department of Health (DH), 2007) focused attention on improvements in care across the stroke pathway. The concept of 'time is brain' increased awareness among commissioners and service providers that rapid access to specialist stroke services saves lives and improves patient outcomes. This chapter will consider the incidence and prevalence of stroke, outline the risk factors for stroke and TIA, and then focus on acute presentation and initial management of stroke. Although initial stroke care is now provided in specialist hyper-acute and acute stroke units, nurses will encounter stroke survivors in emergency departments (ED) and many other inpatient clinical areas. It is important that nurses have a good understanding of stroke and its effects and the ways in which healthcare services and health professionals can make sure that appropriate help and support is provided.

Aim and Learning Outcomes

The Aim

The aim of this chapter is to explore priorities in assessment and management of stroke. The recognition and management of transient ischaemic attack, also known as a 'minor stroke', will also be discussed in the context of stroke-specific assessment and management in the emergency department. The integrated case study provides opportunities to focus on nursing roles and requirements for stroke-specific nursing care in the hyper-acute and acute period post-stroke.

Learning Outcomes

At the end of this chapter the reader will be able to:

1. Recognise that transient ischaemic attack and stroke are medical emergencies requiring rapid specialist assessment and management in the emergency department.
2. Recognise the increased risk of stroke associated with a transient ischaemic attack and appreciate the need for a structured approach to management and secondary prevention following a transient ischaemic attack.
3. Understand the importance of accurate history taking, rapid investigation and accurate diagnosis in determining whether thrombolysis or intra-arterial clot retrieval should be considered as treatment options following stroke.
4. Understand the priorities in initial stroke management including nursing care following administration of thrombolysis.

5. Discuss the rationale for nursing observations and multidisciplinary rehabilitation-focused care in the hyper-acute and acute phases of the stroke pathway.

Incidence and Prevalence

Each year an estimated 152,000 people have a stroke in the UK, one person every 3.5 minutes or so; approximately 110,000 of these are new strokes. Stroke is slightly more common in women than in men. Approximately one in four people can expect to have a stroke if they live to 85 years of age (Stroke Association, 2015). Stroke is commonly assumed to be a disease of old age, but can occur at any point in the lifespan; 25 per cent of people who experience a stroke will be under 65 years of age and about 10,000 people under the age of 30 will have a stroke each year. As many as 1 in 150 strokes occur in those aged less than 20 years, with up to 400 occurring in children and 200 in babies each year (Stroke Association, 2015). The mortality rate at one month after stroke is falling, down from 20–30 per cent in the 1990s to 12–15 per cent in 2008 (Wolfe, 2000; Lee et al., 2011). More than 20,000 transient ischaemic attacks (TIAs) occur each year (National Audit Office, 2010). Stroke is the largest cause of complex disability in the UK where it is estimated that up to 1.2 million people are living with disabilities after stroke.

Risk Factors for Stroke and Transient Ischaemic Attack

These are typically divided into non-modifiable and modifiable risk factors. Non-modifiable risks include genetic inheritance, with single gene disorders associated with increased incidence of ischaemic stroke (Meschia et al., 2011), low birth weight and increasing age. Race-ethnicity is also a factor; those from the black, South Asian and Hispanic communities are reported to have an increased incidence of stroke at a younger age than their white counterparts (Schwamm et al., 2010). The higher incidence of stroke in these populations is associated with known modifiable risk factors. However, the association between race-ethnicity and stroke is proving to be more complex than first thought (Wang et al., 2013). Modifiable risk factors include hypertension, diabetes mellitus, and cigarette smoking; these three factors alone represent 50 per cent of the total risk. Other modifiable factors are atrial fibrillation, left ventricular disorder, hyperlipidaemia, obesity, asymptomatic stenosis of the carotid arteries, and abuse of alcohol or drugs (Alexandrov, 2010a; Stroke Association, 2015) and oestrogen replacement therapy (Boardman et al., 2015). Short-term exposure to high levels of air pollution has also been strongly associated with increased stroke risk in the week following exposure (Shah et al., 2015). Public health efforts to address the risk of stroke in populations thus need to identify and advise those who are at increased risk by virtue of non-modifiable factors and help individuals recognise and manage the health-related effects of modifiable risk factors.

Case Scenario: Presenting Condition

Initial Scenario

Balbir Singh is 58 years old; he works as a journalist for a UK-based Sikh newspaper covering politics and finance on the Indian sub-continent. Balbir was born in India but has lived in England since he was 11 years old. He is married to Jaswir and they have one daughter aged 26 (Manjit) who lives in the USA. Balbir is 5 feet 9 inches tall and weighs 14 stones (96.8 kg), he smoked 20–30 cigarettes a day until 12 months ago when he stopped smoking; he takes no regular exercise. Balbir's father and grandfather both had hypertension and died as a result of myocardial infarction. Balbir has not visited his GP for a number of years, and has not had his blood pressure checked recently; he is not on any prescribed medicines. During an early evening meeting at the newspaper Balbir felt dizzy; when he walked to the water cooler he fell forward onto his knees and was unable to get up from the floor. His colleagues noticed that although he was conscious, Balbir's speech seemed slurred; the left side of his mouth looked different to the right and he could not move his left arm at all. Balbir was made comfortable on the floor supported by cushions. An ambulance was called and Balbir's colleagues stated that they thought he had had a stroke. On arrival the paramedic team assessed Balbir using the FAST (Face, Arms, Speech, Time) test; they asked whether Balbir's fall was witnessed and exactly what time this occurred. The paramedic team recorded his level of consciousness using the Glasgow Coma Scale (GCS), and his temperature, pulse, blood pressure and blood glucose level, as well as assessing whether Balbir could move his arms and legs when prompted, and they noted the clarity of his speech in response to their questions. This initial assessment suggested Balbir may have had a stroke and he was taken by ambulance to the emergency department (ED) of a hospital designated as a hyper-acute stroke centre. The paramedic team would usually pre-alert the ED to mobilise the stroke team.

Before reading the next section consider the following:

1. Which two sets of major blood vessels supply the brain?
2. What is the name of the important vascular structure formed from interconnecting blood vessels that can be found at the base of the brain?
3. The brain requires approximately 750 mL of oxygenated blood each minute; this represents 15 per cent of the cardiac output. There are no reserves of oxygen or glucose (key elements of normal cellular metabolism) within the brain: what are the likely consequences of an interruption in the blood supply to an area of the brain tissue?

Types of Stroke

The presenting signs and symptoms suggest Balbir has probably had a stroke but over the next 15–45 minutes rapid assessment and medical investigations are required in the emergency department (ED). Hankey and Blacker (2015) summarise the key elements of assessment and investigation required to arrive at an accurate diagnosis of stroke in the ED. It is essential to rule out other possible causes for his signs and symptoms (referred to as stroke mimics) and, if he has had a stroke, to establish whether the cause is ischaemic or haemorrhagic. This will determine the most appropriate form of treatment to provide. If Mrs Singh has not been contacted then every effort should be made to arrange for her to come to the ED as treatment options should be discussed with the patient and a close family member wherever possible (Forster et al., 2012).

Brain blood supply

Two sets of major blood vessels supply the brain (see Figure 5.1): the anterior circulation is derived from the right and left internal carotid arteries, and the posterior circulation from the two vertebral arteries. These two sets of blood vessels are connected at the base of the brain to form the circle of Willis; this important structure is made up of the major branches of the anterior and posterior circulation and can, if complete, provide a degree of collateral circulation in the event of arterial occlusion as is seen in the case of ischaemic stroke. However, it is important to note that this compensatory process is not likely to result in arterial blood supply sufficient to maintain normal brain function. More detail on brain anatomy and blood supply can be found in Marieb (2015) and a more applied discussion in Williams et al. (2010). The key point is that interruption of the brain blood supply through ischaemia or haemorrhage will rapidly result in localised and potentially irreversible brain injury. The phrase 'time is brain' is now used internationally to acknowledge that time lost in diagnosing and treating the cause of stroke leads to irreparable damage to the affected brain tissue.

As indicated earlier, there are two main causes of stroke; figures vary but ischaemic strokes (at 75–85 per cent) are more common than haemorrhagic strokes (at 15–25 per cent). The primary cause of ischaemic stroke and TIA is vessel occlusion resulting from large artery thrombosis, or embolism. Embolism is usually cardiac in origin, for example in association with atrial fibrillation which often goes undiagnosed, or associated with prosthetic heart valves. Ischaemic stroke can also occur post myocardial infarction or following arterial dissection (a separation of the layers of the artery wall)

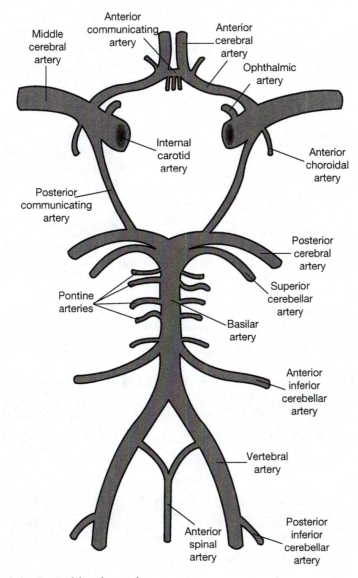

Figure 5.1 Brain blood supply

Source: https://commons.wikimedia.org/wiki/File:Circle_of_Willis_en.svg (accessed 30 January 2016).

as in carotid artery dissection, a common cause of stroke in younger adults (Stein et al., 2015). Haemorrhagic stroke is caused by intraparenchymal (intracerebral) haemorrhage commonly associated with hypertension. A rupture of an arterio-venous malformation or aneurysm can also result in haemorrhagic stroke; a subarachnoid haemorrhage is a third kind of haemorrhagic stroke. See Figure 5.2 for a graphic representation of the mechanism of action of the two main types of stroke and Figures 5.3–5.4 for an outline of the mechanisms of brain injury following stroke.

An ischemic stroke occurs when a blood vesel supplying the brain becomes blocked, as by a clot.

A hemorrhagic stroke occurs when a blood vessel bursts, leaking blood into the brain.

Figure 5.2 Stroke types

Source: US Department of Health and Human Services National Institute of Neurological Disorders and Stroke National Institutes of Health (2009). http://stroke.nih.gov/documents/NINDS_StrokeChallenge_Brochure.pdf (accessed 30 January 2016).

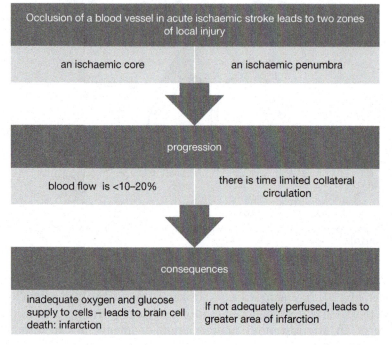

Occlusion of a blood vessel in acute ischaemic stroke leads to two zones of local injury

| an ischaemic core | an ischaemic penumbra |

progression

| blood flow is <10–20% | there is time limited collateral circulation |

consequences

| inadequate oxygen and glucose supply to cells – leads to brain cell death: infarction | If not adequately perfused, leads to greater area of infarction |

Figure 5.3 Mechanism of injury following acute ischaemic stroke

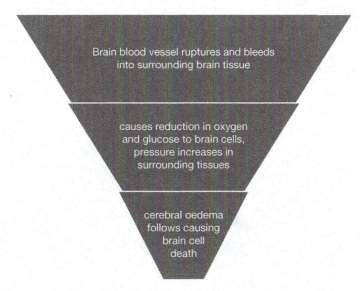

Figure 5.4 Mechanism of injury following haemorrhagic stroke

Brain Injury in Stroke

Brain structure and overall functions are described in Chapter 4 (Table 4.1). To understand stroke it is important to be familiar with the functions of the cerebral cortex and also the cerebellum and brain stem. See Figure 5.5 for a representation of the four lobes (frontal, temporal, parietal and occipital) that make up the cerebral cortex. Figure 5.6 identifies the overall motor and sensory functions associated with different areas of the cerebral cortex; these include cognitive functions including thinking, problem solving, decision making and memory, as well as speech, vision and movement.

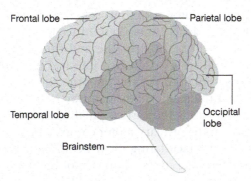

Figure 5.5 Lobes of the brain

Source: Cancer Research UK/Wikimedia Commons. https://commons.wikimedia.org/wiki/File:Diagram_showing_the_lobes_of_the_brain_CRUK_308.svg (accessed 30 January 2016).

Figure 5.6 Motor and sensory regions of the cerebral cortex

Source: Blausen.com staff. 'Blausen gallery 2014'. *Wikiversity Journal of Medicine.* DOI:10.15347/wjm/2014.010. ISSN 20018762. https://commons.wikimedia.org/wiki/ File:Blausen_0102_Brain_Motor%26Sensory.png#/media/File:Blausen_0102_Brain_ Motor%26Sensory.png (accessed 30 January 2016).

Posture, balance and fine motor control are associated with the cerebellum. Figure 5.7, known as the sensory homunculus, graphically represents the distribution of sensory functions associated with the amount of nervous tissue in the cerebral cortex related to a particular region of the body; a similar distribution can be seen in the motor homunculus (Marieb, 2015). The pictorial representation of body regions here is proportional to how richly innervated a particular region is, not to its actual size; see, for example, the face and the hands, both richly innervated. In recognising how post-stroke impairments are related to brain structure and functions it is important to remember the cerebral cortex is divided into two hemispheres which in general terms control functions on the opposite side of the body. In the central nervous system the major motor pathway responsible for control of the majority of the muscles is the corticospinal tract. The neurons making up this tract originate in the primary motor cortex, and project through the brain into the spinal cord, facilitating movement. The neurons controlling the left side of body originate in the right side of the brain in the primary motor cortex area. The axons of these neurons stay on that side of the brain through the internal capsule, and the cerebral peduncle (in the midbrain), to

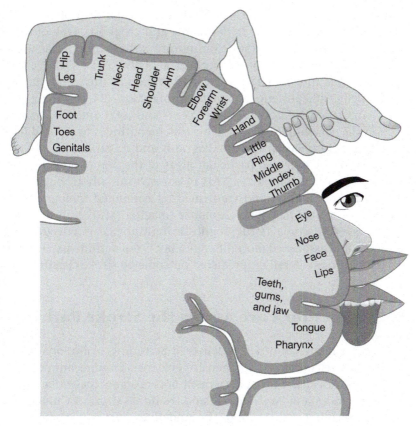

Figure 5.7 Primary sensory cortex (homunculus)
Source: Anatomy & Physiology, Connexions Web site. http://cnx.org/content/col11496/1.6/.
https://commons.wikimedia.org/wiki/File:1421_Sensory_Homunculus.jpg (accessed 30
January 2016).

the medullary pyramid. At this point, the axons cross over from one side to
the other, known as decussation, continuing down the corticospinal tract in
the spinal cord. It is this decussation in the medullary pyramid that means
one side of the brain controls the opposite side of the body (Marieb, 2015).

Some functions or abilities appear to be localised to one hemisphere.
In most people the left hemisphere appears to be dominant; for these
individuals language and mathematical abilities are localised in the left
hemisphere, whilst music and visual–spatial processing are localised in the
right hemisphere. However, this division is not true of all functions, so for
example each hemisphere processes vision for the opposite side. The short-
and long-term impairments seen in stroke are associated with damage to
specific functional areas of the brain. Whilst accurate predictions cannot

always be made, a stroke associated with a particular area of the brain is often associated with specific impairments and prognosis. One of the best known indicators is the Oxford Community Stroke Project classification (OCSP) system developed by Bamford et al. (1991). The OCSP classifies ischaemic stroke into four types: lacunar infarction (frequency of occurrence 25 per cent), posterior circulation infarction (24 per cent), partial anterior circulation infarction (34 per cent) and total anterior circulation infarction (17 per cent). In this system, which continues to be used locally, nationally and internationally, the diagnosis and classification is based on the location of the stroke in particular areas of the brain and the patient's presenting signs and symptoms. This is assessed initially through clinical neurological examination and confirmed by computed tomography (CT) or diffusion-weighted magnetic resonance imaging (MRI) scan techniques. The OCSP is regarded as a useful prognostic indicator, i.e. it indicates level of dependence and associated mortality rates, but is not definitive (see Bamford et al., 1991 for more detail on predicted outcome by stroke classification).

Guidelines for Care Across the Stroke Pathway

Stroke care in many countries is delivered according to National Clinical Guidelines; these contain comprehensive evidence-based recommendations for service provision and for management of care across the stroke pathway. In England, Wales and Northern Ireland, National Clinical Guidelines for Stroke have been in use since 2000. The guidelines, currently in a fourth edition (2012) are prepared by the Intercollegiate Stroke Working Party (ISWP) and published by the Royal College of Physicians (ISWP, 2012). Similar guidelines can be found in Europe, Australia, Canada and the United States.

Assessment and Management of Transient Ischaemic Attacks

Transient ischaemic attack, or TIA, is commonly referred to as a minor stroke. The risk factors for TIA are the same as those outlined for stroke. TIAs are characterised by their sudden onset, and there is typically a focal cerebral or monocular deficit. However, what differentiates TIA from stroke is that the symptoms can resolve quickly and will last less than 24 hours. TIA is not a minor event; there is a high risk of stroke following TIA (Giles et al., 2007; Dutta et al., 2015). Early assessment and treatment in the ED and associated stroke services can reduce this risk by as much as 80 per cent (Wilson et al., 2014). Unfortunately, most people experiencing a TIA do not seek medical attention quickly enough to take advantage of this. Mass media campaigns including, in the UK, the FAST (Face, Arms, Speech, Time) campaign have had some effect in increasing public awareness of stroke and TIA but have not proved effective in changing behaviour (Dombrowski et al., 2013, 2014). Only a small number of people experiencing TIA call an ambulance; many wait to make an appointment with their GP. In the BEATS study (Wilson et al., 2014), and in qualitative studies (e.g. Jones, 2013), reasons given for not seeking urgent medical attention included non-recognition of symptoms and uncertainty about the appropriateness of seeking urgent help, especially when symptoms were mild or transient. National Institute for Health and Care Excellence (NICE, 2008) guidelines recommend those at high risk of stroke should be assessed by a specialist within 24 hours of symptom onset and those at lower risk within a week. This recommendation has led to the establishment of rapid access TIA clinics across the UK with some international evidence that such clinics significantly reduce risk of subsequent stroke (Luengo-Fernandez et al., 2009; Dutta et al., 2015). It has been estimated that this approach could prevent about 10,000 strokes annually. Table 5.1 summarises the treatment pathway that should be followed for people presenting with TIA (ISWP, 2012; NICE, 2008).

Table 5.1 Recommendations for management of transient ischaemic attack

Service provision

Commissioners of stroke services should ensure that people presenting with transient ischaemic attacks can be seen by or referred to an acute neurovascular service. This service should provide care based on the current National Clinical Guidelines for Stroke (Intercollegiate Stroke Working Party (ISWP), 2012) and NICE CG:68. These require that all investigations and treatments to reduce the risk of stroke should be completed within 24 hours for high-risk cases (see below) or within one week for all other cases.

Specific assessment and management recommendations for TIA

Pre-hospital assessment should include the FAST tool. However, there are two important considerations relating to the use of this tool in those suspected of TIA:
• The symptoms reported by patients in a call to an ambulance service or general practitioner may have resolved by the time the assessment is undertaken, and
• The FAST tool may not identify symptoms such as sudden onset visual disturbance. In these cases, despite the negative FAST, the patient should be referred to the acute neurovascular service for investigation in a specialist TIA clinic.

In those who, at the time of assessment in the GP surgery or ED, have no neurological symptoms (that is the symptoms have resolved within 24 hours) an assessment to

(Continued)

Table 5.1 (*Continued*)

---

determine subsequent risk of stoke must be performed using a validated risk assessment tool such as the ABCD² before referral to a TIA clinic.

ABCD² Score for TIA: Total score from 0 (lowest risk) to 7 (highest risk).

- **A** (Age); 1 point for age > 60 years,
- **B** (Blood pressure > 140/90 mmHg); 1 point for hypertension at the acute evaluation,
- **C** (Clinical features); 2 points for unilateral weakness, 1 for speech disturbance without weakness, and
- **D** (symptom duration); 1 point for 10–59 minutes, 2 points for > 60 minutes.
- **D** (Diabetes); 1 point

Stroke risk at 2 days, 7 days, and 90 days:

- Scores 0–3: low risk
- Scores 4–5: moderate risk
- Scores 6–7: high risk

Based on the risk score then the following treatment is normally instigated:

ABCD² score of 4 or more:

- commence aspirin or clopidogrel (300 mg as a loading dose and 75 mg daily thereafter) immediately
- commence a statin e.g. simvastatin at 40 mg, immediately
- undergo specialist assessment and investigation (ideally including diffusion-weighted magnetic resonance imaging) within 24 hours of symptom onset in specialist TIA clinic or on a stroke unit
- provide information on driving – in the UK, those experiencing a TIA must not drive for 28 days
- provide information on and introduce secondary prevention measures such as blood pressure monitoring and treatment for hypertension, dietary change, exercise prescription.

ABCD² score of 3 or below:

As above except that specialist assessment and investigation should occur as soon as possible and not later than one week after symptom onset.

For people presenting with TIA and atrial fibrillation (which further increases risk of subsequent stroke) an anticoagulant therapy (e.g. Warfarin or one of the newer novel oral anticoagulants e.g. Dabigatran) should be commenced provided that investigations rule out intracranial haemorrhage and there are no other contraindications.

People who had a TIA, and who after assessment in a TIA clinic are considered to be suitable for carotid endarterectomy, should have carotid imaging undertaken urgently to facilitate carotid surgery which should be undertaken within 7 days of symptom onset.

The information in this table has been adapted from and summarises guidance which can be found in the National Clinical Guidelines for Stroke (Intercollegiate Stroke Working Party (ISWP), 2012) and NICE CG:68 (2008).

Assessment and Management of Acute Stroke in the Emergency Department

The stroke specialist team will coordinate and undertake assessment and management of the immediate care in the ED; recall that 'time is brain'. Priorities for the first hour in the ED are accurate history taking and neurological examination, brain imaging and blood investigations; associated nursing roles include vital signs recording using the ABCDE approach and information provision to the patient and family. The stroke specialist team will try to establish the exact time when stroke symptoms were noted; in Balbir's case this is clear. In an unwitnessed event, they will establish

---

Case Scenario Update

On arrival in ED Balbir is conscious, he has dysarthria and although he is trying to communicate it is difficult to comprehend what he is saying. Balbir has a left-sided paralysis (hemiplegia) involving both his left arm and his left leg; he cannot move either when requested to do so but he appears to understand the request and shakes his head and sighs. The paramedics report a positive FAST test and that Balbir's Glasgow Coma Scale score is 10 (E=4, M=3, V=3) on admission. Balbir is accompanied by a colleague from his workplace who is trying to contact Balbir's wife and daughter. The ED admitting doctor immediately rings the dedicated line for the hyper-acute stroke unit to notify them of the admission and requests the stroke specialist nurse attend ED.

Vital signs

Balbir's blood pressure is 160/100, his pulse is 90 and regular, respirations 18 breaths per minute, temperature 37.0 °C; he is pale but not cyanosed. Oxygen saturation = 97 per cent. He appears to confirm that he takes no prescribed medications, but it is unclear whether he takes any over-the-counter medicines. Weight and past medical history are indicated above. A Recognition of Stroke in the Emergency Room (ROSIER) (Nor et al., 2005) test is completed and a score of +4 is recorded; this indicates that acute stroke is the likely diagnosis (see p.126).

Before reading the next section consider the following:

1. Review Balbir's vital signs recorded on arrival in ED. Make a note of whether these are within expected normal ranges and whether any would raise cause for concern.
2. Consider why it is important that ED nursing staff encourage Balbir's wife to attend the ED immediately.
3. Consider the information needs of Balbir and his wife and family in the first hour in the ED.

when the person was last observed to be symptom free. This information is pivotal to determining immediate treatment options. The Recognition Of Stroke In the Emergency Room (ROSIER) score (Nor et al., 2005) is a simple and rapidly conducted scoring system which includes assessment of symptom onset, the date/time, and determines whether there has there been loss of consciousness or syncope scoring, -1 for yes and 0 for no. Similarly, whether there has been any seizure activity, whether there was new acute onset (or on awakening from sleep) of the following: asymmetrical facial weakness, asymmetrical arm weakness, asymmetrical leg weakness, speech disturbance and visual field defect (each scoring -1 or 0). The total score range is: -2 to +5; stroke is likely if total scores are >0. Stroke is unlikely but not completely excluded if total score is < or = to 0 (Nor et al., 2005).

The ROSIER score has indicated the likelihood of stroke in Balbir's case; rapid primary clinical neurological assessment will follow. This will normally be supported by completion of the National Institutes of Health Stroke Scale (NIHSS). The NIHSS provides a score of between 0, indicating no neurological deficit, and 42, indicating a severe neurological deficit. Hypoglycaemia is a stroke mimic; if the capillary glucose (BM stix) recording is <3.5 mmol/L this should be treated and the patient reassessed. Thereafter, monitoring is essential to maintain blood glucose within the range 4–11 mmol/L as hyperglycaemia is associated with poorer neurological outcomes and increases the risk of bleeding in those who receive thrombolysis (Rowat, 2009).

Brain Imaging

A key priority immediately after the rapid ED assessments outlined above is to proceed to brain imaging within one hour of ED admission for people with acute stroke symptoms (ISWP, 2012). CT remains the most common form of brain imaging in the UK due to availability and ease of access. However, there is good evidence that diffusion-weighted MRI has greater diagnostic accuracy than CT for acute ischaemic stroke (Schellinger et al., 2010). The primary purpose of brain imaging is to exclude intracerebral haemorrhage and determine whether administration of thrombolysis and/or intra-arterial clot retrieval should be considered. Evidence of cerebral ischaemia may be difficult to detect at this stage but radiologists and stroke physicians will examine the CT images; this will also help rule out stroke mimics including tumours, sub-dural haematoma and cerebritis. If intracerebral haemorrhage is ruled out by brain imaging, the patient's suitability for treatment with the thrombolytic agent Alteplase® will be considered. See comments later in this chapter about intra-arterial clot retrieval. These investigations should all take place within one hour of arrival at ED or sooner.

Importance of Reperfusion in Ischaemic Stroke

Following occlusion of a blood vessel in an ischaemic stroke, two zones of local injury occur. These are described as the core and the ischaemic penumbra, which is often described as an area of moderately ischaemic brain tissue surrounding an area of more severe ischaemia, the core. In the core, blood flow can be less than 10–25 per cent and the severe reduction in oxygen and glucose results in death of the neurons and glial cells. However, the cells within the ischaemic penumbra, although at risk, will remain viable for a short period of time as some oxygen and glucose is provided by the collateral circulation. This is a time sensitive period because, unless reperfusion is successfully achieved, a wider area of infarction will develop with the consequent risk of more severe disability and death. In order to ensure thrombolysis is indicated and poses minimal risk the stroke team will establish Balbir's past medical history. This includes checking for a history of hypertension and cardiovascular events or problems, e.g. atrial fibrillation or a history of bleeding or coagulation disorders and a medication history which includes anti-coagulants (both of which could rule out use of thrombolysis) (Table 5.2). They will also rapidly assess stroke and cardiovascular risk factors including family history, diabetes, smoking, dietary intake, weight, alcohol intake and exercise.

It is clear that in Balbir's case he can provide only a limited history and so it is essential that every attempt is made to ensure his wife attends the ED. Assessment will continue with a 12-lead ECG to check for cardiac arrhythmias including atrial fibrillation, which is associated with an increased risk of stroke; full blood count, biochemical profile, cardiac enzymes, and clotting screen. Physical assessment will be undertaken, focusing firstly on neurological assessment including testing of motor, sensory and cognitive functioning, followed by a standard physical examination. Balbir's weight will be recorded using a trolley scale. For more detail on physical and neurological assessment in stroke see Alexandrov (2010b) and Stein et al. (2015).

Thrombolysis for Ischaemic Stroke

Thrombolysis is a reperfusion therapy designed to recanalise obstructed arterial vessels. Thrombolytic agents (such as Alteplase®) are serine proteases that work by converting plasminogen to the natural fibrinolytic agent plasmin. Plasmin breaks down the fibrinogen and fibrin contained in a clot. The use of Alteplase® is limited to a narrow therapeutic window during which the treatment is known to be maximally effective. Provided there are no contraindications, clinicians should consider administration

Table 5.2   Reasons why thrombolysis is not appropriate for some stroke survivors

i)	Outside the time window of 3–4.5 hours
ii)	Outside the (**within**) 3-hour time window and over 80 years of age
iii)	Known coagulation disorder
iv)	On anticoagulants
v)	Intracerebral haemorrhage

of Alteplase® within 3 hours of known symptom onset for people of all ages. The IST-3 (2012) trial results indicated no increased risk to the over 80s during that time period but reported that efficacy of treatment reduced significantly after 3 hours. National Clinical Guidelines for Stroke ISWP (2012: 46) recommend clinicians consider administration of Alteplase® between 3 and 4.5 hours for people under 80. Between 3 and 6 hours (ISWP, 2012: 46) recommend that clinicians should review patients on an individual basis but note that benefits of treatment with Alteplase® 'are likely to be smaller than for those treated within 3 hours but that the risk of worse outcomes including death will not on average be increased'.

Table 5.3   Mechanical clot retrieval

Recent research has demonstrated that mechanical clot retrieval (intra-arterial thrombectomy) can improve the outcomes for some people who have experienced an ischaemic stroke caused by occlusions in the proximal anterior cerebral circulation. Patients in this group have poorer outcomes at 90 days and have been shown to benefit less from reperfusion treatment with Alteplase® alone. Mechanical clot retrieval is also designed to recanalise obstructed arterial vessels in order to reperfuse the ischaemic penumbra. Results from four randomised controlled trials have found improved functional independence at three months with no significant increase in mortality in those treated using mechanical clot retrieval devices when compared to standard treatment (Berkhemer et al., 2015; Goyal et al., 2015; Campbell et al., 2015; Saver et al., 2015). At the time of writing intra-arterial clot retrieval with or without the addition of thrombolytic agent is only performed in specialist neurological centres. This form of intervention may become a more mainstream therapeutic technique in the next three to five years. However, it seems clear that more research is required to address the remaining uncertainties relating to this form of intervention; these include questions about the benefits for patients with more distal occlusions, the most appropriate time window for the intervention, and the influence of the type of mechanical retrieval device used.

Case Scenario Update

Balbir is considered suitable for thrombolysis; after discussion between the stroke consultant, Balbir and his wife, tissue plasminogen activator (tPA) in the form of Alteplase® (0.9 mg tPA per 1 kg of patient weight to a maximum dose of 90 mg) is prescribed. Administration is 10 per cent as an IV bolus dose over 1 minute then the remainder infused over 1 hour. He is then transferred to the hyper-acute stroke unit for monitoring. Hyper-acute stroke care is defined as the healthcare activities that take place between the time of first contact with a potential stroke patient and either admission to hospital or outpatient management in the community. Hyper-acute stroke units in the UK tend to take admissions direct from the ED and care for stroke survivors for between two and five days (this figure continues to fall and is often 72 hours or less).

Alexandrov (2010b) notes the importance of accurate blood pressure monitoring and control prior to and post administration of thrombolysis. This is because poorly controlled hypertension is the most common reason associated with symptomatic intracerebral haemorrhage in patients treated with intravenous (IV) tPA. ISWP (2012: 53) guidelines state that 'blood pressure reduction to 185/110 mmHg or lower should be considered in people who are candidates for thrombolysis'. However, reducing blood pressure too low can reduce cerebrovascular blood flow and reduce the perfusion in the already compromised ischaemic penumbra; therefore any changes in blood pressure from Balbir's baseline recording of 160/100 would be reported to the lead physician immediately. Nurses play a key role in management of post-thrombolysis care. In most hyper-acute units the patient is nursed one to one for the first 6 hours. Balbir would be nursed in a bed where continuous observation is possible. The standard approach to monitoring is outlined below.

Post-thrombolysis Care

During the IV administration period and immediately thereafter the primary concern is to detect anaphylaxis (rare) and oro-lingual angioedema (quite rare, 1–2 per cent incidence). If an urticarial rash, peri-orbital swelling or oro-lingual angioedema are evident the IV tPA should be stopped and the patient reviewed by a doctor urgently. Tachypnoea, dyspnoea, tachycardia are also seen in anaphylactic reactions. Swelling of the tongue is seen in oro-lingual angioedema and may require emergency intubation or tracheostomy. It is important to observe for any signs of extracranial haemorrhage; in the event of bleeding pressure would be applied to the sites and medical staff informed immediately. If there are other signs of haemorrhage (fall in blood pressure, tachycardia) medical staff should be contacted and will order an immediate non-contrast CT scan. Taking arterial or intravenous blood samples and intravenous line insertion should be avoided for 24 hours unless the patient is critically ill. To further reduce the risk of bleeding, insertion of urinary catheters and nasogastric tubes should be avoided for 24 hours. All anti-thrombotic medications (anti-platelet and anti-coagulation medications) will be omitted for at least 24 hours. Thereafter, unless contraindicated, aspirin 300 mg daily will be prescribed for two weeks and then Clopidogrel 75 mg daily (ISWP, 2012).

Vital Signs

Blood pressure and pulse should be recorded every 15 minutes for the first two hours after completion of the tPA infusion, then every 30 minutes for six hours, then hourly for 16 hours. Manual sphygmomanometers may be recommended, particularly in patients with atrial fibrillation because of significant beat-to-beat variability (Middleton et al., 2015); in this case the average of three consecutive systolic and diastolic measurements should be recorded. Continuous cardiac monitoring should occur; nurses should note any aberrant cardiac rhythms (see Chapter 6) and document and report these if they are evident. The NIHSS should be recorded two hours after IV tPA administration and will normally be repeated at 12 and 24 hours; with an increase in frequency of scoring if deterioration occurs. Assessment of neurological status using the Glasgow Coma Scale is included in some post-thrombolysis care pathways but is not recommended for ongoing monitoring after ischaemic stroke as scores of 15 (normal) have been recorded despite evidence of significant disability on NIHSS scoring (Middleton et al., 2015).

Oxygen saturations should be monitored every four hours but supplemental oxygen therapy is not recommended for people with acute stroke unless saturations drop below 95 per cent and hypoxia is evident. Pyrexia is associated with poorer outcomes after stroke; therefore temperature should be monitored every four hours. Treatment with paracetamol or cooling blankets may be considered where high temperature (>37.5°C) persists (Rowat, 2009; Middleton et al., 2015). Similarly, patients with post-stroke hyperglycaemia, but not known to have diabetes mellitus, have a higher risk of death when compared with those (not known to have diabetes mellitus) whose blood glucose is within normal range after stroke. Therefore, six-hourly capillary blood glucose motoring is recommended with the intention to maintain blood glucose between 4.0 to 11.0 mmol/L.

Swallowing Assessment

Dysphagia is common after stroke with up to 65 per cent of patients experiencing swallowing difficulties (Martino, 2005). Balbir should remain nil by mouth until he is screened by a dysphagia trained nurse or a Speech and Language Therapist (SALT). Disruptions to the swallowing mechanism are common after stroke. The risk of aspiration of fluid or foodstuffs into the lungs is high; this results in aspiration pneumonia which can significantly impair recovery and threaten survival. The risk of aspiration pneumonia is increased threefold in those with dysphagia. Swallowing should be assessed using a validated screening tool (Donovan et al., 2013). During the test careful observation of oro-motor control and laryngeal phases of the attempted swallow is undertaken. This test should occur within four hours of admission to ED (ISWP, 2012). If there is evidence of swallowing difficulty (dysphagia), Balbir would be referred to the SALT team and maintained nil by mouth. National Clinical Guidelines for Stroke (ISWP, 2012) recommend specialist swallowing assessment by a SALT ideally within 24 hours and not later than 72 hours. For nurses it is essential to provide mouth care and for the stroke specialist multidisciplinary team (MDT) to consider nasogastric feeding if Balbir's swallow is not safe after 24 hours (Geeganage et al., 2012). No food, fluid or medication should be given orally during this time. If swallowing improves then staged progression to full diet may include supervised thickened fluids, pureed and then soft diet. Specific advice would be required from the SALT team working in conjunction with dieticians and nurses caring for Balbir. Studies assessing the natural history of swallowing function after acute stroke suggest that many patients with dysphagia recover their swallowing within the first week and the majority will have improved by the end of the second week (Donovan et al., 2013).

Middleton et al. (2011) have shown that introducing protocols focused on pyrexia, hyperglycaemia and swallowing, and associated training for nurses into stroke unit care can significantly improve outcomes. Balbir will be nursed at bed rest for 24 hours. There is no agreed international standard for positioning in the first 24 hours post-ischaemic stroke. Practice varies between countries. In the UK patients are usually nursed with the head of bed at 30 degrees, whereas in some countries, the patient is nursed flat as there is some evidence that this position increases cerebral perfusion. Regular position change is essential to reduce the risk of pressure ulcer formation; this is important as Balbir will have reduced mobility and reduced sensation.

A large international crossover randomised controlled trial will commence in late 2015. The HeadPoST trial will compare outcomes for patients nursed flat with those for patients nursed at 30 degrees in the first 24 hours post-stroke. See Table 5.4 for a summary of the HeadPoST trial.

Table 5.4   HeadPoST trial

HeadPoST is a multicentre, prospective, cluster randomised crossover blinded outcome assessment study to compare the effectiveness of the lying flat (0°) head position with the sitting up (≥ 30°) head position, in the first 24 hours of admission to hospital for patients with acute stroke, on the outcome of death or disability over the subsequent 90 days. For more details see:

www.georgeinstitute.org.au/projects/head-position-in-stroke-trial-headpost

Depending on whether presenting symptoms improve or not, patients may be discharged direct to an early supported discharge team (Fearon and Langhorne, 2012), to an acute stroke unit or combined acute and rehabilitation stroke unit. Sentinel Stroke National Audit (SSNAP) (Royal College of Physicians (RCP), 2015) data for October to December 2014 indicated that 59.8 per cent (improving but still short of target) were admitted to a stroke unit within four hours of arrival at ED and 85 per cent spent >90 per cent of their hospital stay on a stroke unit (up from 63 per cent in 2010). There is strong evidence from the Stroke Unit Trialists' Collaboration Cochrane Systematic Review findings (updated 2013) that, compared with conventional care, organised inpatient stroke unit care resulted in long-term reduction in death, dependency and the need for institutional care; similar outcomes have been reported for early supported discharge (Fearon and Langhorne, 2012).

Ongoing Rehabilitative Care

This begins in the acute stage and the areas of care identified should be considered when providing nursing care of any kind. Whether or not patients receive thrombolysis there are other aspects of stroke care in which nurses play a key role as members of stroke-specialised MDTs. In addition to the elements of care outlined above these include appropriate positioning, mobilisation, assessment of continence and ongoing communication. Multidisciplinary working is central to high quality stroke practice; stroke unit nurses should be working with therapists in the areas identified below.

Positioning and Early Mobilisation

Correct limb positioning is important to maintain muscle tone, to avoid joint injury and pain (especially the shoulder joint on the affected side, the hand and wrist and the foot). Physiotherapists will demonstrate how to use pillows/towels or blankets as 'scaffolding' to maintain good posture and position. Family members can also be taught these skills. After 24 hours and following assessment by physiotherapists Balbir would be sat out of bed for a short period in a specialist stroke chair with support for his left arm and hand and left leg; hoist use may be necessary to achieve this initially. ISWP (2012) recommendations indicate that all patients should be mobilised within 24 hours. The AVERT trial (very early mobilisation within 24 hours of stroke onset) compared very early mobilisation provided by physiotherapist and nurses with usual care (Bernhardt et al., 2015). The initial findings of this large international trial (n = 2,104) reporting on outcomes at three months were published in early 2015. These indicated that patients in the usual care group had a more favourable outcome at three months than those who received higher dose very early mobilisation (Bernhardt et al., 2015). Further interpretation of the AVERT trial findings is needed; these will inform clinical guidelines going forward. At present, guidance supports early mobilisation but at a lower level of intensity than in the AVERT trial intervention.

Deep vein thrombosis (DVT) and pulmonary embolism (PE) are common complications of reduced mobility post-stroke, particularly in the first month, with up to 50 per cent of patients having thrombus in either the calf or thigh of the paretic limb (Dennis et al., 2013). The CLOTS3 trial (2013) reported that intermittent pneumatic compression (using thigh-length compression sleeves) reduced the risk of DVT and may improve survival in patients who are immobile after stroke. Earlier trials (CLOTS1&2, Dennis et al., 2013) found no benefit associated with use of compression stockings (knee or thigh length); ISWP (2012) recommend that compression stockings should not be used with stroke patients.

Continence

Getliffe and Brooks (2010) note that between 32 and 79 per cent of stroke survivors will experience urinary incontinence, and as many as 30 per cent of people will experience faecal incontinence, largely due to functional disability, up to 7–10 days after stroke. There is a clear association between urinary incontinence and poorer outcomes, including increased incidence of depression, admission to long-term care and increased mortality (Getliffe and Brooks, 2010; Thomas, 2005). Individual assessment is key to determining the likely cause of incontinence post-stroke. ISWP (2012) guidance indicates urinary catheters should not be inserted unless there is evidence of retention of urine. Monitoring of fluid intake and output, support and assistance to use a beside commode or to access the toilet using a wheelchair should all be considered alongside noting patterns of continence/incontinence and any signs such as frequency and urgency which will require investigation. The ICONS feasibility trial (Thomas et al., 2014) provided some indication that a structured approach to assessment and management of post-stroke urinary incontinence, allied to staff training, may be beneficial, particularly for certain types of incontinence (urge and stress); however, further large-scale randomised controlled trials of such interventions are required before definitive guidance can be provided.

Communication

Whilst meeting the need for information is consistently one of the highest priorities for stroke survivors and their families, it is one of the areas of stroke care where there is most need for effective strategies to provide clear and consistent information at a time when it is needed (Forster et al., 2012; Cameron et al., 2013; ISWP, 2012). Core elements of effective communication include provision of information regarding the nature of the stroke event experienced; an explanation of the initial impairments evident after the stroke and how these will be treated; clear explanations of planned interventions; and the purpose of processes of care. Family members of stroke survivors may wish to support elements of personal care and help with hydration and nutrition; this can be encouraged but requires structured information provision and some skills training provided by nurses and therapists (Forster et al., 2012). Information needs change over time and nurses and other members of the stroke MDT must be prepared to reiterate and repeat information on a frequent basis (Cameron et al., 2013). Stroke is typically a sudden and distressing event for the survivor and their family; psychological support is another key element of post-stroke care with the ISWP (2012) recommending a stepped care approach to providing this kind of support. This is a responsibility for the whole stroke team and not just for clinical psychologists.

Case Scenario Update

After 12 hours it is clear that Balbir's symptoms have not improved significantly although he has some evidence of improvement in motor function in his left arm and leg. His speech is improving but his swallow is regarded as unsafe. Thrombolysis is not effective in achieving reperfusion and improvement in function in all cases. Balbir's Barthel score is 2 (out of 20) at this stage. The Barthel Index consists of 10 items that measure a person's daily functioning, specifically the activities of daily living and mobility (Mahoney and Barthel, 1965). The items include feeding, moving from wheelchair to bed and return, personal grooming, transferring to and from a toilet, bathing, walking on level surface, going up and down stairs, dressing, and continence of bowels and bladder.

Management of Haemorrhagic Stroke

Diagnosis is established following CT; treatment then depends largely on the type of haemorrhage seen (Alexandrov, 2010b). Initially all patients would be nursed with the head of the bed at 30 degrees to reduce the likelihood of increased intracranial pressure secondary to intracranial haemorrhage. The most common type seen is intraparenchymal haemorrhage, often associated with a history of hypertension. At present there is no indication that surgical treatments for haemorrhagic stroke are more effective than non-invasive management (Alexandrov, 2010b). Brain imaging and coagulation studies are important investigations to determine the likely cause of the haemorrhagic stroke and along with the clinical signs and progress will determine possible interventions (for example aneurysmal repair, or management of clotting disorder). The main focus for acute management is blood pressure monitoring and control and again nurses will play a key role in this process. The ongoing nursing observations and care for patients presenting with acute intracerebral haemorrhage are as outlined above; variations to the care management would be directed based on individual need by the stroke physicians.

Summary

This chapter has reviewed the key aspects of stroke care in the first 72 hours of the hyper-acute period and identified the ways in which nurses are integrally involved as members of the stroke-specific multidisciplinary team. Stroke and TIA are now regarded as medical emergencies and health professionals understand that 'time is brain'. Stroke services have been radically reorganised in recent times so that stroke survivors have the opportunity to receive evidence-based care. The stroke care pathway spans more than the hyper-acute, acute and inpatient rehabilitation periods. The longer-term rehabilitation and support needed by stroke survivors is another area of importance but beyond the scope of this chapter; see further reading for more information.

Further Reading

Middleton, S., R. Grimley and A. W. Alexandrov. 'Triage, Treatment and Transfer: Evidence-based Clinical Practice Recommendations and Models of Nursing Care for the First 24 Hours of Admission to Hospital for Acute Stroke', *Stroke*, **46**(2) 2015, e18–e25. doi: 10.1161/STROKEAHA.114.006139.

National Institute for Health and Care Excellence. *Acute Stroke Pathway* (2015) [Online]. Available from: http://pathways.nice.org.uk/pathways/stroke (accessed 14 April 2015).

Williams, J., L. Perry and C. Watkins (eds). *Acute Stroke Nursing* (Oxford: Wiley-Blackwell, 2010).

Care Quality Commission. 'Supporting Life After Stroke: A Review of Services for People Who Have Had a Stroke and Their Carers' (2011) [Online]. Available from: www.cqc.org.uk/sites/default/files/documents/supporting_life_after_stroke_national_report.pdf (accessed 30 March 2015).

References

Alexandrov, A. W. (2010a) 'What is a Stroke?', Chapter 3 in J. Williams, L. Perry and C. Watkins (eds), *Acute Stroke Nursing* (Oxford: Wiley-Blackwell, 2010a).

Alexandrov, A. W. 'Acute Stroke Nursing Management', Chapter 4 in J. Williams, L. Perry and C. Watkins (eds), *Acute Stroke Nursing* (Oxford, Wiley-Blackwell, 2010b).

Bamford, J. P., M. Sandercock, C. Dennis, J. Warlow and J. Burn. 'Classification and Natural History of Clinically Identifiable Subtypes of Cerebral Infarction', *Lancet*, 337(8756) (1991), 1521–6.

Berkhemer, O. A., P. S. S. Fransen, D. Beumer et al.. 'A Randomized Trial of Intraarterial Treatment for Acute Ischemic Stroke', *New England Journal of Medicine*, 372 (2015),11–20.

Bernhardt, J. and the AVERT Trial Collaboration Group. 'Efficacy and Safety of Very Early Mobilisation within 24 hours of Acute Stroke Onset (AVERT): A Randomized Controlled Trial', *Lancet* (2015). doi: http://dx.doi.org/10.1016/S0140-6736(15)60690-0.

Boardman, H. M. P., L. Hartley, A. Eisinga, et al.. 'Hormone Therapy for Preventing Cardiovascular Disease in Post-menopausal Women', *Cochrane Database of Systematic Reviews 3* (2015), CD002229.

Cameron, J. I., G. Naglie, F. L. Silver and M. A. M. Gignac. 'Stroke Family Caregivers' Support Needs Change Across the Care Continuum: A Qualitative Study Using the Timing It Right Framework', *Disability and Rehabilitation*, 35(4) (2013), 315–24.

Campbell, B. C. V., P. J. Mitchell, T. J. Kleinig et al.. 'Endovascular Therapy for Ischemic Stroke with Perfusion-Imaging Selection', *New England Journal of Medicine*, 372 (2015), 1009–18.

CLOTS (Clots in Legs Or sTockings after Stroke) Trials Collaboration 2013. 'Effectiveness of Intermittent Pneumatic Compression in Reduction of Risk of Deep Vein Thrombosis in Patients Who Have Had a Stroke (CLOTS3): A Multicentre Randomised Controlled Trial. *Lancet*, 382(9891) (2013), 516–24. doi: 10.1016/S0140-6736(13)61050-8.

Dennis, M., P. Sandercock, J. Reid, C. Graham, G. Murray, G. Venables, A. Rudd, G. Bowler. 'The CLOTS Trials Collaboration. The Effect of Graduated Compression Stockings on Long-term Outcomes After Stroke. The CLOTS Trials 1 and 2', *Stroke*, 44 (2013), 1075–9. doi: 10.1161/STROKEAHA.111.680298.

Department of Health. *National Stroke Strategy* (London: Department of Health, 2007).

Dombrowksi, S. et al.. 'The Impact of the UK "Act FAST" Stroke Awareness Campaign: Content Analysis of Patients, Witness and Primary Care Clinicians' Perceptions', *BMC Public Health*, 13 (2013), 915. doi: 10.1186/1471-2458-13-915.

Dombrowski S., M. White, J. Mackintosh, P. Gellert, V. Arraujo-Soares, R. Thomson, H. Rodgers, G. Ford and F. Sniehotta. 'The Stroke "Act FAST" Campaign:

Remembered But Not Understood?', *International Journal of Stroke*, **10**(3) (2014), 324–30. doi: 10.1111/ijs.12353.

Donovan, N. J., S. K. Daniels, J. Edmiaston, J. Weinhardt, D. Summers and D. Mitchell on behalf of the American Heart Association Council on Cardiovascular Nursing and Stroke Council Dysphagia Screening. 'State of the Art Invitational Conference Proceeding from the State-of-the-Art Nursing Symposium, International Stroke Conference 2012', *Stroke*, **44** (2013), e24–e31. doi: 10.1161/STR.0b013e3182877f57.

Dutta, D., E. Bowen and C. Foy. 'Four Year Follow Up of Transient Ischemic Attacks, Strokes, and Mimics: A Retrospective Transient Ischemic Attack Clinic Cohort Study', *Stroke*, **46** (2015), 1227–32. doi: 10.1161/STROKEAHA.114.008632.

Fearon, P. and P. Langhorne. 'Early Supported Discharge Trialists. Services for Reducing Duration of Hospital Care for Acute Stroke Patients', *Cochrane Database of Systematic Reviews* **9** (2012), art. no.: CD000443. doi: 10.1002/14651858. CD000443.pub3.

Forster, A., L. Brown, J. Smith, A. House, P. Knapp, J. Wright and J. Young. Information Provision for Stroke Patients and Their Caregivers. *Cochrane Database of Systematic Reviews*, **11** (2012), art. no.: CD001919. doi: 10.1002/14651858.CD001919.pub3.

Geeganage, C., J. Beavan, S. Ellender and P. M. W. Bath. Interventions for Dysphagia and Nutritional Support in Acute and Subacute Stroke. *Cochrane Database of Systematic Reviews*, **10** (2012), art. no.: CD000323. doi: 10.1002/14651858. CD000323.pub2.

Getliffe, K., and W. Brooks. 'Promoting Continence', Chapter 6 in J. Williams, L. Perry and C. Watkins (eds), *Acute Stroke Nursing* (Oxford: Wiley-Blackwell, 2010).

Giles, M. F., P. M. Rothwell. 'Risk of Stroke Early after Transient Ischaemic Attack: A Systematic Review and Meta-Analysis. *Lancet Neurology*, **6** (2007), 1063–72.

Goyal, M., A. M. Demchuk, B. K. Menon et al.. 'Randomized Assessment of Rapid Endovascular Treatment of Ischemic Stroke', *New England Journal of Medicine* **372** (2015), 1019–30.

Hankey, G. and D. J. Blacker. 'Is It a Stroke?' *British Medical Journal*, **350** (2015), h56. doi: 10.1136/bmj.h56.

Intercollegiate Stroke Working Party (ISWP). *National Clinical Guidelines for Stroke*. 4th edn (London: Royal College of Physicians, 2012) [Online]. Available from: www. rcplondon.ac.uk/sites/default/files/national-clinical-guidelines-for-stroke-fourth-edition.pdf (accessed 15 April 2015).

The IST-3 Collaborative Group. 'The Benefits and Harms of Intravenous Thrombolysis with Recombinant Tissue Plasminogen Activator within 6 h of Acute Ischaemic Stroke (The Third International Stroke Trial [IST-3]): A Randomised Controlled Trial', *Lancet*, **379**(9834) (2012), 2352–63. doi: 10.1016/S0140-6736(12)60768-5.

Jones, S. *Acute Stroke and the Public's Response to Symptoms*. Unpublished PhD. University of Central Lancashire, 2013).

Lee, S., A. C. E. Shafe and M. R. Cowie. 'UK Stroke Incidence, Mortality and Cardiovascular Risk Management 1999–2008: Time-trend Analysis From the General Practice Research Database', *BMJ Open* (2011) 1:e000269. doi: 10.1136/bmjopen-2011-000269.

Lincoln, N. B., I. I. Kneebone, J. A. B. McNiven and R. Morris. *Psychological Management of Stroke* (Chichester: Wiley-Blackwell, 2012).

Luengo-Fernandez, R., A. M. Gray and P. M. Rothwell. Effect of Urgent Treatment for Transient Ischaemic Attack and Minor Stroke on Disability and Hospital Costs (EXPRESS study): A Prospective Population-based Sequential Comparison', *Lancet Neurology*, **8** (2009), 235–43. doi: 10.1016/ S1474-4422(09)70019-5.

Mahoney F. I. and D. Barthel. 'Functional evaluation: the Barthel Index.' *Maryland State Med Journal* **14** (1965), 56–61.

Marieb, E. N. *Essentials of Human Anatomy & Physiology*, 11th edn. (Harlow: Pearson Education, 2015).

Martino, R., N. Foley, S. Bhogal, N. Diamant, M. Speechley and R. Teasell. 'Dysphagia After Stroke: Incidence, Diagnosis, and Pulmonary Complications', *Stroke*, **36** (2005), 2756–63. doi: 10.1161/01.STR.0000190056.76543.eb

Meschia, J. F., B. B. Worrall and S. S. Rich. 'Genetic Susceptibility to Ischaemic Stroke', *Nature Reviews Neurology*, **7**(7) (2011), 369–78. doi: 10.101038/nrnneurol.2011.80

Middleton, S., P. McElduff, J. Ward, J. M. Grimshaw, S. Dales, C. D'Este et al.. 'QASC Trialists Group. Implementation of Evidence Based Treatment Protocols to Manage Fever, Hyperglycaemia and Swallowing Dysfunction in Acute Stroke (QASC): A Cluster Randomized Controlled Trial. *Lancet*, **378** (2011), 1699–1706. doi: 10.1016/S0140-6736(11)61485-2.

Middleton, S., R. Grimley and A. W. Alexandrov. 'Triage, Treatment and Transfer: Evidence-based Clinical Practice Recommendations and Models of Nursing Care for the First 24 Hours of Admission to Hospital for Acute Stroke. *Stroke* **46**(2) (2015), e18–e25. doi: 10.1161/STROKEAHA.114.006139.

National Audit Office. *Department of Health: Progress in Improving Stroke Care* (London: The Stationery Office, 2010) [Online]. Available from: www.nao.org.uk/report/ department-of-health-progress-in-improving-stroke-care/ (accessed 15 April 2015).

National Institute for Health and Clinical Excellence (NICE). *National Clinical Guideline for Diagnosis and Initial Management of Acute Stroke and Transient Ischaemic Attack (TIA). CG:68.* (2008) [Online]. Available from: http://publications.nice.org. uk/stroke-cg68 (accessed 15 April 2015).

National Institute for Health and Care Excellence (NICE). *Stroke Rehabilitation: Long-Term Rehabilitation after Stroke. CG:162.* (2013) [Online]. Available from: www. nice.org.uk/CG162 (accessed 15 April 2014).

Nor, A. M., J. Davis, B. Sen, D. Shipsey, S. J. Louw, A. G. Dyker et al.. 'The Recognition of Stroke in the Emergency Room (ROSIER) Scale: Development and Validation of a Stroke Recognition Instrument', *Lancet Neurology*, **4** (2005), 727–34.

Rowat, A. 'Using the Mnemonic "Brain Attack" in the Management of Acute Stroke. *Nursing Standard*, **24**(6) (2009), 50–7.

Royal College of Physicians (RCP). *Sentinel Stroke National Audit Programme. Clinical Audit Results: October to December 2014* (London: Royal College of Physicians, 2015) [Online]. Available from: www.strokeaudit.org/results/Clinical-audit/National-Results.aspx (accessed 15 March 2015).

Saver, J. L., M. Goyal, A. Bonafe et al.. 'Stent-retriever Thrombectomy after Intravenous t-PA vs. t-PA Alone in Stroke', *New England Journal of Medicine* (2015). doi: 10.1056/NEJMoa1415061.

Schellinger, P. D. R. Bryan, L. R. Caplan, J. A. Detre, R. R. Edelman, C. Jaigobin, C. S. Kidwell, J. P. Mohr et al.. 'Evidence-based Guideline: The Role of Diffusion and Perfusion MRI for the Diagnosis of Acute Ischemic Stroke. Report of the Therapeutics and Technology Assessment Subcommittee of the American Academy of Neurology', *Neurology* **75**(2) (2010), 177–85. doi: 10.1212/ WNL.0b013e3181e7c9dd

Schwamm, L. H., M. J. Reeves, W. Pan, E. E. Smith, M. R. Frankel, D. Olson, X. Zhao, E. Peterson and G. Fonarow. 'Race/Ethnicity, Quality of Care and Outcomes in Ischaemic Stroke', *Circulation*, **121** (2010), 1492–1501.

Shah, A. S. V., K. K. Lee, D. A. McAllister et al.. 'Short Term Exposure to Air Pollution and Stroke: A Systematic Review and Meta-analysis', *British Medical Journal* **350** (2015), h1295.

Stein, J. L., R. Harvey, C. J. Weinstein, R. D. Zorowicz and G. Wittenberg (eds). *Stroke Recovery and Rehabilitation.* 2nd edn (New York: Demos Medical, 2015).

Stroke Association. *State of the Nation Stroke Statistics* (London: Stroke Association, 2015) [Online]. Available from: www.stroke.org.uk/tags/women?key=state+of+the+nation (accessed 30 March 2015).

Stroke Unit Trialists' Collaboration. 'Organised Inpatient (Stroke Unit) Care for Stroke', *Cochrane Database of Systematic Reviews*, 9 (2013), art. no.: CD000197. doi: 10.1002/14651858.CD000197.pub3.

Thomas L. H., J. Barrett, S. Cross, B. French, M. Leathley, C. Sutton and C. Watkins. Prevention and Treatment of Urinary Incontinence after Stroke in Adults. *Cochrane Database of Systematic Reviews 3* (2005). Art. No.: CD004462. doi: 10.1002/14651858.CD004462.pub2.

Thomas, L. H., C. L. Watkins, C. J. Sutton, D. Forshaw, M. J. Leathley, B. French, C. R. Burton, F. Cheater, B. Roe, D. Britt, J. Booth, E. McColl and The ICONS Project Team and the ICONS Patient, Public and Carer Involvement Groups. 'Identifying Continence Options after stroke (ICONS): A Cluster Randomised Controlled Feasibility Trial. *Trials*, **15** (2014), 509. doi: 10.1186/1745-6215-15-509.

Wang, Y. A. G. Rudd, C. Wolfe. 'Trends and Survival Between Ethnic Groups after Stroke', *Stroke*, **44** (2013), 380–7. doi: 10.1161/strokeaha.112.680843.

Williams, J., L. Perry and C. Watkins (eds). 2010 *Acute Stroke Nursing* (Oxford: Wiley-Blackwell, 2010).

Wilson, A. D. et al.. 'Delay Between Symptom Onset and Clinic Attendance Following TIA and Minor Stroke: The BEATS Study', *Age and Ageing*, **43**(2) (2014), 253–6.

Wolfe, C. D. A. 'The Impact of Stroke', *British Medical Bulletin*, **56**(2) (2000), 275–86.

World Health Organisation (WHO) *Cardiovascular Diseases (CVDs): Fact Sheet No. 317* (2015) [Online]. Available from: www.who.int/mediacentre/factsheets/fs317/en/ (accessed 30 March 2015).

6

Acute Coronary Syndrome

Alison Malecki-Ketchell

Introduction: Coronary Heart Disease in Context

Despite a fall in mortality rates, cardiovascular disease (CVD) remained the leading cause of death in men and women in 2010 in the UK, accounting for almost 180,000 deaths with persistent regional, socio-economic and behavioural variation and associated increases in some risk factors such as type 2 diabetes and obesity. Overall UK death rates from CVD remain relatively high compared to many Western European countries, though are significantly lower than many Eastern European countries (Townsend et al., 2012). CVD manifests as a range of conditions including coronary heart disease (CHD), stroke, hypertension, hypercholesterolaemia, diabetes, chronic kidney disease, peripheral arterial disease and vascular dementia, all of which are usually associated with atherosclerosis and are linked by common risk factors (DH, 2013). Mortality from CHD has seen a steady decline across most of Europe, decreasing in the UK by 45 per cent between 1998 and 2008 while the incidence of myocardial infarction (MI) fell by almost one-third in England between 2002 and 2010, by 25 per cent in Scotland between 2000 and 2009 and the death rate following acute MI in England almost halved since 2002 (Townsend et al., 2012). However, the trend is not universal, with a notable slowing in the decline among younger age groups (Bertuccio et al., 2011); a continued UK North–South divide, with higher prevalence in Scotland and the North of England; and increased incidence among lower socio-economic groups and men of South Asian and Eastern European descent (Townsend et al., 2012). The Cardiovascular Disease Outcomes Strategy (DH, 2013) identified that, despite the continual decline in annual mortality from CHD, attributed to pharmacological and technological advances and lifestyle improvements, CHD still accounted for approximately 80,000 deaths in 2010 in the UK (Townsend et al., 2012) (Table 6.1).

Table 6.1 UK death rates by sex (all ages) in 2010

	Men	Women	Total
Cardiovascular disease (CVD)	85,528	91,550	179,078 1/3rd of all UK deaths
Coronary heart disease (CHD)	46,591 1 in 5 male deaths	33,977 1 in 10 female deaths	80,568
All cancer	84,373	76,802	161,175

Source: Adapted from Coronary Heart Disease Statistics, British Heart Foundation (Townsend et al., 2012)

In March 2000, the Department of Health published a set of targets within the National Service Framework for Coronary Heart Disease (NSF CHD), which aimed to reduce mortality and morbidity from CHD (DH, 2009). Acute coronary syndrome (ACS) is an umbrella term used to describe a range of acute cardiac events associated with CHD, ranging from unstable angina (UA) to non-ST segment elevation myocardial infarction (NSTEMI) and ST segment elevation myocardial infarction (STEMI). In response to overwhelming evidence of the survival benefit of reperfusion therapy for acute STEMI, the National Infarct Angioplasty Project (NIAP) recommends primary percutaneous coronary intervention (PCI) as the preferred coronary reperfusion strategy if presentation is within 12 hours of symptom onset and it can be delivered within 120 minutes of the time when pharmacological thrombolysis could have been given (DH, 2008; NICE, 2013a). If PCI cannot be performed within 120 minutes of the patient's call for help ('call-to-balloon' time) and they are within 12 hours of onset of symptoms, pharmacological thrombolysis should be given (NICE, 2013a). The optimal benefit afforded by both PCI and pharmacological reperfusion is time dependent, hence the government target times set for 'call-to-balloon' time is within 120 minutes (NICE 2013a) or pharmacological thrombolysis within 60 minutes of 'call-to-needle' and 30 minutes of hospital arrival (DH, 2000). There has been significant improvement in the accurate and prompt management, care and subsequent outcomes of patients presenting with ACS, with 92 per cent of eligible STEMI patients receiving PCI within 90 minutes in 2011–12 across England (DH, 2013). However, geographical variation exists and patients presenting with NSTEMI and unstable angina do not always receive the desired level of care (DH, 2013). The immediate management of NSTEMI and unstable angina, recommended by NICE guidelines, differs and is dependent upon reaching a definitive diagnosis and an assessment of risk for MI and death (NICE, 2013b). Therefore achieving set targets necessitates prompt and accurate assessment of all chest pain patients in order that a definitive working diagnosis can be established to inform the most appropriate and timely treatment strategy. In line with NICE clinical guidance 95 (NICE, 2010), emphasis upon the importance of a full clinical assessment, monitoring and management of a patient presenting with chest pain during the acute phase is the focus of this chapter (DH, 2013).

Aim and Learning Outcomes

The Aim

The aim of this chapter is to explore the priorities of early accurate assessment and management of the individual presenting acutely with sudden onset of central chest pain. The main focus of the chapter is acute coronary syndrome with a specific emphasis upon acute STEMI. The case scenario provides the basis for the application of evidence-based theoretical rationale to clinical practice.

Learning Outcomes

At the end of this chapter the reader will be able to:

1. Define acute coronary syndrome and distinguish between the differing manifestations of ACS.
2. Identify and explain the pathophysiological basis of the presenting signs and symptoms of acute ST elevation myocardial infarction.
3. Recognise the immediate assessment, specific monitoring and key investigations required to enable an accurate and timely diagnosis.
4. Explore the evidence underpinning immediate priorities of management with a particular focus upon pharmacological and invasive interventions.
5. Appreciate the role of different health professionals in acute assessment and management of ACS.
6. Be aware of the common complications associated with acute MI.

The Case Scenario: The Presenting Complaint

Jon Kowalski is a 55-year-old, previously fit and well gentleman of Polish descent who was admitted to the accident and emergency (A&E) department at 09.00 hours, complaining of severe crushing central chest pain, which awoke him at

The Case Scenario *continued*

07.30 hours that morning. At 08.30 hours Gaviscon® had not relieved the pain and so Jon called 999. The paramedic ambulance crew gave Jon 300 mg of soluble aspirin orally and a 3 mg Suscard buccal® tablet was placed between his upper lip and gum during the journey to hospital. On admission Jon continues to complain of pain with radiation into his left arm and neck and he looks pale and sweaty, feels nauseous, appears to be restless and agitated and reports never having experienced pain like this before. Jon is divorced and lives alone though his partner and two children who are both married live locally. Jon is a bus (PSV) driver; he smokes 20 cigarettes per day; drinks five to six units of alcohol a week; enjoys walking and swimming and has a body mass index (BMI) of 26. A provisional diagnosis of acute coronary syndrome (ACS) is made.

Consider the following:

1. With reference to the underlying pathophysiology describe what is meant by acute ACS.
2. What are the common signs and symptoms associated with ACS?
3. List the known modifiable and non-modifiable risk factors for heart disease and identify those that appear to directly affect Jon.

Coronary Heart Disease

The Coronary Circulation

An explanation of normal coronary anatomy is a useful prerequisite to understanding the pathological disease process associated with coronary artery disease. The function of the heart requires a continuous supply of nutrients and oxygen to the myocardium, which is supplied via a network of coronary arteries and veins. There are two main coronary arteries – the right and left – which originate from the right and left coronary sinus of valsalva, respectively, just above the aortic valve.

The right coronary artery (RCA) follows the right atrioventricular groove, eventually dividing into two large branches: the posterior descending (PD) and marginal (M) branches (Figure 6.1). In most hearts, the RCA and its branches are responsible for supplying oxygenated blood to the right atrium, the right ventricle (RV) and the inferior surface of the left ventricle (LV), the sinus node (about 70 per cent of cases), atrioventricular node (about 90 per cent of cases) and the common bundle of the conduction system. The left coronary artery (LCA) leaves the aorta as the left main stem (LMS) before almost immediately dividing into two major coronary arteries: the left anterior

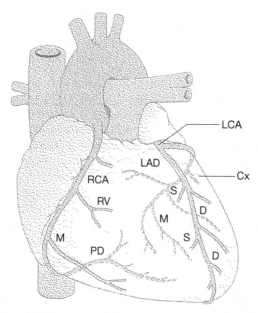

Figure 6.1 The normal coronary circulation

descending (LAD) and the circumflex (Cx) (Figure 6.1). The LAD descends along the interventricular septum, further dividing into large septal (S) and diagonal (D) branches, which supply oxygenated blood to the anterior surface of the left ventricle and most of the left and right bundle branches of the conduction system. The Cx follows the left atrioventricular groove, supplying the lateral and posterior aspects of the left ventricle, the sinus node (about 25 per cent of cases, with the RCA and Cx jointly responsible in the remaining 5 per cent) and the atrioventricular node (about 10 per cent of cases). The major vessels lie on the epicardial surface of the myocardium before further dividing to form a perfuse system of smaller branches that perforate the entire thickness of the muscle wall. The arteries then divide to form arterioles and a massive capillary network, which surrounds and supplies each muscle fibre with essential nutrients and oxygen and from which almost all the oxygen is extracted by the myocardial fibres. Collateral connections of less than 200 micrometres (µm) in diameter exist between the branches of the coronary arteries at subarteriolar level, though under normal circumstances very few collateral vessels are visible. Venules and veins join to form large venous channels, which return the deoxygenated blood, carbon dioxide and waste products of cellular metabolism to the right atrium via the anterior cardiac veins (right coronary blood) and the coronary sinus (left coronary blood).

The coronary artery lining is composed of an outer collagenous layer (tunica adventitia) for protective strength, a thicker medial layer of elastic fibres and smooth muscle (tunica media) enabling contraction and relaxation and an endothelial lining of simple squamous cells (tunica intima) to promote a laminar flow of blood along the vessel (Figure 6.2). The endothelium is normally a metabolically active barrier between circulating blood and the vessel lining which is responsible for secreting a range of protective vasoactive substances that promote a non-thrombogenic and non-adherent surface.

Coronary Artery Disease (CAD)

Coronary artery disease describes a pathological process affecting the coronary artery. The commonest cause of coronary artery disease is **atherosclerosis**, though other pathological disorders of the coronary arteries do exist (Table 6.2). CAD may exist for a number of years without affecting myocardial function and is therefore not necessarily synonymous with coronary (ischaemic) heart disease.

The Development of Coronary Atherosclerosis

CAD is largely attributed to the presence of atherosclerotic plaque between the inner (intima) and muscle (medial) linings of the walls of large and medium sized arteries (Figure 6.2). The development of atherosclerotic plaque is thought to begin with a 'fatty streak', commonly found within the intimal lining at a very young age. Excess circulating low density lipoproteins (LDLs) infiltrate and accumulate within the inner lining of the artery where they become oxidised and engulfed by macrophagic monocytes to form 'foam cells'. Circulating T cell lymphocytes move into the space, activating an inflammatory response. The foam cells, macrophages and lymphocytes form the 'fatty streak' (Figure 6.2). Fatty streaks are relatively innocuous in themselves; however, they may increase in frequency between 8 and 18 years

Table 6.2 Pathological disorders of the coronary arteries

- Congenital deformities, e.g. arterio-venous fistulae, anomalous origin of pulmonary artery
- Coronary embolism, e.g. arising from left atrium, left ventricle, mitral or aortic valve disorders, infective endocarditis
- Syphilitic aortitis
- Dissecting aortic aneurysm occluding coronary artery
- Connective tissue disorders, e.g. polyarteritis, pseudoxanthoma elasticum, systemic lupus erythematosus
- Coronary artery spasm of normal or diseased arteries
- Atherosclerosis is the commonest cause

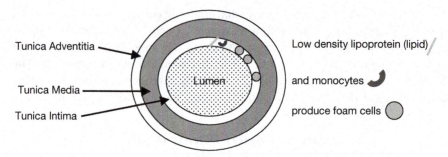

Figure 6.2 The fatty streak

and exist in the aorta and coronary arteries of most individuals by the age of 20 (Lilly, 2011), and may develop into a more injurious atherosclerotic lesion.

Progression of the fatty streak into an atherosclerotic lesion known as 'fibro-lipid plaque' is dependent upon its location within the coronary artery and the presence of predisposing risk factors (Table 6.3). It may

Table 6.3 Predisposing risk factors associated with development of atherosclerotic plaque

Pathophysiological factors
Epicardial section of the coronary artery especially at bends and bifurcations
Increased C-reactive protein (CRP) (AHA, 2003) or elevated homocysteine (Yusuf et al., 2001a)
Infection, e.g. *Chlamydia pneumoniae, Helicobacter pylori*, herpes, cytomegalovirus have been implicated though their role remains unclear (Ross, 1999)

Non-modifiable risk factors
Genetic predisposition (family history of early CHD)
Increasing age
Gender – male more susceptible
Personality type D, anger, hostility (Denollet et al., 2006)
Ethnic origin e.g. South Asian (Yusuf et al., 2001b); Eastern European (Bertuccio et al., 2011)

Modifiable risk factors
Smoking
High serum cholesterol levels, i.e. elevated low density lipid (LDL) and low high density lipids (HDL)
High glucose levels, diabetes and/or insulin resistance
High saturated fat diet
Hypertension
Overweight and obesity
Physical inactivity and sedentary lifestyle
Chronic work-related stress
Social isolation and depression (Barth et al., 2004)

develop as young as 15 years, with a propensity to progress rapidly between 15 and 35 years in susceptible individuals (Jowett and Thompson, 2007). Risk factors, regardless of their modifiability, interact in a synergistic manner and therefore the more risk factors that Jon has the more susceptible he is to the development of coronary artery atherosclerotic disease.

Jon's evident risk factors are his age, gender and Polish descent, smoking and possible stress related to his occupation as a PSV driver, and are sufficient to have increased Jon's susceptibility to atherosclerotic development. The pathological progression of fatty streak to fibro-lipid plaque is a complex process mediated by endothelial dysfunction and foam cell activity. Increased endothelial permeability facilitates further entry of lipid into the intima and failure to secrete normal anti-thrombotic molecules attracts platelets to the area and increases the potential for localised platelet aggregation and adhesion. Foam cells, activated platelets and endothelial cells also secrete a number of factors that stimulate the migration and proliferation of smooth muscle cells into the intima, which then engulf lipid to form more foam cells. A highly thrombogenic necrotic core encased within a fibrous cap develops (Figure 6.3).

It is thought that plaque enlargement may be further augmented by small recurrent ulcerations within the cap, which expose plaque contents to the circulation, attracting further aggregation and adhesion of activated platelets, which become incorporated into the lesion. Initially most atherosclerotic plaque expands away from the vessel lumen. However, as it increases in size plaque may begin to project inwards, causing progressive narrowing of the lumen. Many individuals live unknowingly with coronary artery disease for a number of years as the degree of narrowing is not thought to be of significance until it obstructs approximately 70 per cent of the luminal diameter. Once atherosclerotic plaque produces significant stenosis of the vessel it may impair sufficient blood flow to the serving myocardium, leading to clinical symptoms of coronary (ischaemic) heart disease.

Figure 6.3 The fibro-lipid plaque

Coronary (Ischaemic) Heart Disease

The Joint International Society and Federation of Cardiology and World Health Organization Task Force have described CHD as myocardial impairment caused by an imbalance between coronary blood flow and myocardial demand directly associated with changes in the coronary circulation. In practice it is often referred to as ischaemic heart disease (IHD). Early symptoms are often precipitated by exercise when a narrowed coronary artery fails to increase blood supply in response to increased myocardial demand. Insufficient oxygen supply leads to myocardial cell ischaemia, which most often presents as chest pain or chest discomfort, known as 'angina'. Stable angina describes chest pain that is triggered by exercise and usually responds to rest and coronary vasodilation with rapid-onset, short-acting nitrate therapy in various forms such as glyceryl trinitrate (GTN) spray, a GTN tablet below the tongue or Suscard buccal® between the lip and gum. A provisional diagnosis of stable angina based upon symptom presentation may be confirmed by a non-invasive exercise tolerance test demonstrating ischaemic electrocardiographic (ECG) changes or invasive coronary angiography. It is often managed by GPs with beta blockers (e.g. Atenolol® or Metoprolol®), which slow the heart rate and therefore reduce the demand for myocardial oxygen, and a daily anti-platelet agent such as aspirin 75 to 150 mg daily. Prophylactic use of GTN prior to exercise or in response to chest pain should also be advised. Stable angina is generally considered to be a warning sign of CHD rather than an acute event in itself. Some individuals presenting acutely will have a history of stable angina; however, as in Jon's case the acute event may be the first sign of coronary artery disease.

Acute Coronary Syndrome

The acute coronary event is now thought to be a consequence of sudden rupture or erosion of the plaque cap and thrombus formation rather than vessel occlusion caused by progressive plaque enlargement. The fate of the plaque may in part be dependent upon the composition of the plaque cap and contents. Plaque composed of a high proportion of smooth muscle cells and connective tissue and covered in a thick fibrous cap tends to be more prominent on angiography yet often appears to be relatively stable and less likely to rupture. In contrast, plaques rich in lipid with a thin fibrous cap are considered to be 'vulnerable' and much more susceptible to rupture despite their often minor appearance on angiography (Lilly, 2011). Current theory suggests that the presence of factors such as excessive smoking, hyperlipidaemia, diabetes, infection, stress and hypertension may cause sudden changes in coronary blood pressure or vascular tone, which may predispose plaque rupture leading to further plaque enlargement or an acute coronary event.

Unstable Angina

Unstable angina results from superficial fissuring of plaque and collagen exposure to the circulation, which attracts activated platelets to the area, enabling platelet aggregation, adhesion and platelet deposition, commonly known as 'white clot'. Partial occlusion of the vessel severely restricts flow of blood and oxygen to the myocardium beyond the narrowing, leading to cell ischaemia. Ischaemic myocardium classically presents as a sudden onset of chest pain at rest that is not easily resolved with nitrate therapy, a normal or abnormal ST segment and T wave on ECG and negative serum troponin at 12 hours post onset of symptoms. Approximately 10 to 20 per cent of patients diagnosed with unstable angina will progress to MI within the ensuing days or weeks if they fail to respond well to medical therapy. Jon's chest pain presentation could indicate unstable angina as a possible differential diagnosis; however, given his minimal response to nitrate therapy (Suscard buccal®) further investigation is required before a definitive diagnosis can be made.

Myocardial Infarction

Angiographic evidence suggests that approximately 15 per cent of MIs occur as a result of severe (> 90 per cent) stenosis of the artery but the majority are as a direct consequence of plaque rupture and total coronary occlusion with thrombus. In most cases the site of platelet deposition facilitates the clotting mechanism, leading to the conversion of soluble prothrombin and fibrinogen into insoluble thrombus formation and fibrin deposition, known as 'red clot', at the site of rupture (Figure 6.4).

The subsequent total coronary occlusion causes abrupt cessation of blood and oxygen to the serving myocardium, resulting in patchy areas of ischaemia, injury and infarction. Myocardial injury is reversible damage caused by temporary blood and oxygen deprivation, which may be resolved if blood flow is restored within 30 to 45 minutes. If the sudden cessation of blood flow is not limited to less than 45 minutes MI (cell necrosis) ensues from endocardium to epicardium in a time-dependent manner with permanent necrotic damage to affected cells leading to cell fibrosis, electrical inactivity and loss of contractility. The extent of necrosis and resulting size

Platelet adhesion provides the platform for the clotting cascade to activate clotting factor X (CFX)

⟹ CFXa necessary for the final common pathway of clotting

CFXa converts prothrombin (CFII) to thrombin (CFIIa)

Thrombin (CFIIa) converts soluble fibrinogen to insoluble fibrin = 'red clot' formation

Figure 6.4   Clot formation

of infarction may be restricted to patchy areas of muscle or may affect the full thickness of myocardium, and is dependent upon the length of time of absent blood flow, the degree of diminution of blood flow affected by localised vasomotor changes and the extent of collateral flow. In the presence of atherosclerotic coronary artery obstruction, collateral connections may become larger and functionally capable of restoring some blood flow to a distal portion of an obstructed vessel from a non-obstructed neighbour. In some individuals the collateral coronary circulation may play a significant role in myocardial damage limitation and greatly improve long-term prognosis. MI typically manifests as a sudden onset of chest pain unrelieved by nitrate, with (STEMI) or without (NSTEMI) ST segment elevation on ECG, and is associated with elevated serum troponin levels. The risk of mortality and morbidity remains a significant threat for Jon without immediate assessment, primary intervention and secondary prevention and rehabilitation.

Assessment and Reaching a Diagnosis

For the sake of narrative fluency each aspect of the preliminary assessment will be discussed separately; however, in practice it is the integration of assessment information that is essential for the accurate and prompt definitive diagnosis required for appropriate symptom relief and life-saving intervention. Secondary assessment involves a more detailed history, examination and further investigation once the patient is stabilised.

The Case Scenario: Assessment and Reaching a Diagnosis

Jon's chest pain was not relieved despite the Suscard buccal® and he began to complain of headache. 24 per cent oxygen therapy via a face mask was commenced and venous access was secured with a 14G cannula inserted into his left antecubital fossa. The Suscard buccal® was removed and IV diamorphine 5 mg and IV metoclopramide 10 mg was administered.

Immediate Assessment
1. What are the immediate assessment priorities in Jon's case and what is the rationale for each measure?
2. Describe the common cardiac and non-cardiac causes of chest pain.
3. Identify the common characteristics which help distinguish different causes of chest pain.
4. Describe the underlying pathophysiology of ischaemic chest pain.
5. How would a definitive cause and diagnosis for the chest pain be established?
6. Describe the rationale for the treatment received so far.

The Preliminary Assessment

Myocardial ischaemia, injury and infarction alters cell membrane permeability to essential ions for normal electrophysiological and contractile function and may predispose life-threatening arrhythmias such as ventricular tachycardia (VT), ventricular fibrillation (VF) and atrio-ventricular (AV) node conduction defects, as well as adversely affecting contractile strength. Bennett (2013) offers further explanation and ECG interpretation of a range of common arrhythmias. Death from MI is most likely to occur within the first hour of onset of symptoms and the usual cause is VF. The incidence of primary VF post acute MI is approximately 4.7 per cent (Dubois et al., 1986; Thompson et al., 2000; Henkel et al., 2006) and therefore the ABC approach to assessment is essential to establish Jon's immediate haemodynamic status.

Airway

Most patients like Jon are fully conscious and able to maintain a patent airway; however, the risk of cardio-respiratory arrest is sufficiently significant to warrant continuous vigilance. In the event of clinical deterioration the 'look, listen and feel' method of airway assessment should be employed (see Chapter 1) and basic life support measures including insertion of adjunct airway management must be instigated in the event of inadequate airway maintenance.

Breathing

Breathing assessment will include respiratory rate, depth, regularity and noise observed for 30 seconds and thereafter every four hours if findings fall within normal parameters (Table 6.4). The presence and characteristics of a cough and sputum should be documented and a sample of expectorant collected for microbiology if infection is suspected. Provided peripheral perfusion is adequate, continuous non-invasive oxygen saturation (SpO$_2$) monitoring measures the adequacy of respiration and should be maintained above 95 per cent. Adequacy of peripheral perfusion can be assessed by capillary refill time: normal capillary refill time is less than two seconds. Measurement of arterial blood gases are not usually necessary unless airway and breathing assessment thus far have revealed respiratory abnormalities. It is usual for individuals with chest pain to receive supplementary oxygen such as 24 per cent via face mask or in some cases a high (60 to 100 per cent) concentration via a non-rebreathe bag to maintain SpO$_2$ within normal limits until a full assessment of breathing has been undertaken. However, unless the patient is breathless, is in heart failure and/or saturation levels are below 95 per cent, there is no evidence to suggest that routine supplementary O$_2$ provides any real benefit (O'Driscoll et al., 2008). McNulty et al. (2005) concluded that high flow oxygen aimed at maintaining oxygen saturation levels at 100 per cent may increase coronary vascular resistance and reduce coronary blood flow, adversely affecting myocardial oxygen supply. Therefore some caution with routine administration of supplementary oxygen should be applied and if saturation is above 94 per cent and the mask exacerbates feelings of nausea, sweating and claustrophobia then it is reasonable to remove the mask. However, maintenance of close observation and monitoring of breathing and SpO$_2$ levels to ensure they remain within normal limits is imperative. Saturation levels below

Table 6.4 Normal physiological parameters

- Heart rate: 60–95 beats/min
- Heart rhythm: regular PQRST sinus rhythm
- Systolic BP: 100–140 mmHg
- Diastolic BP: 60–90 mmHg
- Respiration: 12–16/min, noiseless and effortless
- Oxygen saturation: >95%

95 per cent may indicate hypoxaemia and the need for supplementary O_2 therapy to ensure adequate oxygenation of coronary flow to the myocardium. It should be remembered that oxygen dose, method of delivery and target saturation should be based upon accurate assessment and prescribed by a medical practitioner.

Circulation

Circulation assessment via cardiac monitoring (three or five lead) provides a continuous recording of Jon's heart rate, regularity and rhythm and enables prevention or early detection and treatment of potentially life-threatening atrial and ventricular arrhythmias (see Bennet (2013) for further explanation and ECG interpretation). Jon's radial pulse should be palpated for 30 seconds to assess pulse volume and skin temperature, which provide a useful indication of perfusion. A regular sinus rhythm between 60 and 95 beats/min is expected. A sinus tachycardia up to approximately 140 beats/min might indicate pain, anxiety or a physiological response to low blood pressure (BP) to maintain an adequate cardiac output. A heart rate below 60 beats/min may be within Jon's normal range, particularly if he participates in regular vigorous exercise. Alternatively it may indicate a conduction defect in electrical activity across the heart and a potential fall in cardiac output. Jon's BP may be within normal limits (Table 6.4) or a high BP may be indicative of pain, anxiety or underlying hypertension. A low BP may be normal for Jon or indicative of failure of his heart to maintain an adequate cardiac output during the acute event. If Jon's observations are within normal parameters it is safe to record them and reassess four hours later, during intervention or in response to other evidence of deterioration. Observations that are outside normal parameters should be observed continuously, recorded and reported to medical staff for intervention and repeated as frequently as every ten minutes until a stable trend is established.

A slight rise in Jon's four-hourly temperature recording between 37 and 38 °C during the first 24 hours might be expected as a sign of the acute inflammatory process. A marked increase in temperature above 38 °C may indicate active infection and should be further investigated. During observation and recording of vital signs a brief verbal history of the presenting signs and symptoms can be ascertained from Jon.

Signs, Symptoms and Symptom Relief

Patients experiencing ACS most commonly present with severe chest pain, although this can vary significantly from one individual to the next as gender (female), age (> 65) and the presence of diabetes can alter pain perception and symptom presentation. At a cellular level an insufficient supply of oxygen to meet myocardial demand provokes anaerobic respiration as a means of energy production, with the consequent accumulation of the by-product lactic acid and excess unused adenosine within the cell. Adenosine and lactic acid stimulate cardiac nociceptors, which transmit pain signals to the medulla via sympathetic afferent fibres located in the upper thoracic and lower cervical spinal cord, giving rise to the experience of chest and arm pain, and cardiac vagal afferent fibres, which convey a feeling of neck and jaw pain (Foreman, 1999). As a consequence ischaemic pain is typically described as diffuse rather than localised central chest pain with radiation into the arms, jaw and neck. Jon presented with classic characteristics of ischaemic cardiac pain, which include common descriptors such as 'crushing', 'heavy', 'bandlike' and 'squeezing'. Ischaemic pain is not 'stabbing' in nature, though occasionally some individuals may describe it as 'sharp' (referring to the intensity rather than knife-like quality) or 'burning'. A localised left or right sided 'sharp' or 'stabbing' chest pain is more likely to be associated with a respiratory cause (Table 6.5).

Stable angina may be precipitated by a number of factors, such as exercise, emotional states, a heavy meal, cold weather or an autonomic sympathetically mediated tachycardia. However, severe unstable angina or an acute MI can occur at rest. Although some individuals experience maximal pain from the onset, many describe an increase in intensity over minutes or hours that becomes constant and eventually recedes with intervention. Often the history of the preceding weeks reveals increasing episodes of similar though less severe pain. Ischaemic pain is not aggravated or relieved by hunger or food (gastric origin) movement or respiration (pericarditic, pleuritic or musculoskeletal) or non-steroidal anti-inflammatory agents such as

Table 6.5 Common causes of chest pain

Cardiac	*Non-cardiac*
• Ischaemia: stable angina; unstable angina • Non ST elevation MI (NSTEMI) • ST elevation MI (STEMI) • Dissecting aortic aneurysm • Pericarditis • Myocarditis	• Respiratory: infection, pulmonary embolus, pneumothorax, pleuritis • Gastro-intestinal: oesophagitis, gastritis, spasm, gastric/duodenal ulcer, acute cholecystitis, pancreatitis • Muscular-skeletal • Herpes zoster (shingles) • Anxiety • Referred pain

ibuprofen (Table 6.5). Ischaemia is usually relieved by the coronary vasodilating properties of nitrate drugs, though unstable episodes may require successive treatment to secure complete pain relief. Some patients may complain of a consequent headache with continued nitrate therapy due to the associated cerebral vasodilation. If pain persists beyond 30 minutes despite nitrate therapy then MI should be suspected. Pain from myocardial injury and infarction will only respond to opiate therapy such as intravenous (IV) diamorphine (2.5 to 5 mg) or morphine sulphate (10 mg) and for this reason Suscard buccal® was removed and Jon was given intravenous (IV) diamorphine 5 mg. A verbal measure, usually on a 0 to 10 verbal rating scale with 0 being 'no pain' and 10 being 'the worst pain ever', enables Jon to provide a subjective assessment of his pain and may inform the need for repeated IV diamorphine until complete pain relief is achieved. Continuous assessment of respiratory effort can alert practitioners to the potential depressive effects upon the respiratory centre, in which case IV Naloxone® may be required to reverse the opiate effects.

A full assessment, including a range of questions pertaining to chest pain symptoms (Table 6.6), should be performed in the first instance, followed by a reassessment of Jon's perception of pain on a 0 to 10 scale until it has completely subsided or with recurrence.

Questions related to the locality and characteristics of the pain established during history taking, assessment and clinical examination may reveal the differential diagnosis. However, not all patients experience chest pain, those who do may not always describe the classic descriptive features discussed and caution with over-reliance upon patient history is advised, as a degree of overlap in location and symptom description between patients with cardiac pain and those with non-cardiac chest pain has been suggested

Table 6.6   Assessment of descriptive features of chest pain

Site – Where is the pain?
Onset – When did the pain start? Was it sudden or gradual, progressive or regressive?
Character – What is the pain like? Describe the pain
Radiation – Does the pain radiate anywhere?
Associated signs – Are there any other signs and symptoms such as nausea, sweating, pallor?
Time – How long has the pain lasted? Has it changed over time?
Exacerbating / Precipitating / Relieving factors – Does anything start, stop or change the pain?
Severity – How bad is the pain on a 0 to 10 scale?
SOCRATES provides a useful mnemonic acronym to prompt evaluation of the nature of the pain

---

(Eslick, 2005). Moreover, for some, chest pain may be overshadowed by other associated symptoms such as nausea, vomiting, breathlessness and syncope. Nausea and vomiting is a common response to pain, hypotension and opiate therapy. It has been specifically associated with infarction of the inferior aspect of the left ventricular myocardium (Culi et al., 2001), though it has also been suggested that infarct size rather than location may be the key factor (Herlihy et al., 2004). The mechanism remains unclear, though stimulus of autonomic receptors in close proximity to the ischaemic zone may trigger the vomiting centre within the medulla. It is therefore customary to administer an anti-emetic such as IV metoclopramide 10 mg in conjunction with opiate therapy and ensure that vomit bowls, tissues and mouthwash are readily available to Jon. Dyspnoea or shortness of breath may be indicative of left ventricular failure, respiratory disease such as chronic obstructive pulmonary disease or anxiety, and should be thoroughly evaluated as part of the initial ABC assessment. Although they are not definitive physical signs of MI, most patients experience evidence of autonomic sympathetic nervous activation and peripheral vasoconstriction such as profuse diaphoresis (sweating) and pallor mediated by pain and anxiety, which may excite an associated tachycardia and a consequent undesirable increase in cardiac workload. A number of strategies may be employed to help to alleviate some of Jon's anxiety and tension associated with the gravity of the situation from his perspective (Table 6.7).

Other accompanying signs, such as palpitations, syncope (transient loss of consciousness), dizziness or light headedness, are less common, though they may reflect altered cardiac output, excess vagal stimulation, bradycardia or arrhythmia and should be further observed and investigated. Myocardial ischaemia (insufficient oxygen) and infarction (oxygen deprivation) alter the electrical activity of the affected cells and may be visualised by the ECG.

Table 6.7 Strategies that might help to reduce anxiety during the acute phase

---

1. Adequate, timely pain assessment and relief.
2. Constant reassurance through simple, repetitive, clear, here and now information regarding current treatment and care. Provide careful explanation in answer to questions posed by John.
3. Visibility, approachability and presence enabling John to attract attention easily.
4. Promotion of a professional but compassionate competent manner.
5. Close monitoring may provide a sense of safety for some, though once the intensity of observation is relaxed stress levels may increase.

Specific Investigations

The ECG provides a pictorial image of the electrical activity of the heart. Electrodes (red upper right, yellow upper left, green lower left, black lower right) strategically positioned on the upper and lower limbs or chest sense and transmit cardiac electrical activity via leads to a monitor (Figure 6.5).

Cardiac monitoring is commonly set to rely upon the green lower left electrode (lead II) to record the heart rate and rhythm. The cardiac monitor interprets, augments and converts the signal into a wave form on the screen. A flat isoelectric line corresponds with absent electrical activity within the heart. An electrical impulse travelling across the heart towards an electrode is transformed into an upright deflection above the baseline and conversely an electrical impulse travelling away from an electrode is transcribed as a downward deflection below the baseline.

Figure 6.6 depicts the normal PqRST complex in lead II of the ECG. The small, upright, rounded P wave represents the electrical impulse as it travels across the atria (atrial depolarisation) (Figure 6.7).

The PR interval, measured from the beginning of the P wave to the beginning of the R wave, represents the time it takes for the electrical impulse to cross the atria and conduct down through the AV node. As conduction through the AV node is slow and the electrode at the skin surface is not sufficiently sensitive to detect it the PR interval is represented as a short flat line after the P wave. The q point or small negative physiological q wave that follows the PR interval represents the impulse as it travels across the upper ventricular septum in a left to right direction. The qRS represents the electrical impulse as it conducts rapidly down the right and left ventricles (ventricular depolarisation) towards the electrode (R wave). Once the electrical impulse has conducted across the entire ventricular muscle mass,

EARTH

Figure 6.5 Limb lead electrode positions

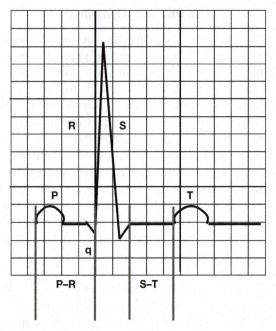

Figure 6.6 The normal PqRST complex

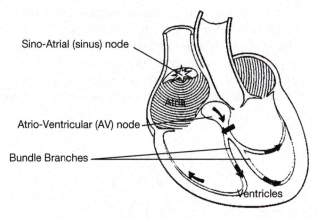

Figure 6.7 Electrical conduction across the heart

ventricular depolarisation is complete and electrical activity momentarily suspended to allow the ventricles time to fully contract in response to the electrical impulse. As the electrode can no longer detect electrical activity the wave returns to the baseline (S wave) to form the flat isoelectric ST segment. In order that the cardiac cells may respond to another electrical impulse they must return to their original electrical state (repolarisation).

**4 limb electrodes
termed I, II and III**

**6 chest electrodes termed
V1, V2, V3, V4, V5 and V6**

Figure 6.8   The 12-lead ECG electrode positions

Atrial repolarisation is not sensed by the surface ECG; however, ventricular repolarisation gives rise to a small, upright, rounded T wave. The 12-lead ECG utilises 10 electrodes placed across the chest (Figure 6.8) to provide a PqRST image of the electrical impulse from 12 different viewpoints.

As the muscle mass of the left ventricle (LV) is the greater and tends to sit uppermost in the chest and the majority of electrodes are positioned around the left chest wall, the qRS complexes largely reflect LV depolarisation in most leads (Figure 6.9).

The 12-lead ECG offers visual images of electrical depolarisation and repolarisation of difference aspects of the LV (Table 6.8).

The ECG provides a non-invasive, widely accessible, inexpensive test for the evaluation of chest pain. Ischaemia (insufficient oxygen) and injury (oxygen starvation) initially delay repolarisation of affected cardiac cells,

Figure 6.9   Normal 12-lead ECG

Table 6.8 Twelve ECG leads, corresponding coronary artery and affected area of myocardium

II, III, AVF	Right coronary artery (RCA)	Inferior wall: usually left ventricle (LV). 25% affect the right ventricle inferior wall visualised in V4R, V5R and V6R
I, AVL, V1 to V6	Proximal left anterior descending (LAD)	Left ventricle: extensive anterior region
V1, V2, V3	Left anterior descending (LAD)	Left ventricle: antero septal region
I, AVL, V4, V5, V6	Distal left anterior descending (LAD) or circumflex (Cx)	Left ventricle: antero lateral region
AVR	Right coronary artery (RCA)	Overlooks the right atrium and may be largely ignored

which may translate into an altered ST segment and/or T wave changes on ECG. Depression of the ST segment more than 2 mm below the baseline in more than two associated (anterior or inferior) leads may be indicative of severe ischaemia and unstable angina (Figure 6.10).

Inversion of the T wave in the opposite direction to the qRS is also an indication, though less reliable, of ischaemia (Figure 6.11). ST segment

Figure 6.10 ST segment depression

Figure 6.11 T wave inversion

depression and T wave inversion are relatively non-specific ECG changes that may evolve into a partial thickness non-Q wave MI in approximately 15 per cent of cases or represent unstable or stable angina, though in some instances they may be associated with non-cardiac chest pain.

Elevation of the ST segment more than 2 mm above baseline in more than two associated (anterior or inferior) leads indicates acute myocardial injury and is often the first witnessed ECG sign of acute MI, occurring within minutes of injury and lasting for up to 48 hours (Figure 6.12). The T wave may be superimposed within the elevated ST segment. ST segment changes are transient and will return to the base line as either sufficient oxygen is restored to the cells or cells necrose and become permanently damaged and electrically inert due to cessation of oxygen supply.

As injured cells infarct during the following 24 hours infarct tissue, which extends throughout the full thickness of the left ventricle, may create a pathological Q wave that deflects downwards immediately after the PR interval and whose depth is usually at least one-third of the height of the following R wave to reach significance (Figure 6.13).

Q waves usually develop as the ST segment begins to return to the baseline at 12 to 24 hours post symptom onset and are permanent indicators of MI. T wave inversion in the same leads often occurs at approximately 48 hours post symptom onset as the ST segment returns to the baseline (± Q waves) and may remain on the ECG for up to one year (permanently in some cases). Changes to the qRST complex will occur in the ECG leads

Figure 6.12 ST segment elevation

Figure 6.13 Q wave formation

Figure 6.14 Jon's 12-lead ECG

that overlook the affected area of the heart. Thus the area of ischaemia or infarction of myocardial muscle and the offending coronary artery can be identified through changes to the qRST complex in the corresponding ECG (Table 6.8). Jon's 12-lead ECG taken on admission confirmed ST segment elevation in leads I, AVL and V2, V3, V4, V5 and V6 (Figure 6.14), with no Q waves and upright T waves suggesting acute myocardial injury in the anterior region of the left ventricle caused by left anterior descending occlusion. Reciprocal ST segment depression can also be seen in the opposite leads II, III and AVF, which represents an electrical mirror image of the ST elevation. Coronary angiography is, however, necessary to definitively establish the affected coronary artery.

A Diagnosis of STEMI

Jon's signs, symptoms and clinical presentation suggest that he has experienced an acute anterior STEMI. At this stage, a decision regarding Jon's immediate management and care should be reached, which will determine his transfer from A&E either to a coronary care unit or to the cardiac catheter laboratories if available on-site. Enforced bed rest is initially instigated for Jon to promote a reduction in cardiac workload, optimise the balance between myocardial oxygen demand and supply, and enable continuous cardiac monitoring and further investigation to confirm the diagnosis and treatment. Jon is unlikely to have experienced continuous cardiac ECG monitoring and regular 12-lead ECG recording before. His lack of knowledge and experience and the associated enforced restriction in independence may provoke or exacerbate feelings of uncertainty and loss of control and self-esteem, and further raise anxiety and stress. This may promote further sympathetic nervous activity with the undesirable physiological consequence of increased heart rate and BP and thus cardiac workload. Bed rest should therefore be limited to the initial assessment and treatment period and be relaxed as soon as Jon is pain free, has no evidence of rhythm or heart failure complications and has had any invasive arterial devices removed. Once Jon is pain free, he should be encouraged to attend to his toilet and hygiene needs as independently as possible and full mobility should be gradually restored. It is equally imperative that an explanation in clear and simple terms of the equipment, monitor tracings and his mobility limits is offered and reinforced if necessary. A full understanding of the method and necessity of close observation can provide a sense of security for some individuals.

Diagnosing a NSTEMI

The ECG has provided a definitive diagnosis in Jon's case; however, this is not always the case. Although oxygen deprivation is likely to interfere with normal electrical repolarisation of the affected cells, the ECG lacks sensitivity and cannot always be relied upon to provide conclusive evidence of myocardial injury or infarction. ST elevation or new left bundle branch block is a highly reliable indicator (95 per cent) of acute STEMI; however, not all patients present with classic ECG changes and therefore a more substantive diagnosis may be obtained from serum troponin measurement. Three subtypes of troponin (troponin C (TnC); troponin T (TnT); troponin I (TnI)), a protein component of the contractile filaments, are present in smooth muscle and cardiac muscle. Oxygen deprivation causes the immediate release of troponin, which is serum detectable from small amounts of myocardial necrosis. As the composition of cardiac TnT and TnI is different to smooth muscle they both provide a sensitive and specific biochemical marker of myocardial damage. The sensitivity of troponin has resulted in a substantial increase in the annual number of diagnosed MIs.

In the UK an estimated 103,000 people have an MI per year, of whom approximately 12 per cent will die within 30 days (Townsend et al., 2012). A diagnosis of acute MI with symptoms of ischaemic chest pain unrelieved by nitrate can be made if the serum troponin level is raised, irrespective of whether there is ST segment elevation (STEMI) or not (NSTEMI) on the 12-lead ECG (Fox et al., 2004). Highly sensitive cardiac Troponin (hs-cTn) T or I measurement has become the gold standard for diagnosis of MI and different laboratory assays will produce local Trust parameters for negative, borderline and positive results (Table 6.9).

Table 6.9   ACS categories based upon TnI : TnT levels

ACS with UA	=	TnI < 0.06 µg/L : TnT < 0.1 µg/L
ACS with myocardial necrosis	=	TnI > 0.06–0.5 µg/L : TnT 0.18–1.5 µg/L
ACS with clinical MI	=	TnI > 0.5 µg/L : TnT > 1.5 µg/L

(or CK twice upper limit: 160 U/L on normal reference range)

Normal values differ between men and women and local laboratory test procedures
Source: Adapted from British Cardiac Society (Fox et al., 2004)

Table 6.10   Limitations of troponin measurement

1. Biochemical markers are not detectable early after onset of necrosis and therefore a negative sample at admission cannot exclude MI
2. Peak troponin elevation can be up to 12 hours post symptom onset
3. Troponin may remain elevated for two to three weeks, prohibiting use for detecting repeated episodes of myocardial injury
4. Troponin cannot be used to diagnose ischaemia
5. A negative troponin may identify the patient as lower risk but not low or no risk for MI

Negligible myocyte necrosis may release borderline levels of troponin and NSTEMI and STEMI are associated with a positive rise; however, troponin measurement is not without limitations (Table 6.10).

Although troponin is the gold standard biomarker for myocardial injury and may be used in conjunction with creatine kinase-MB (CK-MB) and myoglobin to enable a rapid diagnosis of ACS, in an effort to overcome some of the limitations of current troponin assays and establish a more reliable and accurate diagnostic tool, the validity, sensitivity and specificity of several biochemical markers to detect evidence of myocardial injury are currently being studied. B-type natriuretic peptides, copeptin, ischaemia-modified albumin, heart-type fatty-acid-binding protein (hFABP), myeloperoxidase, C-reactive protein, choline, placental growth factor and growth-differentiation factor-15 remain the subject of ongoing investigation (Kehl et al., 2012). However, until more conclusive evidence exists, the routine use of these biochemical markers in the diagnosis of ACS is not currently recommended by NICE.

Venous blood sampling for a range of tests (Table 6.11) should be undertaken, though results may not be readily available for several hours.

Elevated levels of serum creatine phosphokinase myocardial band (CK-MB) released during cell necrosis can also diagnose MI; however, the peak elevation time of six to twelve hours post symptom onset limits its use for

Table 6.11   Routine venous blood sampling

1. Full blood count (FBC): low Hb (anaemia), raised WBC (infection)
2. Clotting screen: if indicated by current medication, e.g. warfarin
3. Urea and electrolytes (U&E): electrolyte balance and renal function
4. Cholesterol: > 5.0 mmol/L will be treated with statin therapy
5. Random serum blood glucose: > 11 mmol/L may be treated with IV dextrose and insulin (Digami 1 & 2 trials: Malmberg et al. 1999, 2005; Weston et al. 2007)
6. Capillary blood glucose if high or low glucose is suspected, e.g. diabetic patient
7. Liver function tests (LFT): baseline prior to statin therapy, which may alter liver function
8. Creatinine phosphokinase (CK): raised levels indicate the extent of myocardial damage

early definitive diagnosis and necessitates serial sampling at eight to twelve hour intervals. As it is relatively more expensive to test and considered to be slightly less sensitive than troponin for myocardial necrosis it has largely fallen out of use as an early diagnostic tool. Once the patient is stabilised and early intervention and management have been initiated a more detailed secondary assessment may be elicited (Table 6.12).

A definitive diagnosis of STEMI is based upon:

1. History of severe chest pain lasting more than 20 minutes and not relieved by nitrate.
2. ST elevation (or new left bundle branch block pattern) on ECG.
3. Elevated serum cardiac troponin (though treatment should not be delayed awaiting results) means that appropriate treatment and care can be safely initiated for Jon.

Table 6.12   Secondary assessment

- Past medical history (PMH): cardiac and systemic
- Family history (FH)
- Social history (SH)
- Systemic enquiry: general, gastric, urinary, central nervous systems
- Risk factor evaluation (RF)
- Drug history: prescribed, over the counter and recreational
- Full clinical examination: peripheral pulses, jugular venous pressure (JVP), heart and lung sounds, systemic examination
- Chest X-ray and echocardiography

The Case Scenario: Medical Management and Care Issues

At 09.30hrs and within ten minutes of receiving opiate analgesia Jon reported complete relief from his chest pain. His vital signs were observed and recorded as follows:

> Continuous cardiac rhythm monitoring 86 to 92 b/min regular sinus rhythm
> BP systolic 90 to 100 mmHg, diastolic 55 to 60 mmHg
> 4-hourly respirations 12 to 16 per min
> Continuous O_2 saturation 96 to 98 per cent (24 per cent oxygen via mask commenced by the paramedic crew was discontinued)
> 12-lead ECG shows ST elevation in leads I, AVL, V2 to V6

A definitive diagnosis of anterior STEMI approximately two hours from onset of symptoms is reached. Medical treatment should be instigated immediately and the continuous monitoring, recording and reporting of vital signs during the acute phase of illness remains an essential aspect of nursing care (NICE 2007a). Symptom relief, effective communication with Jon, his close friends and relatives and provision of simple comfort measures are equally important care issues.

Immediate Medical Management
1. What are the current treatment options for an acute STEMI?
2. What factors might inform the choice of immediate management?
3. Explore your local policy regarding immediate treatment for STEMI.
4. What are Jon's main care issues?

Medical Management Strategies

Accurate and effective assessment and management of acute MI is a multi-professional responsibility. In the UK a range of pre-hospital assessment and treatment initiatives exist across different geographical locations, including specially trained paramedic crews and rapid response and telemetry systems enabling transfer of ECGs to local A&E or coronary care departments for interpretation to facilitate optimal 'call to treatment time'. Paramedic crews are increasingly expected to record and interpret the 12-lead ECG in order that the patient can be transferred to the most appropriate hospital site for immediate management. Jon's timely arrival in A&E within two hours of onset of ischaemic-sounding chest pain and ST elevation on 12-lead ECG make him an ideal candidate for reperfusion therapy. Individuals presenting with a good clinical history and new bundle branch block masking ST segment elevation on ECG are also considered suitable for reperfusion therapy (FTT, 1994). However, not all individuals experience chest pain or have

ECG changes and must await confirmation from troponin results to peak at 12 hours post symptom onset, taking them out of the reperfusion treatment zone. Therefore, many A&E departments will now measure the troponin level on admission and if there are signs of early elevation concordant with patient history, the patient may be referred for reperfusion therapy. Furthermore, many with chest pain delay seeking help and fail to present for treatment early enough to benefit from reperfusion therapy. A number of factors, including gender, age, culture, socio-economic status, experience and misinterpretation of symptoms, transport issues or failing to contact the emergency services, may explain this (Horne et al., 2000; Bird et al., 2009). National campaigns and local initiatives to educate and encourage individuals to report chest pain as soon as possible by contacting 999 aim to improve this situation. The overall aim of immediate reperfusion strategies is to dissolve fibrin rich clot, restore coronary artery patency to limit infarct size and so improve mortality and long-term morbidity.

Primary Percutaneous Coronary Intervention

Jon should receive an invasive catheter-based reperfusion commonly referred to as primary PCI or primary angioplasty. Large randomised controlled trials have revealed that PCI confers a reinfarction, stroke and 2 per cent short-term mortality benefit over thrombolytic therapy (Keeley et al., 2003). This benefit was further emphasised with the advent of stent implantation into the offending coronary artery following balloon angioplasty (Nordmann et al., 2004). Consequently primary PCI is the current treatment of choice for patients presenting with STEMI to a hospital with on-site PCI facilities (cardiac catheter lab and cardiac surgical backup), 24-hour interventionalist cover and technical expertise (Antman et al., 2007). PCI requires the immediate transfer of Jon to the cardiac catheter labs where it can be performed under local anaesthesia with radiographic control. Jon will receive an oral loading dose of a $P2Y_{12}$ adenosine diphosphate (ADP) receptor antagonist, either 60 mg Prasugrel® (Montalescot et al., 2009; NICE, 2014) or 180 mg Ticagrelor® for their anti-platelet properties (Lindholm et al., 2013; NICE 2011b). PCI involves passing a small balloon at the tip of a catheter, introduced into the arterial system via the femoral, brachial or radial artery, into the occluded coronary artery. The femoral artery was the dominant approach for a number of years, however difficulties with compression at the site and risk of bleeding has led to advances in alternative insertion points. The brachial and more recently the radial approach have become more popular, as the artery lies closer to the skin enabling ease of arterial compression following the procedure and thus reduced bleeding problems. However, the small arterial diameter necessitating the use of

narrow gauge catheters does create other technical challenges and is therefore not favoured by all interventionalists for all procedures. The balloon
is inflated to re-open the coronary artery and then removed leaving a bare
metal or drug-eluting stent in place to maintain a rigid support within the
artery wall and so resume vessel patency and blood flow (Figure 6.15). During PCI reperfusion a weight-adjusted IV bolus dose and infusion of either
a glycoprotein IIb/IIIa inhibitor such as Abciximab®, Tirofiban®, or in Jon's
case Bivalirudin® (a direct thrombin inhibitor), is usually administered during and not before the procedure (DeLuca et al., 2005; NICE 2011a).

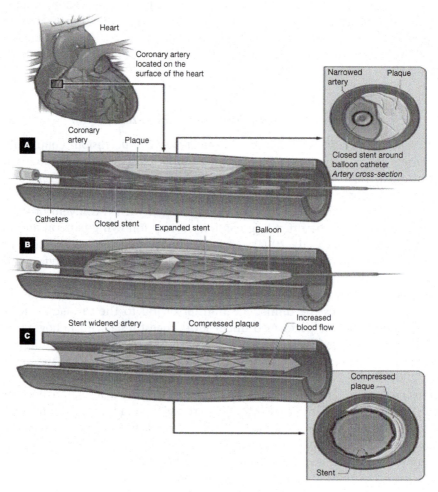

Figure 6.15 Coronary angioplasty and stent insertion

Source: National Institutes of Health and the US Department of Health and Human
Services/National Heart, Lung and Blood Institute. Reproduced with permission.

Meta-analyses of randomised clinical trials demonstrated that PCI was superior to pharmacological thrombolysis, with lower rates of mortality, reinfarction and stroke, but only when the additional time taken to deliver PCI relative to fibrinolysis was not excessive (Hartwell et al., 2005). Thus, the mortality benefit afforded by PCI over pharmacological thrombolysis is time dependent and a delay beyond the recommended 'call-to-balloon' time of 120 minutes may negatively affect survival benefit (Betriu and Masotti, 2005). Following a national roll-out programme of PCI services across the UK that commenced in 2009 many centres now provide on-site primary PCI enabling direct patient transport to, or immediate transfer from, primary or secondary care to tertiary centres. The DANAMI-2 trial, to ascertain whether patients should receive IV thrombolysis on-site or be transferred to the nearest centre for PCI, accepting the risk of a time to reperfusion delay, revealed that the notable reduction in mortality, reinfarction and stroke with primary PCI for patients admitted directly to invasive treatment centres was equally applicable to patients transferred to referral hospitals (Anderson et al., 2003). Transfer for primary PCI should always

The Case Scenario: Ongoing Care Issues

A brief past medical history and clinical examination revealed that Jon was previously fit and well and had no apparent contraindications to treatment. Jon was transferred immediately to the cardiac catheter labs for primary PCI with IV Bivalirudin® (an aggressive anti-platelet agent). The procedure revealed occlusion of the proximal left anterior descending artery which was dilated and implanted with a bare metal stent. The circumflex and right coronary arteries were normal. He had a pre-procedure stat dose of oral Prasugrel® 60 mg followed by a daily 10 mg maintenance dose for up to 12 months and weight-adjusted subcutaneous Enoxaparin® was commenced until discharge from hospital. The medical plan was to commence a daily maintenance dose of aspirin 75 mg, Metoprolol® on day one post MI, a loading dose of oral Enalapril® on day one post MI if BP stable and Simvastatin® 40 mg at night. Bed rest and continuous cardiac monitoring for arrhythmia detection were maintained and a detailed social, family and risk factor assessment was completed.

Nursing Care Issues
1. Consider the appropriate ongoing assessment, monitoring and care required for Jon, particularly during initial intervention.
2. Explore the potential psychological and social needs for Jon and his family.
3. Consider what secondary prevention, educational information and advice Jon will require during the cardiac rehabilitation phase.
4. What complications may arise in the hours post STEMI?

be considered for all high-risk patients thought to have large infarctions, those in cardiogenic shock, those with failed thrombolysis and those with a prolonged time from symptom onset to presentation.

Ongoing Care Issues and the Role of the Nurse

Immediate Nursing Issues

Following PCI, Jon's immediate care revolves around monitoring his haemodynamic status and careful observation of the arterial puncture site and distal pulses for signs and symptoms of post procedural complications every 30 minutes until stable. If radial artery access is used, Jon will have a transradial 'TR Band™' or similar compression device in place to assist haemostasis of the radial artery. It is a transparent band which allows direct visualisation of the puncture site for bleeding. At approximately 90 minutes post procedure, the pressure is gradually reduced in preparation for removal. Alternatively a femoral arterial puncture site may be sutured or sealed at the end of the procedure using devices such as the collagen plus angioseal, consisting of an anchor inserted into the artery, a collagen plug that seals the outside and a suture that unites both elements. The angioseal would allow Jon to sit up immediately post procedure; however, it is relatively expensive and sometimes difficult to deploy. Alternatively, the arterial catheter sheath may remain inserted in the femoral artery post PCI to be removed approximately four to six hours post procedure, with prolonged manual or mechanical pressure applied to the puncture site to ensure adequate stasis. Manual pressure that relies upon direct 'digit to groin' pressure for approximately ten minutes can be physically arduous and time consuming; therefore mechanical devices such as a 'fem-stop', involving application of an inflatable dome secured over the puncture site with a belt, are often employed. Jon's arterial sheath and puncture site post removal must be closely observed every 30 minutes for signs of bleeding and the presence of pedal pulses on the affected side noted. Removal of the sheath may induce a vasovagal response, leading to a transient bradycardia, sudden hypotension and feeling faint, though this is not common and can be overcome with IV Atropine®. Nevertheless, observation and continuous monitoring of heart rate, rhythm, BP and signs of chest pain or discomfort should continue at least every 30 minutes for the first two hours post procedure and removal of arterial sheath. Jon must be reminded to inform the nurse if he experiences any chest pain or discomfort during his stay in order that reassessment and appropriate management can be promptly initiated.

The majority of patients remain haemodynamically stable post reperfusion; however, on occasion some individuals experience a profound hypotension immediately post PCI and may require additional temporary cardiac support from an intra-aortic balloon pump inserted via the arterial catheter sheath, with the same close monitoring for the duration of the therapy. Skin colour and warmth provides a useful visual guide of systemic perfusion and as the kidneys are particularly sensitive to decreased perfusion pressure, urinary output measurement provides a valuable clinical indicator of cardiac output and BP. A 70 kg individual would normally produce at least 0.5 mL/kg/hour and so if Jon produces less than 35 mL/hour, low cardiac output and BP or in a minority of cases urinary retention due to a reaction to the dye used during PCI, requiring bladder catheterisation, should be suspected.

Aside from immediate coronary angiography a definitive clinical measure of reperfusion success is not currently available. Chest pain relief is affected by a variety of factors, not least opiate therapy and fluctuation in coronary blood flow post infarction, and is therefore not a helpful guide. A repeat ECG at 60 to 90 minutes post reperfusion therapy to assess ST segment resolution may provide some indication of tissue-level reperfusion and prognosis, as patients who have ≥70 per cent ST resolution are thought to have a better prognosis. Following PCI, approximately 20 to 30 per cent of patients do not demonstrate ST resolution despite TIMI flow grade 3 at the end of the procedure and are more likely to have an unfavourable prognosis (Claeys et al., 1999); however, isolated reliance upon ST segment resolution as an indicator is not recommended. There is some correlation between accelerated idioventricular rhythm and restoration of vessel patency. Therefore a combination of sudden or near complete relief from chest pain, ST segment resolution and accelerated idioventricular rhythm is highly specific for successful reperfusion, though this tends to be evident in only approximately 10 per cent of individuals (see Bennett, 2013, for further explanation of idioventricular rhythm). Further venous blood sampling for troponin or creatine phosphokinase (CK) is not routinely necessary following a history and ECG diagnosis of STEMI. However, local policies differ and some hospitals may measure one or both biochemical markers at 12 hours post admission as an indication of infarct size. The frequency of observation of vital signs will be determined by the current trend but may be reduced to four-hourly once Jon is pain free, thrombolysis is successfully infused or four hours post removal of the PCI arterial sheath with no obvious signs of complication (Table 6.13).

Alternative Pharmacological Reperfusion Therapy

In the absence of a local PCI service in some districts, pharmacological thrombolytic reperfusion remains the mainstay treatment for STEMI; however, it is estimated that only approximately 5 per cent of patients diagnosed with STEMI now receive pharmacological thrombolysis. Thrombolysis therapy should be initiated if immediate PCI within the 120-minute time frame

Table 6.13 Potential complications post-STEMI

---

1. Tachyarrhythmia, bradyarrhythmia or conduction defects (see Bennett, 2013).
2. Post infarction ischaemia/angina.
3. Reinfarction – incidence ranges from less than 5 per cent post reperfusion therapy to 16 per cent of non reperfused patients.
4. Acute left ventricular failure – acute pulmonary oedema ± decreased stroke volume and cardiac output.
5. Congestive cardiac failure – raised pulmonary and systemic venous pressure leading to pulmonary and systemic congestion and decreased cardiac output.
6. Mitral regurgitation – frequency of a new murmur is between 20 and 55 per cent.
7. Pericarditis – sterile inflammation of the pericardium usually associated with Q wave anterior myocardial infarction causing sharp chest pain, a pericardial rub and effusion and concave ST segment elevation across multiple ECG leads. Incidence has fallen dramatically with reperfusion therapy.
8. Cardiogenic shock – usually signifies severe coronary artery disease and occurs when more than 40 per cent of the left ventricular mass is infarcted and ischaemic.
9. Cardiac rupture – rupture of left ventricular free wall, ventricular septum leading to a ventricular septal defect, the papillary muscle or chordae tendinae.
10. Left ventricular aneurysm – severe persistent infarct expansion and scar tissue development lead to a discrete bulge of the left ventricle.
11. Left ventricular thrombus – usually associated with anterior region infarction and occurs at the site of infarct expansion or apical aneurysm.
12. Left ventricular remodelling – structural and functional changes of the left ventricle which commence during the acute myocardial infarction and may continue to evolve over months or years and follow a sequence of events. Infarct expansion – thinning and dilation of the infarct zone which may lead to left ventricular remodelling; dilation of the uninfarcted myocardium leading to hypertrophy; fibrosis and contractile impairment; global change of shape of left ventricle from elongated to spherical.

---

from onset of symptoms is not locally available. A decline in 30-day mortality post STEMI from 25–30 per cent in the 1960s and 18 per cent in the mid-1980s to 8–9 per cent in 2002 was largely attributed to the widespread use of thrombolytic therapy, aspirin and coronary interventions (Van de Werf et al., 2003). A wealth of randomised controlled trials has firmly established the use of fibrinolytic therapy (thrombolysis) to treat STEMI since the early 1980s; however, the mortality benefit is also time dependent, with no convincing evidence of benefit beyond 12 hours (GUSTO Investigators, 1993; Boersma et al., 1996). Patients treated within the first hour, frequently referred to as the 'golden hour', have the highest absolute and relative mortality benefit. This well-established time-dependent factor for thrombolysis supports the 60-minute 'call-to-needle time' and 30-minute 'door-to-needle

Table 6.14 Thrombolytic agents for STEMI

Agent	Routine use	Administration	Adjunct therapy
Streptokinase® (SK): relatively cheap. Once only use as streptococcal derivative induces antibody response	Acute inferior STEMI and/or > 75 years old unless absolutely contraindicated (Table 6.15)	15,000,000 units in 100 ml of 5% dextrose or 0.9% saline infused over 60 minutes	None (though subcutaneous s/c enoxaparin® is often prescribed until mobility restored)
Alteplase® (tPA) tissue plasminogen activator – approximately 4 times the cost of SK	Acute anterior STEMI, ≤75 years old and all those previously treated with streptokinase unless contraindicated (Table 6.15)	Accelerated regime: 15 mg IV bolus; 50 mg infused over 30 minutes; 35 mg infused over 60 minutes	IV heparin®, s/c enoxaparin® weight adjusted 48 to 72 hours or fondaparinux®
Tenecteplase® (TNK-tPA) – similar cost to tPA	As tPA	Single weight adjusted IV bolus	S/c enoxaparin® weight adjusted 48 to 72 hours or fondaparinux®

time' set by the CHD NSF thrombolysis standards (DH, 2000). Several large studies (GISSI 2, 1990; ISIS 3, 1992; GUSTO, 1993) have compared different thrombolytic agents (Table 6.14).

The ease and speed of administration of IV TNK® with adjunct IV Heparin® or weight-adjusted doses of subcutaneous low molecular weight heparin (LMWH) such as Clexane® or Enoxaparin® makes this the usual drug of choice. LMWH, a sub-fraction of standard heparin that has demonstrated a number of clinical benefits, not least removing the need for close aPTT monitoring, has largely superseded IV heparin therapy (ASSENT 3, 2001; Antman et al., 2006). Alternatively in some centres, a single bolus subcutaneous injection of 2.5 mg of Fondaparinux®, which selectively inactivates clotting factor Xa and thus reduces the opportunity for further red clot formation, may be preferred (Figure 6.4).

Thrombolysis is not without risk; hypotension, usually relieved by temporary cessation of the infusion and elevation of the feet, and rarely requiring IV Atropine® or volume expansion, and severe allergic reactions are occasionally associated with IV Streptokinase®. Bleeding post thrombolysis with all agents is a major potential complication and observation and early detection is of paramount importance in reducing long-term associated

Table 6.15 Contraindications to thrombolysis

Absolute contraindications	*Relative contraindications*
• Haemorrhagic stroke or stroke of unknown origin • Ischaemic stroke within previous 6 months • Central nervous system damage or neoplasm • Recent (within 3 weeks) major surgery/head injury • Gastrointestinal bleed within 1 month • Known bleeding disorder • Aortic dissection	• Transient ischaemic attack within 6 months • Oral anticoagulant therapy (check clotting) • Pregnancy or within 1 week post-partum • Non compressible vascular punctures • Traumatic or prolonged resuscitation • Refractory hypertension (systolic > 180 mmHg) • Advanced liver disease • Infective endocarditis • Active peptic ulcer

morbidity. The worst outcome is intracerebral haemorrhage, which occurs in 0.5 per cent and may be detected by headache, acute confusional state, visual disturbance, seizure or other new neurological signs. Unfortunately, despite early recognition, diagnosis and possible surgical intervention, there is approximately 75 per cent risk of mortality or a permanent neurological deficit, particularly in older adults >70 years receiving tPA or TNK. There is a 3–13 per cent risk of major non-cerebral bleeding associated with all three agents. Gastrointestinal, retroperitoneal or trauma site bleeding affects less than 5 per cent, though it may be life threatening if undetected, whereas the commonest site around intravenous access is usually self-limiting. Continuous monitoring of heart rate and rhythm, BP recording and general observation, particularly of venous puncture sites, should be reported every 30 minutes for the first two to three hours. Superficial bleeding is the most common problem encountered in practice and with vigilance and care is usually limited to localised bruising.

Adjunct Pharmacological Treatment Following Either Reperfusion Therapy

NICE (2007b) guidance 48 recommends prescription of a range of cardiac drugs, physical activity, lifestyle modification of diet, smoking habit and alcohol consumption, and invitation onto cardiac rehabilitation programmes for all patients following MI to minimise the risk of further acute events. ISIS 2 confirmed an additional mortality benefit associated with adjunct aspirin therapy with all reperfusion therapies, and it is now standard therapy given to virtually all patients with acute coronary syndrome (ISIS 2, 1988). This explains why Jon received a stat oral dose of 300 mg of dispersible aspirin for its anti-platelet properties in an effort to disperse the offending platelet-rich 'white clot' rather than for its more traditional analgesic effect. A daily maintenance dose of 75 mg of oral aspirin should be continued indefinitely. The CLARITY trial found that in addition to aspirin, concomitant early oral Clopidogrel® therapy for patients with STEMI appeared to confer further benefits in terms of mortality, patency and reinfarction over aspirin alone (Sabatine et al., 2005; NICE, 2007b). Clopidogrel® also provides an effective alternative for individuals who are unable to tolerate the potential gastric irritation sometimes caused by aspirin. In Jon's case, 10 mg daily of an alternative thioendopyridine, Prasugrel® (NICE, 2014) or twice daily 90 mg Ticagrelor® will be prescribed for up to one year. On day one post acute presentation Jon is likely to be prescribed a low dose beta blocker such as Metoprolol®; Atenolol® or Carvedilol® might be considered for patients with poor LV function assessed on echocardiography. A significant survival benefit is afforded by angiotensin-converting enzyme inhibitors (ACEI) such as Ramipril®, Enalapril® or Captopril® for post MI patients with evidence of left ventricular dysfunction (Cleland et al., 1993; GISSI 3, 1994; ISIS 4, 1995). Assuming blood pressure was within normal parameters Jon would commence a graded dose on day one post MI, with 30-minute BP recording for approximately two hours after the first dose to observe for signs of hypotension. Angiotensin receptor 2 antagonists such as Losartan® or Valsartan® may be substituted for patients unable to tolerate the side effects of ACE inhibitors, a tickly cough being a common complaint. Statins (3-hydroxy-3-methylglutaryl coenzyme A (HMG-CoA) reductase inhibitors) such as Pravastatin®, Simvastatin® and Atorvastatin® profoundly reduce plasma cholesterol levels and are instrumental in reducing the incidence of recurring coronary events and improving outcomes post MI (Armitage, 2010). The current national threshold for statin intervention is 5.2 mmol/L but in practice if Jon's admission serum cholesterol level was found to be more than 4 mmol/L he is most likely to commence a large nightly dose (at least 40 mg) of a statin in view of his evident coronary artery disease. As statins may adversely affect liver function a baseline liver function test is advisable prior to initiation of therapy. Both GISSI 3 (1994) and ISIS 4 (1995) trials failed to establish any benefit from intravenous nitrates or long-acting oral nitrates during the acute MI phase. However, intravenous nitroglycerin preparations are used in the treatment of post MI heart failure and recurrent ischaemic pain. Similarly, calcium channel blockers have not demonstrated benefit and are not routinely prescribed post MI. Nifedipine®

is generally contraindicated post MI and Diltiazem® and Verapamil® are reserved for specific treatment of post-infarction angina or supraventricular arrhythmias. Opie and Gersh (2013) focus upon the pharmacological action of cardiac drugs in detail.

Psychosocial Concerns

The psychological consequence of the acute and continuing phases of care post STEMI have been well documented and should not be underestimated. A lack of knowledge can lead to misunderstanding and misinterpretation of the situation, and worries and uncertainty related to the implications of having had a 'heart attack', now and in the future, exacerbating fears of the unknown, are common concerns that Jon may experience. The very speed of symptom onset, diagnosis and intervention during the acute episode exacerbated profound feelings of emotional shock for a group of PCI patients interviewed by Astin et al. (2009). This was further compounded by an apparent mismatch between expectations and reality, which appeared to affect the ability of these patients to make sense of their condition in a coherent manner. This led to a degree of misconception that the condition was 'acute' and treatment 'curative', evading the necessity for longer-term self-management for a chronic condition (Astin et al., 2009). Sudden loss of close communication and contact with family and significant others contributes to feelings of fear, isolation and hopelessness, which may further intensify anxiety. Elevated levels of fear and anxiety during the acute phase may not only prompt the undesirable physiological cardiac effects already mentioned but if overlooked lead to depression and adversely affect long-term rehabilitation and survival (Jowett and Thompson, 2007). Major depression has been reported in up to 20 per cent of patients hospitalised with MI; a further 10 to 17 per cent display significant symptoms of depression and the majority of these patients remain depressed one to four months later (Bush et al., 2005). It is therefore imperative that assessment and management of Jon's emotional response and adjustment to the immediate phase remain a central aspect of his acute care. Reassurance and appropriate information giving are imperative at all stages of care. Clear, concise, timely and reinforced communication and explanation regarding immediate treatment can help to restore some sense of control over the situation, promote informed decision making, reduce anxiety and enhance compliance with care. Visibility, approachability, empathy and an air of professional competence by health professionals involved in Jon's care can further endorse this.

Once Jon has recovered from the acute event, the first of four phases of structured cardiac rehabilitation should be commenced (Table 6.16). The

Table 6.16 Four phases of cardiac rehabilitation

Phase 1 initiates information and advice giving by a cardiac rehabilitation nurse with patient and family prior to discharge and includes:

1. Emotional assessment, reassurance and stress management
2. Risk factor assessment and modification planning
3. Assessment of patient knowledge and understanding of heart disease
4. Accurate, consistent, relevant educational advice about:
   - Coronary heart disease
   - Individual risk factors
   - Drug therapy and chest pain management
   - Healthy diet
   - Smoking cessation
   - Return to usual activities of daily living
   - Return to work
   - Return to sexual activity and issues related to erectile dysfunction
   - Return to driving
   - Holidays, flying and travel abroad
5. Verbal discussion may be supplemented by written leaflets, videos and the Heart Manual (6 week programme)

Phase 2: home visits facilitated by the specialist community cardiac rehabilitation team immediately post discharge for approximately 3 months and including:

1. Pulse and blood pressure monitoring
2. Reinforce lifestyle risk factors and modification
3. Monitor anxiety and depression levels
4. Support patient and family with individual needs

Phase 3: structured exercise programme facilitated by cardiac rehabilitation nurses and trained fitness instructor or physiotherapist 6 to 8 weeks post discharge, including:

1. Educational and psychological support
2. Advice on risk factors

Phase 4: long-term maintenance by primary care practitioners

Cardiovascular Disease Outcomes Strategy (DH, 2013) recommends that all heart patients be invited to participate in multidisciplinary secondary prevention and cardiac rehabilitation programmes, which offer comprehensive individualised support to change their lifestyle, involving education and psychological input, as well as exercise training.

Phase 1 aims to teach, advise, support and promote Jon's understanding of the MI and treatment received, his return to full independence and behavioural changes he may wish to adopt in order to restore a full, healthy and happy lifestyle that minimises the risk of further acute cardiac events. However, the average length of hospital stay following PCI is three to four days (slightly longer post thrombolysis). This and frequent transfers between and within hospitals restrict the available time for healthcare practitioners to offer sufficient, relevant explanation, information and advice on healthy lifestyles, potential behaviour modification and structured exercise programmes to return Jon to full physical activity, or to discuss his psychosocial and spiritual needs. Further to this the emotional shock of having had a 'heart attack' may influence Jon's ability to absorb, retain and recall information given. Astin et al. (2008) recommend that information giving be 'staged' to better reflect patient priorities and specific needs and be offered and reinforced prior to and immediately post hospital discharge in the home by specialist nurses to enhance continuity of care and address further information needs. Prior to discharge Jon specifically needs to:

- be fully informed of all medications prescribed and to receive a Clopidogrel®/Prasugrel® card;
- know how to deal with future episodes of chest pain and how to use his GTN spray effectively, and be advised to seek professional help if the chest pain is not resolved within 15 minutes;
- know what constitutes a 'healthy heart' diet and exercise regime and be introduced to opportunities to stop smoking in an effort to help him make healthy life choices in the future.

Social support is an essential aspect of physical and psychosocial recovery and so Jon's home circumstances must also be considered. Although driving a car is permitted one month after a STEMI, Jon will require a negative exercise stress test before he may be able to resume employment as a bus driver. This will usually be arranged as an outpatient visit once Jon has been discharged into the care of the GP and community-based cardiac rehabilitation team. All stages of heart patients' care rely upon a multidisciplinary approach including doctors, nurses, pharmacists, physiotherapists, dieticians, smoking cessation teams, social workers and clinical psychologists in some instances. Comprehensive cardiac rehabilitation programmes are a clinical and cost-effective intervention as important as drug therapy in secondary prevention after MI and should be offered to all patients post MI regardless of age, gender, ethnicity, co-morbidity or cardiac function (NICE, 2007b). Evidence suggests that they can reduce mortality by as much as 20 to 25 per cent over three years and can improve health outcomes and quality of life for people with CHD (DH, 2000), yet less than half of eligible patients in the UK access cardiac rehabilitation (Beswick et al., 2005). Cardiac rehabilitation begins before discharge from hospital, though it is largely provided as either home- or community-based programmes where there is an increasing emphasis upon employing strategies to enhance access, participation and retention of participants.

Summary

Early, accurate assessment, timely intervention and care during the acute phase and entry into a comprehensive cardiac rehabilitation programme should enable Jon to return to a happy, healthy and active work, social and personal life.

Further Reading

Bennett, D. H. *Cardiac Arrhythmias*, 8th edn (London: Wiley-Blackwell, 2013).

Epstein, O., G. D. Perkin, J. Cookson, I. S. Watt, R. Rakhit, A. W. Robbins and G. A. W. Hornett. *Clinical Examination*, 4th edn (London: Mosby International Ltd, 2008).

Gamon, R., T. Quinn and B. Parr. *Emergency Care of the Patient with a Heart Attack* (Edinburgh: Churchill Livingstone, 2006).

Lilly, L. S. (ed.). *Pathophysiology of Heart Disease: A Collaborative Project of Medical Students and Faculty*, 5th edn (Baltimore, MD: Lippincott, Williams & Wilkins, 2011).

Opie, L. H. and B. J. Gersh. *Drugs for the Heart*, 8th edn (Philadelphia: Elsevier Saunders, 2013).

References

American Heart Association (AHA). 'Markers of Inflammation and Cardiovascular Disease'. *Circulation*, 107 (2003), 499–511.

Anderson, H. R., T. T. Nielson, K. Rasmussen et al.. 'For the DANAMI-2 Investigators. A Comparison of Coronary Angioplasty with Fibrinolytic Therapy in Acute Myocardial Infarction', *New England Journal of Medicine*, 349 (2003), 733–42.

Antman, E. M., M. Hand, P. W. Armstrong et al.. 'Focused Update of the ACC/AHA 2004 Guidelines for the Management of Patients with ST Elevation Myocardial Infarction: A Report of the American College of Cardiology/American Heart Association Task Force on Practice Guidelines', *Journal of the American College of Cardiology*, 51 (2007), 210–47.

Antman, E. M., D. A. Morrow, C. H. McCabe et al.. 'Enoxaparin versus Unfractionated Heparin with Fibrinolysis for ST Elevation Myocardial Infarction', *New England Journal of Medicine*, 354 (2006), 1477–88.

Armitage, J., L. Bowman, K. Wallendszus et al.. 'Intensive Lowering of LDL Cholesterol with 80 mg versus 20 mg Simvastatin Daily in 12,064 Survivors of Myocardial Infarction: A Double-blind Randomised Trial', *Lancet*, 376 (2010), 1658–69.

Assessment of the Safety and Efficacy of a New Thrombolytic Regimen (ASSENT) 3 Investigators. 'Efficacy and Safety of Tenecteplase in Combination with Enoxaparin, Abciximab or Unfractionated Heparin: The ASSENT-3 Randomised Trial in Acute Myocardial Infarction', *Lancet*, **358** (2001), 605–13.

Astin, F., S. J. Closs, J. McLenachan, S. Hunter and C. Priestley. 'The Information Needs of Patients Treated with Primary Angioplasty for Heart Attack: An Exploratory Study', *Patient Education and Counselling*, doi: 10 1016/j. pec.2008.06.013 (2008).

Astin, F., S. J. Closs, J. McLenachan, S. Hunter and C. Priestley. 'Primary Angioplasty for Heart Attack: Mismatch between Expectations and Reality?', *Journal of Advanced Nursing*, 65(1) (2009), 72–83.

Barth, J., M. Schumacher and C. Herrmann-Lingen. 'Depression as a Risk Factor for Mortality in Patients with Coronary Heart Disease: A Meta-analysis', *Psychosomatic Medicine*, **66** (2004), 802–13.

Bennett, D. H. *Cardiac Arrhythmias*, 8th edn (London: Wiley-Blackwell, 2013).

Bertuccio, P. F. Levi, F. Lucchini, L. Chatenoud, C. Bosetti, E. Negri and C. La Vecchia. 'Coronary Heart Disease And Cerebrovascular Disease Mortality In Young Adults: Recent Trends In Europe', *European Journal Of Cardiovascular Prevention And Rehabilitation*, **18** (4) (2011). 627–34.

Beswick, A. D., K. Rees, R. R. West, F. C. Taylor, M. Burke, I. Griebsch, R. S. Taylor, J. Victory, J. Brown and S. Ebrahim. 'Improving Uptake and Adherence in Cardiac Rehabilitation: Literature Review', *Journal Of Advanced Nursing*, **49**(5) (2005), 538–55.

Betriu, A. and M. Masotti. 'Comparison of Mortality Rates in Acute Myocardial Infarction Treated by Percutaneous Coronary Intervention versus Fibrinolysis', *American Journal of Cardiology*, **95** (2005), 100–1.

Bird, M. W., A. G. Woods and N. A. Warren. 'Factors Influencing Treatment Delays for Acute Myocardial Infarction', *Critical Care Nursing Quarterly*, **32**(1) (2009), 19–23.

Boersma, E., A. Mass, J. Deckers and M. Simoons. 'Early Thrombolytic Treatment in Acute Myocardial Infarction: Reappraisal of the Golden Hour', *Lancet*, 348 (1996), 771–5.

Bush, D. E., R. C. Ziegelstein, U. V. Patel, B. D. Thombs, D. E. Ford, J. A. Fauerbach, U. D. McCann, K. J. Stewart, K. K. Tsilidis, A. L. Patel, C. J. Feuerstein and E. B. Bass. *Post-Myocardial Infarction Depression* (Rockville: Agency for Healthcare Research and Quality (AHRQ) 310, 2005).

Claeys, M. J., J. Bosmans, L. Veenstra et al.. 'Determinants and Prognostic Implications of Persistent ST Segment Elevation after Primary Angioplasty for Acute Myocardial Infarction: Importance of Microvascular Reperfusion Injury on Clinical Outcome', *Circulation*, **99** (1999), 1972–7.

Cleland, J. G., L. Erhardt, G. Murray, A. S. Hall and S. G. Ball. 'Effect of Ramipril on Mortality and Morbidity of Survivors of Acute Myocardial Infarction with Clinical Evidence of Heart Failure. The Acute Infarction Ramipril Efficacy (AIRE) Study Investigators', *Lancet*, **342** (1993), 821–8.

Culi, V., D. Miri and D. Eterovi. 'Correlation Between Symptomatology and Site of Acute Myocardial Infarction', *International Journal of Cardiology*, **77**(2/3) (2001), 163–8.

DeLuca, G., H. Suryapranata, G. W. Stone et al.. 'Abciximab as Adjunctive Therapy to Reperfusion in Acute ST Segment Elevation Myocardial Infarction: A Meta Analysis of Randomised Trials', *JAMA*, **293** (2005), 1759–65.

Denollet, J., S. S. Pederson, C. J. Vrints and V. M. Conraads. 'Usefulness of Type D Personality in Predicting Five Year Cardiac Events Above and Beyond Concurrent Symptoms of Stress in Patients with Coronary Heart Disease', *American Journal Cardiology*, **97** (2006), 970–3.

Department of Health (DH). *National Service Framework for Coronary Heart Disease* (London: HMSO, 2000).

Department of Health (DH). *Treatment of Heart Attack National Guidance: Final Report of the National Infarct Angioplasty Project (NIAP)*. (London: Department of Health, 2008). Available from: www.dh.gov.uk/en/Publicationsandstatistics/Publications/PublicationsPolicyAndGuidance/DH_089455 (accessed 11 November 2014) *(Guideline Ref ID DOH2008)*.

Department of Health (DH). *Coronary Heart Disease National Service Framework: Building on Excellence, Maintaining Progress* (London: HMSO, 2009).

Department of Health (DH). *Cardiovascular Disease Outcomes Strategy. Improving Outcomes For People With Or At Risk From Cardiovascular Disease* (London: HMSO, 2013).

Dubois, C., J. Smeets and C. Demoulin. 'Incidence, Clinical Significance and Prognosis of Ventricular Fibrillation in the Early Phase of Myocardial Infarction', *European Heart Journal*, **7**(11) (1986), 945–51.

Eslick, G. D. 'Usefulness of Chest Pain Character and Location as Diagnostic Indicators of an Acute Coronary Syndrome', *American Journal of Cardiology*, **95**(10) (2005), 1228–31.

Fibrinolytic Therapy Trialists (FTT) Collaborative Group. 'Indications for Fibrinolytic Therapy in Suspected Acute Myocardial Infarction: Collaborative Overview of Early Mortality and Major Morbidity Results from All Randomised Trials of More than 1000 Patients', *Lancet*, **343** (1994), 311–22.

Foreman, R. D. 'Mechanisms of Cardiac Pain', *Annual Review of Physiology*, **61** (1999), 143–67.

Fox, K. A. A., J. Birkhead, R. Wilcox, C. Knight and J. Barth. 'British Cardiac Society Working Group on the Definition of Myocardial Infarction', *Heart*, **90** (2004) 603–9.

GISSI 2 International Study Group. 'In Hospital Mortality and Clinical Course of 20,891 Patients with Suspected Acute Myocardial Infarction Randomised between Alteplase and Streptokinase with or without Heparin', *Lancet*, **336** (1990), 71–5.

GISSI 3. 'Effects of Lisinopril and Transdermal Glyceryl Trinitrate Singly and Together on Six Week Mortality and Ventricular Function after Acute Myocardial Infarction', *Lancet*, **343** (1994), 1115–22.

GUSTO Investigators. 'An International Randomised Trial Comparing Four Thrombolytic Strategies for Acute Myocardial Infarction', *New England Journal of Medicine*, **329** (1993) 1615–22.

Hartwell, D., J. Colquitt, E. Loveman, A. J. Clegg, H. Brodin, N. Waugh et al.. 'Clinical Effectiveness and Cost-Effectiveness of Immediate Angioplasty for Acute

Myocardial Infarction: Systematic Review and Economic Evaluation. Health Technology Assessment', 9 (17) (2005), 1–114.

Henkel, D. M., B. J. Witt, B. J. Gersh, S. J. Jacobsen, S. A. Weston, R. A. Meverden and V. L. Roger. 'Ventricular Arrhythmias after Acute Myocardial Infarction: A 20 Year Community Study', *American Heart Journal*, 151(4) (2006), 806–12.

Herlihy, T., M. E. McIvor, C. C. Cummings, C. O. Siu and M. Alikahn. 'Nausea and Vomiting During Acute Myocardial Infarction and Its Relation to Infarct Size and Location', *American Journal of Cardiology*, 60(1) (2004), 20–2.

Horne, R., D. James, K. Petrie, J. Weinman and R. Vincent. 'Patients' Interpretation of Symptoms as a Cause of Delay in Reaching Hospital during Acute Myocardial Infarction', *Heart*, **83** (2000), 388–93.

ISIS 2 (Second International Study of Infarct Survival) Collaborative Group. 'Randomised Trial of Intravenous Streptokinase, Oral Aspirin, Both, or Neither Among 17,187 Cases of Suspected Acute Myocardial Infarction', *Lancet*, **ii** (1988), 349–60.

ISIS 3 (Third International Study of Infarct Survival) Collaborative Group. 'A Randomised Comparison of Streptokinase versus Tissue Plasminogen Activator versus Anistreplase and of Aspirin plus Heparin versus Aspirin Alone among 41,299 Cases of Suspected Acute Myocardial Infarction', *Lancet*, **339** (1992), 753–70.

ISIS 4 (Fourth International Study of Infarct Survival) Collaborative Group. 'A Randomised Factorial Trial Assessing Early Captopril, Oral Mononitrate and Intravenous Magnesium Sulphate in 58,050 Patients with Suspected Acute Myocardial Infarction', *Lancet*, **345** (1995), 669–85.

Jowett, N. I. and D. R. Thompson. *Comprehensive Coronary Care*, 4th edn (London: Bailliere Tindall, 2007).

Keeley, E. C., J. A. Boura and C. L. Grines. 'Primary Angioplasty versus Intravenous Thrombolytic Therapy for Acute Myocardial Infarction: A Quantitative Review of 23 Randomised Trials', *Lancet*, **361**(9351) (2003), 13–20.

Kehl, D. W., N. Iqbal, A. Fard, B. A. Kipper, A. De La Parra Landa, and A. S. Maisel. 'Biomarkers in Acute Myocardial Injury', *Translational Research* **159** (4) (2012), 252–64.

Lilly, L. S. (ed.). *Pathophysiology of Heart Disease: A Collaborative Project of Medical Students and Faculty*, 5th edn (Baltimore: Lippincott, Williams & Wilkins, 2011).

Lindholm, D., C. Varenhorst, C. Cannon, R. Harrington, A. Himmelmann, J. Maya, S. Husted, H. Katus, P. Steg, R. Storey, L. Wallentin, and S. K. James. 'Ticagrelor Versus Clopidogrel in Patients with Non-ST-elevation Acute Coronary Syndrome: Results from the Plato Trial', *Journal Of American College Of Cardiology*, **61**(10_S) (2013) [Online]. Available at: http://content.onlinejacc.org/article.aspx?articleid=1664148 (accessed 1 September 2014).

Malmberg, K., A. Norhammar, H. Wedal et al.. 'Glycometabolic State at Admission: Important Risk Marker of Mortality in Conventionally Treated Patients with Diabetes Mellitus and Acute Myocardial Infarction: Long Term Results from the Diabetes and Insulin-Glucose Infusion in Acute Myocardial Infarction (DIGAMI) Trial', *Circulation*, **99** (1999), 2626–32.

Malmberg, K., L. Ryden, H. Wedel et al.. 'Intense Metabolic Control by Means of Insulin in Patients with Diabetes Mellitus and Acute Myocardial Infarction (DIGAMI 2). Effects on Mortality and Morbidity', *European Heart Journal*, **26** (2005), 650–61.

McNulty, P. H., N. King, S. Scott, G. Harlman, J. McCann, M. Kozak, C. E. Chambers, L. M. Demers and L. I. Sinoway. 'Effects of Supplemental Oxygen Administration on Coronary Blood Flow in Patients Undergoing Cardiac Catheterisation', *American Journal of Physiology – Heart and Circulatory Physiology*, **288**(3) (2005), H1057.

Montalescot, G., S. D. Wiviott, E. Braunwald, S. A. Murphy, C. M. Gibson, C. H. McCabe, E. M. Antman and the TRITON-TIMI 38 investigators. 'Prasugrel Compared with Clopidogrel in Patients Undergoing Percutaneous Coronary Intervention for ST-elevation Myocardial Infarction (TRITON-TIMI 38): Double-blind, Randomised Controlled Trial', *Lancet*, **373** (2009), 723–31.

National Heart, Lung and Blood Institute (Part of the National Health Institutes of Health and the US Department of Health and Human Services). *Coronary Heart Disease* (2010) [Online]. Available from www.nhlbi.nih.gov/health/dci (accessed 14 February 2015).

National Institute for Health and Care Excellence (NICE). *Acutely Ill Patients in Hospital: Recognition of and Response to Acute Illness in Adults in Hospital*. NICE Clinical Guideline 50 (London: HMSO, 2007a).

National Institute for Health and Care Excellence (NICE). *Secondary Prevention in Primary and Secondary Care for Patients Following a Myocardial Infarction*. NICE Clinical Guideline 48 (London: HMSO, 2007b).

National Institute for Health and Care Excellence (NICE). *Chest Pain of Recent Onset: Assessment and Diagnosis of Recent Onset Chest Pain or Discomfort of Suspected Cardiac Origin*. NICE Clinical Guideline 95 (London: HMSO, 2010).

National Institute for Health and Care Excellence (NICE). *Bivalirudin for the Treatment of ST Segment Elevation Myocardial Infarction*. NICE Technology Appraisal Guidance 230. (London: HMSO, 2011a).

National Institute for Health and Care Excellence (NICE). *Ticagrelor for the Treatment of Acute Coronary Syndromes* NICE Technology Appraisal Guidance 236 (London: HMSO, 2011b).

National Institute for Health and Care Excellence (NICE). *Myocardial Infarction with ST-Segment Elevation. The Acute Management of Myocardial Infarction with ST-Segment Elevation*. NICE Clinical Guideline 167 (London: HMSO, 2013a).

National Institute for Health and Care Excellence (NICE). *Unstable Angina and NSTEMI: The Early Management of Unstable Angina and Non-ST-Segment Elevation Myocardial Infarction*. NICE Clinical Guideline 94 (London: HMSO, 2013b).

National Institute for Health and Care Excellence (NICE). *Prasugrel with Percutaneous Coronary Intervention for Treating Acute Coronary Syndromes*. NICE Technology Appraisal Guidance 317 (London: HMSO, 2014).

Nordmann, A. J. P. Hengstler, T. Harr et al.. 'Clinical Outcomes of Primary Stenting versus Balloon Angioplasty in Patients with Myocardial Infarction: A Meta Analysis of Randomised Controlled Trials', *American Journal of Medicine*, **116** (2004), 253–62.

O'Driscoll, B. R., L. S. Howard and A. G. Davison. 'British Thoracic Society Guideline for Emergency Oxygen Use in Adults', *Thorax*, 63(suppl. 6) (2008), 1–68.

Opie, L. H. and B. J. Gersh. *Drugs for the Heart*, 8th edn (Philadelphia: Elsevier Saunders, 2013).

Ross, R. 'Atherosclerosis – an Inflammatory Disease', *New England Journal Medicine*, **340** (1999), 115–26.

Sabatine, M. S., C. P. Cannon, C. M. Gibson et al.. 'Addition of Clopidogrel to Aspirin and Fibrinolytic Therapy for Myocardial Infarction with ST Segment Elevation', *New England Journal of Medicine*, **352** (2005), 1179–89.

Thompson, C. A., J. Yarzebski, R. Goldberg, D. Lessard, J. Gore and J. Dalen. 'Changes Over Time in the Incidence and Case Fatality Rates of Primary Ventricular Fibrillation Complicating Myocardial Infarction: Perspectives from the Worcester Heart Attack Study', *American Heart Journal*, **139**(6) (2000), 1014–21.

Townsend, N., K. Wickramasinghe, P. Bhatnagar, K. Smolina, M. Nichols, J. Leal, R. Luengo-Fernandez and M. Rayner. *Coronary Heart Disease Statistics 2012 Edition* (London: British Heart Foundation, 2012).

Van de Werf, F., D. Ardissino, A. Betriu, D. V. Cokkinos et al.. 'Management of Acute Myocardial Infarction in Patients Presenting with ST Segment Elevation: The Task Force on the Management of Acute Myocardial Infarction of the European Society of Cardiology', *European Heart Journal*, **24** (2003), 28–66.

Weston, C., L. Walker and J. Birkhead. 'Early Impact of Insulin Treatment on Mortality for Hyperglycaemic Patients Without Known Diabetes who Present with an Acute Coronary Syndrome', *British Medical Journal*, **93** (2007), 1542–6.

Yusuf, S., S. Reddy, S. Ounpuu and S. Anand. 'Global Burden of Cardiovascular Diseases. Part 1: General Considerations, the Epidemiologic Transition, Risk Factors and Impact of Urbanisation', *Circulation*, **104** (2001a), 2746–53.

Yusuf, S., S. Reddy, S. Ounpuu and S. Anand. 'Global Burden of Cardiovascular Diseases. Part 2: Variations in Cardiovascular Disease by Specific Ethnic Groups and Geographic Regions and Prevention Strategies', *Circulation*, **104** (2001b), 2855–64.

7

Chronic Obstructive Pulmonary Disease

Liz Cleave

Introduction: Chronic Obstructive Pulmonary Disease in Context (UK focus)

Chronic Obstructive Pulmonary Disease (COPD) is the global term given to a group of respiratory diseases that are characterised by irreversible airflow obstruction, are usually progressive and do not change markedly over time (National Institute of Health and Care Excellence (NICE) 2010). COPD encompasses three different diseases: emphysema, chronic bronchitis and chronic asthma. COPD is a preventable and treatable disease (Global Initiative for Chronic Obstructive Lung Disease (GOLD), 2014) and relies upon an early diagnosis so that appropriate curative and preventative management can be commenced in an attempt to delay the disease process. Preventative measures such as smoking cessation once diagnosis has been confirmed can reduce progression and relieve symptoms (National Centre for Smoking Cessation and Training, 2012). COPD is a complex disease and each person diagnosed with COPD experiences the symptoms and disease course in a unique way, especially the impact the disease has on activities of daily living. Pharmacological intervention is an integral aspect of management and aims to delay airflow obstruction. Management strategies must take account of the individual experience of COPD as far as possible.

Unlike many other common chronic diseases the prevalence of COPD has not declined in recent years and according to data is on the increase (NICE, 2010). A diagnosis should be considered in anyone over the age of 35 years presenting with symptoms of dyspnoea, cough and excessive mucus production (NICE, 2010). COPD is a common disease but it is difficult to be certain of the true mortality rate: some patients die with the disease rather than because of it (Table 7.1). The difficulty in an accurate

185

Table 7.1   COPD statistics

Mortality:
Between 25,000 and 30,000 deaths yearly from COPD in the last 25 years
(Department of Health (DH) 2011a)
27,400 deaths from COPD in 2013 (Office for National Statistics, 2013)

Prevalence:
900,000 diagnosed cases but could be as many as 1.5 million due to under-diagnosis
(DH, 2011a)

Source: Adapted from Department of Health (2011a) and ONS (2013).

mortality rate can also be attributed to under-diagnosis and clinical definitions of COPD (DH, 2011a). However, COPD produces significant morbidity
within the UK and has a huge resource implication for the NHS (in terms of
healthcare cost and resources) (DH, 2011a).

It was recognised that there needed to be a coordinated approach to quality care delivery for patients with COPD; therefore in 2011 the Department
of Health developed *An Outcomes Strategy for Chronic Obstructive Pulmonary
Disease (COPD) and Asthma in England.* To assist with the implementation of
this strategy the NHS (2012) published *An Outcomes Strategy for COPD and
Asthma: NHS Companion Document.* To evaluate the strategies implemented,
the National COPD *Audit Programme* (2013) supports the *Outcome Strategy* in
collating data and suggesting improvements to standards of care. Initially,
this audit has collected data from general practitioners' (GPs') records of
patients who have had a diagnosis of COPD and hospital admissions due to
COPD, and it will be utilised to support further strategies in the support of
patients with COPD.

COPD, when severe, is a complex condition. The importance of a full
clinical assessment and the management of the patient when experiencing
an acute exacerbation of COPD (aeCOPD) set the scene for this chapter.

Aim and Learning Outcomes

The Aim

The aim of this chapter is to explore the priorities for accurate assessment
and management of an individual presenting with aeCOPD. It will briefly
outline the assessment and management of a patient with stable COPD and
then critically explore the management of a patient with aeCOPD. The case
scenario will provide the basis for the application of evidence-based theory
to support management decisions.

Learning Outcomes

At the end of this chapter the student will be able to:

1. Define what is meant by the term COPD and recognise the key elements of assessment and management of a patient with stable COPD.
2. Explore and link the pathophysiology to the presenting symptoms associated with aeCOPD.
3. Appreciate the immediate assessment requirements for a patient who experiences aeCOPD.
4. Consider the management of aeCOPD and appreciate the factors indicating a deterioration in the patient's condition.
5. Explore the role of non-invasive ventilation (NIV) in the management of aeCOPD.
6. Consider how acute exacerbation may be prevented.

The Case Scenario: Stable COPD

Arthur is a 55-year-old gentleman who retired early from his job as a welder 18 months ago. He was diagnosed with moderate COPD two years ago. During the last six months of work he reduced his hours to part time because his exercise tolerance rapidly declined. This was mainly due to exertional dyspnoea and a chronic cough that did not allow him to achieve the fine precision required for welding. He had smoked since the age of 16 but gave up smoking 12 months ago following a smoking cessation course suggested by his GP. During the last year his COPD has been relatively stable and he has actively participated in a self-management plan until four months ago when Arthur experienced aeCOPD. The acute episode was treated by his GP by increasing the frequency of an inhaled bronchodilator, the addition of a long-acting bronchodilator and a two-week course of inhaled corticosteroids. Arthur recovered well from this and has been re-stabilised on his original medication. Six weeks ago Arthur visited the GP practice for his annual influenza vaccination.

Consider the following:

1. Define what is meant by the term COPD.
2. Identify the distinctive features of emphysema, chronic bronchitis and chronic asthma.
3. Explore the pathological changes associated with COPD.
4. Discuss the assessment of a person diagnosed with COPD.
5. Explore the specific management of a person with COPD.

Stable COPD

Respiratory Anatomy and Physiology

A knowledge of the underlying normal physiology, pathophysiology, clinical features and maintenance therapy of stable COPD is helpful in understanding the assessment and management of aeCOPD.

The purpose of the respiratory system is to enable movement of oxygen from atmospheric air into the bloodstream for its delivery to the cells for aerobic energy production and the elimination of the waste product of aerobic respiration – carbon dioxide – from the body (Marieb, 2015). The outer aspect of the respiratory system composed of the nose, pharynx, larynx and trachea represents the first point of air entry into the system. The trachea then divides at the carina forming the right and left main bronchi of each lung which provide a reservoir for inspired oxygen-saturated air (Figure 7.1). The right lung is separated by invaginations of the outer pleural lining into three lobes and the left has two lobes. Each bronchus further subdivides to smaller airways called bronchioles which finally terminate at the single epithelial walled alveolar sacs. There are approximately 300 million alveoli

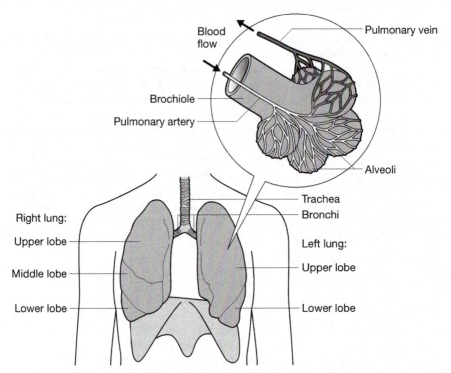

Figure 7.1 The respiratory system

in the human lung providing a massive surface area for oxygen to diffuse from an area of high concentration across the semi-permeable alveolar membrane and capillary walls into the pulmonary circulation where there is a lower concentration of oxygen (Figure 7.1).

Respiration

Respiration is the mechanical process of enabling inspiration of oxygen-saturated atmospheric air (into the lungs) and expiration of carbon dioxide, a waste product of cellular metabolism, from the lungs.

Inspiration is actively controlled by:

1. The movement of the sternum and ribs upwards and outwards under the influence of the intercostal muscles leading to an overall increase in lung volume.
2. The contraction and descent of the diaphragm which is responsible for most of the inspiration in healthy adults (Marieb, 2015).

Expiration results from:

1. A passive relaxation of intercostal muscles, influencing the ribs (and sternum).
2. The relaxation of the diaphragm, allowing the lungs to collapse under the influence of their elastic fibres.

Respiration is controlled by the respiratory centre housed within the medulla oblongata of the brain stem. Nervous impulses arising from the respiratory centre are transmitted via the phrenic and intercostal nerves to respiratory muscles to stimulate a coordinated respiratory movement.

Airway tone is controlled by the autonomic nervous system (Marieb, 2015):

- Adrenoreceptors within the bronchial muscular lining respond to circulating catecholamines such as noradrenaline released from sympathetic nervous activity causing bronchodilation. ß-adrenoreceptor agonists (B2) such as Salbutamol® also cause bronchodilation.

Table 7.2 Definitions

Bronchoconstriction: narrowing of the airway diameter resulting in less airflow available at the alveoli.

Bronchodilation: widening of the airway diameter enabling an increase in airflow.

- Inhaled stimuli such as smoke, dust or cold air can activate cough receptors which trigger reflex bronchoconstriction via vagus parasympathetic nervous activity.

Movement of air in and out of the lungs results from a difference in the pressure in the alveoli and atmospheric pressure. During inspiration atmospheric pressure is greater than alveolar pressure whereas the reverse is true during expiration.

Inspired alveolar oxygen then diffuses across the alveolar membrane into the pulmonary capillary and carbon dioxide moves from the pulmonary capillary back into the alveoli for expiration. Red cell haemoglobin has a high affinity for oxygen which is transported within the arterial circulation as oxyhaemoglobin to the tissues and cells of the body.

Cellular respiration

Cellular respiration describes the process of gaseous exchange at the cells. At a cellular level oxygen is extracted from the capillary blood and utilised by the cell for energy production via anaerobic respiration. The deoxygenated venous circulation transports the waste product of anaerobic respiration, carbon dioxide, back to the lungs for expiration into the atmosphere. Effective respiration must therefore maintain the partial pressure of oxygen (PaO_2) and partial pressure of carbon dioxide ($PaCO_2$) in arterial blood within normal limits (Table 7.3).

Respiration control

Nervous impulses which control respiration are highly influenced by neurogenic and chemical factors (Marieb, 2015). Normal neurogenic influences include:

- a conscious change in respiratory rate and depth;
- impulses from limb receptors in response to exercise and rest;
- impulses from pulmonary receptors sensitive to stretch and irritation;

Table 7.3 Normal arterial blood gas values

Partial Oxygen PaO_2 = 11.0 to 13.0 kPa
Partial Carbon Dioxide $PaCO_2$ = 4.8 to 6.0 kPa
pH = 7.35–7.45
Bicarbonate = 22–26 mmol/L
Base excess = ± 2 mmol/L

impulses from receptors within the respiratory muscles and joints of the chest wall.

Chemical influences occur in response to changes in PaO_2 and $PaCO_2$ detected by peripheral chemoreceptors situated in arterial walls (Marieb, 2015). Chemical influences upon breathing are:

- a rise in $PaCO_2$ is the strongest respiratory stimulant;
- an increase in (hydrogen) H^+ ions in the arterial blood caused by metabolic acidosis will increase ventilation in an effort to remove more CO_2 and therefore reduce arterial pH;
- peripheral chemoreceptors in the carotid and aortic bodies respond to a fall in PaO_2 which in turn stimulate the rate of respiration. However, the stimulus is not strong until the PaO_2 falls below 8 kPa. These receptors also respond to an increase in H^+ ions.

Gaseous Exchange

Efficient gaseous exchange also relies upon adequate ventilation of the alveoli and capillary perfusion (Bourke and Burns 2011). Adequate ventilation is dependent on several complex interactions and a failure in one or more of these can lead to a reduced amount of oxygen being available at the interface and a reduction in the removal of carbon dioxide from the blood. When there is inadequate ventilation or perfusion this can result in a mismatch and leads to ineffective gas exchange either by the transport of oxygen to, or the removal of carbon dioxide away from, the tissues. A ventilation/perfusion mismatch is when there is either inadequate ventilation or perfusion at the alveoli–capillary interface.

Whilst nervous impulses, chemical influences and gaseous exchange all influence the respiratory system these complex interactions include:

1. Airway resistance, i.e. the diameter of the airways which determines the ease of airflow within them.
2. Lung compliance, i.e. the ease of lung expansion.
3. Elasticity, i.e. the stretch and recoil of the lung.

Respiratory failure

Any disruption in the flow of air within the airways can result in respiratory failure. Respiratory failure occurs when there is insufficient oxygen available at the alveoli–capillary interface and results in a decrease in the arterial level of oxygen (hypoxaemia); this is also known as type 1 respiratory

Table 7.4 Key terms defined

Type 1 respiratory failure: $PaO_2 < 8$ kPa and normal (or reduced) $PaCO_2$.
Hypoxaemia = reduced arterial blood oxygen, due to a reduction or lack of inspired
  oxygen. ($PaO_2 < 8$ kPa)

Type 2 respiratory failure: $PaO_2 < 8$ kPa and $PaCO_2 > 6$ kPa.
Hypoxaemia (as detailed above) + hypercapnia (increased arterial carbon dioxide),
  due to increased airways resistance and reduced lung compliance. ($PaO_2 < 8$ kPa
  and $PaCO_2 > 6$ kPa)

---

failure (Table 7.4). Type 2 respiratory failure is when there is an insufficient arterial level of oxygen and a raised level of arterial carbon dioxide known as hypercapnia (Table 7.4). The effectiveness of gaseous exchange can be measured by examining the arterial blood gas (ABG) which measures the arterial level of oxygen (PaO_2) and of carbon dioxide ($PaCO_2$). Blood taken from an artery (normally radial artery) is machine tested to identify the PaO_2 and the $PaCO_2$.

Abnormal arterial blood readings can provide an indication of the degree of respiratory failure the patient is experiencing and how much the body is compensating for the respiratory failure.

Chronic Obstructive Pulmonary Disease

COPD is defined as a slowly progressive disorder characterised by irreversible airflow obstruction that does not change markedly over several months (NICE, 2010). The airway obstruction may be as a result of one or more different disease processes, but results in a loss of normal airway functioning and ineffective gas exchange at the alveoli–capillary interface. The three main diseases that contribute to loss of airflow are chronic bronchitis, emphysema and chronic asthma.

Chronic Bronchitis

Chronic bronchitis is characterised by inflammation and swelling of the lining of the airways leading to airway narrowing and obstruction, airflow reduction and a consequent fall in alveolar ventilation. Pathological changes include hypertrophy of the mucus-secreting glands of the bronchi and an increase in the number of mucus-secreting goblet cells. Inflammation and excess mucus secretion can lead to both airway obstruction and increased likelihood of bacterial infections (Bourke and Burns, 2011). Smoking, particularly the number of cigarettes smoked per day, is a major factor in the development of chronic bronchitis (Chitkara et al., 2012). Climate,

air pollution, socio-economic status and employment have also been implicated. Chronic bronchitis usually is defined clinically as a daily chronic
cough with the production of mucus for at least three months of the year
and for two years in a row (Bourke and Burns, 2011). Chronic bronchitis and
emphysema coexist in many individuals.

Emphysema

Emphysema is defined pathologically as dilatation, permanent enlargement
and destruction of the alveoli. The destruction of the alveolar walls reduces
the elasticity of the lung leading to expiratory airflow limitation and therefore air becomes trapped during expiration. This is directly due to the loss of
elastic recoil within the alveoli, and the trapped air leads to reduced alveolar
space and therefore less oxygen is available for gas transfer (Marieb, 2015).
Further, as a result of the destruction of the alveoli walls, less surface area is
available for gas transfer. Alpha1-antitrypsin deficiency has been associated
with the development of emphysema at a young adult age. Not all individuals born with the deficiency develop the disease (Bourke and Burns 2011).
Cigarette smoking is largely implicated in disease development and progression (Russell et al., 2012).

Chronic Asthma

Asthma is a disease of the airways which results in inflammation of the
airways and a constriction of the muscles surrounding the airways (bronchospasm). Asthma is largely associated with atopy and allergy to common
allergens such as house mites, dust and air pollutants (Bourke and Burns
2011). Airway bronchospasm is reversible by the use of inhaled bronchodilators such as Salbutamol®. In patients with long-standing, poorly controlled
asthma, inflammation can lead to chronic scarring and a reduction in airway diameter, lack of airway reversibility and increasing airway resistance.

Clinical Signs

Although the above disease processes are distinct from each other, COPD is
an amalgamation of different characteristics and shows variation in disease
presentation. Table 7.5 offers a summary of the possible various signs of a
person presenting with COPD.

As a direct result of the physiological changes and effort to achieve alveolar ventilation, the respiratory muscles become weakened by over-inflation
and increased airway resistance. The patient experiencing dyspnoea (difficulty in breathing) uses their rib cage muscles and accessory muscles

Table 7.5　Presenting clinical signs of COPD

Mucus hypersecretion	Airway cell changes resulting in an increased number of goblet cells of the bronchial submucosal glands directly as a result of an irritation.
Ciliary dysfunction	Airway cell changes resulting in an increase in the size and abnormal functioning of the mucociliary escalator – results in a difficulty in expectorating sputum.
Airflow limitation	Loss of bronchial wall and lung elasticity leads to an increase in airway resistance – leading to reduction in force of expiration.
Hyperinflation	With a loss of lung elastic recoil – air becomes trapped within the lungs.

Source: Adapted from Albert et al. (2008)

(sternocleidomastoids) even during quiet respiration. The British Thoracic Society (BTS) and Primary Care Respiratory Society (PCRS-UK, 2012) published the IMPRESS algorithm to give guidance to health professionals on assessment, diagnosis and management of breathlessness. The document also aims to promote best practice and provide clinical leadership in managing patients with COPD. During exercise or, for some patients who struggle for breath, with limited movement the use of accessory muscles to assist breathing becomes even more exaggerated.

Common Clinical Features of COPD

As the disease progresses, changes in pulmonary function will become more evident and an increasing awareness of dyspnoea and sputum production signals the person to seek a consultation with a medical practitioner as in Arthur's case (Kvangarsnes et al., 2013). A diagnosis of COPD should be considered in patients over the age of 35 years who have a risk factor (generally smoking but occupation could be noted) and who present with exertional dyspnoea, chronic cough and regular sputum production.

Breathlessness is a subjective experience for the person and an objective scale can be invaluable in providing an objective assessment of the subjective experience. The MRC dyspnoea scale developed by Fletcher et al. (1959) but still in common use (Russell et al., 2012) may be used to determine the severity of dyspnoea experienced.

It is important that, when reaching a diagnosis of COPD, other respiratory disorders have been considered and excluded (Table 7.6). The most common similar presentation (airway resistance resulting in reduced airflow) is with patients who have asthma. By giving appropriate (inhaled) medication to

Table 7.6 Distinguishing clinical features of COPD and asthma

	COPD	*Asthma*
Current or ex-smoker	Nearly all	Possibly
Symptoms in people under 35 years of age	Uncommon	Common
Chronic productive cough	Common	Uncommon
Breathlessness	Persistent and progressive	Variable
Response to therapy	Partial and incomplete	Good
Nocturnal waking	Uncommon	Common

the patient with asthma, the obstruction within the airways can be reduced by vaso-dilating the airways. Therefore, in asthma airway constriction is reversible. With COPD there is no such reversibility and hence there is decreased alveolar ventilation, the airways are fixed and the airway diameter does not respond to inhaled bronchodilator medication (NICE, 2010).

Specific Assessment and Diagnosis of COPD

The importance of a correct and early diagnosis of COPD cannot be emphasised enough as this will lead to appropriate management (Global Initiative for Chronic Obstructive Lung Disease (GOLD), 2014). Although some debate has emerged about under- or over-diagnosis of COPD, one key measurement supports its diagnosis – spirometry provides an objective measure of the force and volume of expiration. A full respiratory assessment to accompany the spirometry results includes:

1. Assessment of respiratory symptoms – shortness of breath, wheeze, cough and sputum production (consistency, frequency, microscopy culture and sensitivity, cytology).
2. Detailed history of family respiratory problems, smoking patterns, allergies and occupation.
3. Physical assessment of the chest – palpation, percussion and auscultation and noting finger clubbing (bulbous swelling of the soft tissue at the distal end of the fingers) and cyanosis (blue colouration of the skin most noticeable at the peripheries, lips and ears).
4. Assessment of chest X-ray, biochemistry, haematology results.

Spirometry investigation is the most useful in determining the severity of airway obstruction as it measures the volume of air expelled from the lungs

Table 7.7   Spirometry definitions

FEV1 (Forced expired volume in one second): The amount of breath expired in one second following maximal inspiration.

FVC (Forced vital capacity): The amount of forceful breath expired following maximal inspiration.

---

after a maximal inspiration breath. The recording of the forced expiratory volume in one second (FEV1) and forced vital capacity (FVC) give an indication of the degree of airway obstruction (see Table 7.7). The patient recordings obtained are compared to predicted normal values for the patient's height, age and sex. Comparison of FEV1 and FVC with normal predicted values will give an objective measure of the presence of airway obstruction and its degree (Russell et al., 2012).

Airway obstruction refers to a disturbance of the normal physiology indicated by a reduced peak expiratory flow, forced expiratory volume in one second (FEV1) and FEV1/vital capacity (VC) ratio, such that the FEV1 is less than the predicted 80 per cent. The severity of COPD is measured as a percentage as indicated below (Table 7.8).

NICE (2010) recommends post-bronchodilator spirometry to confirm diagnosis of COPD and to assess the severity of the airflow observation the FEV1 reduction from normal should be noted: in patients with mild and moderate airflow obstruction yearly assessment with spirometry, and for severe airflow obstruction twice yearly assessment to determine, monitor and manage disease progression.

Management and Maintenance of Stable COPD

There is strong evidence that COPD is aggravated by air pollution and by dusty occupations (Bourke and Burns, 2011) but the dominant cause

Table 7.8   Severity of airflow obstruction

Severity:	*FEV1 as a % (of predicted FEV1)*
Mild:	> 80%
Moderate:	50–79%
Severe:	30–49%
Very severe:	< 30%

Source: GOLD, 2014

of COPD is cigarette smoking. In stable COPD, the management focus for the health professional is to encourage the patient to stop smoking. The sequence of events in respiratory dysfunction is markedly associated with the duration of smoking, depth of inhalation and the number of cigarettes smoked. Arthur gave up smoking 12 months ago and by doing so may have slowed his rate of airway obstruction.

It is important to prevent frequent exacerbations of COPD; this can be achieved by encouraging the patient to be an active participant in a self-management plan (British Lung Foundation (BLF), 2010). This will detect early signs of deterioration and enable Arthur to maximise the bronchodilator therapy and to commence a dose of oral steroids if symptoms persist (under the guidance of the self-management plan).

Bronchodilators have been used as the principal aspect of medical management. Although these drugs do not significantly improve FEV1, by causing airway dilatation bronchodilators help reduce airway trapping and improve the efficiency of respiratory movements and reduce symptoms of dyspnoea on exertion. To obtain maximum control over the symptoms inhaled medications are essential in the maintenance of respiratory health, and the patient should be assessed in their concordance with their inhaler therapy (NICE, 2010).

Arthur was prescribed short-acting inhaled B2-agonists (SABA) (Salbutamol®) which have a direct effect on the bronchial smooth muscle causing bronchodilation. Although there is no reversibility to airflow obstruction in COPD, short-acting inhaled B2-agonists (SABA) appear to reduce hyperinflation and relieve dyspnoea. If symptoms persist following use of short-acting

---

The Case Scenario: aeCOPD

Arthur had been relatively well until two days ago when he noticed increasing dyspnoea on climbing the stairs. Although he normally had a cough he was aware that he was coughing more often and producing larger amounts of sputum. This morning when he awoke he found his sputum colour had changed to a yellow/green thick consistency and he was finding it difficult to expectorate. He contacted the GP who, during a home visit, found Arthur's condition to have deteriorated since he had seen him previously and Arthur was mildly disorientated in time and place. The GP recorded the following signs:

Respiratory rate 22 breaths per minute
Oxygen saturation 87 per cent on air
Heart rate 102 beats/min
Temperature 38.4 °C

The Case Scenario *Continued*

On the basis of the initial home assessment the GP admits Arthur to the hospital for further assessment.

Consider the following:

1. Describe the common signs of a patient presenting with aeCOPD.
2. Explore the possible causes of the exacerbation.
3. Describe Arthur's immediate assessment priorities and initial investigations in an acute exacerbation.

drugs in stable COPD (NICE 2010), long-acting bronchodilators (LABA) may be used, though this had not yet been so in Arthur's case. These should be discontinued after four weeks if the patient has not experienced benefit from these.

Assessment and Reaching a Diagnosis

The aim of assessment in the home or in the hospital is:

- to provide baseline data from which future observations undertaken can be assessed
- to establish a detailed measure of the success of management
- to evaluate a rationale for the change in management.

Most patients with aeCOPD can be managed at home (NICE, 2010). However, a sudden deterioration in condition or rapid onset of symptoms may need hospital treatment. Arthur's condition is of concern because excessive dyspnoea has confined him to bed; symptom onset was rapid; he shows signs of mild confusion. As Arthur has not experienced this level of dyspnoea and sputum production before and is likely to be anxious and frightened, the GP refers Arthur to the A&E for detailed assessment using the ABCDE approach.

For the purpose of clarity, the observations are discussed separately here. However, in the clinical setting observations would be taken together, and trends and differences would be noted and reported. In mild exacerbations, airflow limitation is frequently unchanged or only slightly increased and could be effectively managed within the primary care setting. Severe exacerbations are associated with a worsening of pulmonary gas exchange because of the inequality between ventilation and perfusion which can be exacerbated by respiratory muscle fatigue. These symptoms should be assessed with other aspects of the disease process such as disease frequency and previous other aeCOPD episodes.

Pathophysiological Changes from COPD to aeCOPD

An exacerbation of COPD can be defined as a worsening of symptoms from an individual's usual stable state (NICE, 2010). In Arthur's case there was evidence of increasing breathlessness and sputum production associated with greater airway inflammation, airflow limitation, mucus hyper-secretion, hyperinflation and impaired ciliary clearance. This means that there is a further increase in airway resistance resulting in reduced gaseous exchange at the alveolar–capillary interface. An inflammatory response may be triggered by a range of factors such as bacterial or viral infection or environmental pollutants. The increased inflammatory response seen with aeCOPD is associated with increased white blood cell activity and the release of neutrophils and eosinophils (Marieb, 2015). Airway inflammation, oedema, mucus hyper-secretion and bronchial vasoconstriction cause a decrease in ventilation and hypoxic vasoconstriction of the pulmonary arterioles which impairs perfusion and leads to an increased ventilation/perfusion mismatch.

The Importance of Reassessment

There is no specific method of assessment of exacerbation severity. Prompt reassessment of reported symptoms is vital for early diagnosis and more intensive treatment of the exacerbation. Patients may experience additional symptoms such as wheeze, chest tightness and increasing fatigue due to the effort of breathing (NICE, 2010).

Airway

Arthur is currently fully conscious and able to maintain his own airway. However, the risk of respiratory arrest must be considered and therefore close continual observation of airway patency should be employed and basic life support must be instigated if airway maintenance deteriorates further (see Chapter 1).

Breathing

Breathing is often the first vital sign to alter in a patient with a deteriorating condition and the potential for respiratory failure. Arthur is described as dyspnoeic which is a sign that should prompt a more detailed assessment

Table 7.9 Arthur's observations

Observations	At home by the GP	On admission to A&E	One hour following admission	One hour following commencement on NIV (non-invasive ventilation)
Temperature (°C)	38.4	39	39.2	39.0
Pulse (beats/min)	102	100	108	98
Respiration (rate/min)	22	24	24	18
SpO_2 (%)	87% (on air)	87% (on air)	86% (on 28% via Venturi mask 4 litres/min)	92% (on entrained air via NIV)
Blood gases				
PaO_2 (normal 11.0–13.0 kPa)		8.2	8.0	10.2
$PaCO_2$ (normal 4.8–6.0 kPa)		6.4	7.4	6.9
pH (normal 7.35–7.45)		7.37	7.34	7.41

of breathing. Respiratory rate, regularity, depth, noise and effort should be observed for one minute and should be repeated every 30 minutes to assess for deterioration and to indicate trend. Normal breathing should be 10 to 18 breaths per minute, noiseless and effortless. Arthur's respiratory rate was initially 22 which can be described as tachypnoea (respiratory rate greater than 18).

Tachypnoea is an early sign of respiratory distress and a deteriorating clinical condition that can be used as an objective measure of trend. Decreased arterial oxygen levels and increased carbon dioxide are detected by arterial sensory chemoreceptors which stimulate the respiratory centre housed within the medulla oblongata to increase stimulation of the intercostal and diaphragmatic muscles which lead to an increase in respiratory rate (Marieb 2015). Rapid breathing may be shallow and an audible wheeze may be heard on auscultation. Wheezing occurs when air is forced through constricted airways. In Arthur's case increased resistance against inspiration caused by obstruction or excess bronchoconstriction may require the use of accessory muscles such as the sternocleidomastoid and scalene muscles for ventilation. Also forced expiration against increased airway resistance may require the additional force of accessory muscles of the abdominal wall to help push the diaphragm upwards to collapse the lungs.

The excessive and deliberate use of accessory muscles signals aeCOPD. Patients who experience difficulty breathing will appear restless and have difficulty finding a comfortable position. Posture is therefore very important and whilst the optimum position to allow maximum air entry would be upright, Arthur may find stability in leaning forward supported by an appropriately positioned table at chest height. Reassurance is essential in gaining the patient's cooperation at a time of respiratory distress. The feeling of dyspnoea and not being able to gain enough breath makes patients panic and feel very anxious. A quiet controlled environment where patients receive reassurance and informed information about immediate management plans and care delivery is essential.

Changes in skin colour may indicate respiratory problems. The consequent fall in available oxygen and rise in carbon dioxide levels may cause skin cyanosis. Initially peripheral cyanosis may be evident as a bluish tinge of the nail beds. Central cyanosis is a sign of worsening respiratory distress and may be visualised as a bluish tinge of the lips, oral mucosa and ears. This is normally detected when the SpO_2 falls below 87 per cent and is considered a late sign of respiratory problems.

The effectiveness of oxygen delivery across the alveolar–capillary divide can be measured using continuous non-invasive O_2 saturation (SpO_2) monitoring via a pulse oximeter. SpO_2 provides information regarding the oxygen level within the peripheral circulation (which can be affected by poor perfusion – see Chapter 1). Airflow limitation and mucus hyper-secretion within the larger airways prevents sufficient O_2 delivery at the alveolar–capillary interface leading to a reduced SpO_2. On admission Arthur's SpO_2 is 87 per cent on air which is below the recommended 88 to 92 per cent saturation level (NICE, 2010) and therefore requires intervention with (titrated) oxygen therapy. An increased concentration of oxygen delivery should result in an improvement in oxygen saturation. Oximetry can reduce the need for invasive ABG analysis. However, it is not the most reliable method of oxygen saturation monitoring, particularly when the patient is severely ill and has poor perfusion. ABG analysis will provide a more detailed evaluation of alveolar ventilation. For respiratory patients the important ABG measures to note are the PaO_2, $PaCO_2$ and pH (Table 7.3). The more serious the interruption of gaseous exchange at the alveolar–capillary interface, the further from normal will be the blood gas measurement. Arthur's initial PaO_2 was low at 8.2 kPa and his $PaCO_2$ was slightly raised at 6.4 kPa. PaO_2 falls reciprocally with an increase in $PaCO_2$ when there is alveolar under-ventilation (Woodrow 2012). Arthur is experiencing a trend towards type 2 respiratory failure (Table 7.4).

Cell metabolism relies upon a normal blood pH value of pH 7.4. (pH is a measurement of the hydrogen (H+) ion concentration in the blood.) A pH <7.35 indicates acidosis and >7.45 indicates alkalosis. The pH is affected by many parameters including the concentration of CO_2 within the blood. An increased $PaCO_2$ can lead to increased blood acidity recognised as a fall in pH below 7.35. Arthur's arterial blood results indicate an altered pH from 7.4 to 7.37 and a drift towards respiratory acidosis (Woodrow, 2012). Generalised hypoxia and respiratory acidosis leads to insufficient delivery of oxygen to all the organs and tissues. Cerebral hypoxia may be displayed in a range of ways from mild disorientation in time and place as in Arthur's case to confusion or loss of consciousness in severe cases. At this stage, although conversation will be difficult for Arthur, regular assessment of time and place should be sufficient. However more formal neurological assessment such as the Glasgow Coma Scale (GCS) (see Chapter 4) should be commenced should his consciousness levels begin to deteriorate.

As a direct result of the increase in inflammation and mucus production within the airway, Arthur has a productive cough and is expectorating copious amounts of sputum. It is important to notice any change in colour or consistency which the patient may report. Colour changes in sputum are important but do not necessarily indicate the level or degree of infection (Bourke and Burns 2011). A sputum pot, tissues and mouthwash should be provided in order to collect sputum carefully and safely and enable the collection of a specimen for analysis of microscopy, culture and sensitivity (MC&S) which will be necessary to detect any bacterial presence and assess the sensitivity and resistance to antibiotic therapy. Arthur's raised temperature of 38.4 °C above normal (37–37.4 °C) indicates pyrexia and provides further evidence of an active infection and inflammation.

Circulation

Arthur's heart rate of 102 beats per minute may be abnormally raised (tachycardia) for a number of reasons, not least as a result of increased sympathetic nervous system activity mediated by feelings of panic and anxiety associated with dyspnoea. It may also indicate one of the body's compensatory mechanisms to circulate oxygenated blood around the body more quickly in response to a low PaO_2 concentration sensed by chemoreceptors situated within the peripheral arterial walls (Marieb, 2015). Although a useful mechanism, the increased myocardial workload will demand an increase in oxygen delivery diverting some of the circulating oxygen away from other organs and tissues and further exacerbating signs of peripheral hypoperfusion. Arthur's blood pressure should be measured at admission and, if within normal parameters, repeated every four hours. A blood pressure of more than 140 mmHg systolic and 90 mmHg diastolic may be associated with stress and anxiety or may indicate underlying hypertension which would require further specific investigation and treatment. A low blood pressure below 100 mmHg systolic may indicate underlying cardiac disease which again should prompt more specific investigation.

Table 7.10 displays a range of routine venous blood sampling tests which Arthur may undergo to provide vital information about the effects of hypoxia on other major organs.

It is important to establish or exclude other potential causes of respiratory distress such as pulmonary embolism (PE), pneumonia, pneumothorax, lung cancer, aspiration or tuberculosis (NICE, 2010). Although the FEV1 was instrumental in an accurate diagnosis of COPD, there is no place for such a measure in an acute exacerbation. A chest X-ray, detailed clinical examination of the respiratory system including palpation, percussion and auscultation with a stethoscope and full secondary assessment (Table 7.11) are useful in determining other pathologies.

Table 7.10   Routine venous blood sampling

1. Full blood count (FBC) – to identify low Hb (anaemia), raised WBC (infection).
2. C-reactive protein (CRP) – when raised suggests active infection.
3. Clotting screen – if indicated by current medication, e.g. warfarin.
4. Urea and electrolytes (U&E) – determines electrolyte balance and renal function.
5. Capillary blood glucose if high or low glucose is suspected, e.g. in a diabetic patient.
6. Liver function tests (LFT) – to establish baseline level function prior to statin therapy which may alter liver function.

Table 7.11   Secondary assessment

1. Past medical history (PMH) – respiratory and systemic.
2. Family history (FH) and social history (SH).
3. Systemic enquiry – general, gastric, urinary, central nervous systems.
4. Evaluation of triggers and risk factors.
5. Drug history – prescribed, over the counter and recreational.
6. Full clinical examination – peripheral pulses, jugular venous pressure (JVP), heart and lung sounds, systemic examination.

The Case Scenario: Medical Management and Care Issues

Arthur's past medical history and symptom presentation reflect aeCOPD. Arthur is commenced on 28 per cent oxygen therapy via a venturi mask, nebulised bronchodilator therapy at four-hourly intervals, bed rest and regular observation of respiratory status including hourly ABGs commenced. The hourly trend following admission in the ABGs reveals a deterioration in PaO_2, $PaCO_2$ and pH levels despite 28 per cent oxygen. The pulse and respiratory rate have increased in compensatory response to worsening respiratory acidosis, decreasing oxygen levels and increasing carbon dioxide levels. A decision to commence Arthur on NIV was made.

Consider the following

1. What was the rationale for the change in pharmacological medication to treat aeCOPD?
2. Assess the role of oxygen therapy in aeCOPD management.
3. Explore the role of NIV in Arthur's management.
4. Identify the key methods employed to prevent further exacerbations.

Medical Management Strategies and Care Issues

The aims of management of a patient with aeCOPD are to:

1. correct hypoxaemia
2. relieve airway obstruction
3. treat the presenting infection
4. manage any co-morbidities.

Early and effective management to prevent the frequency of aeCOPD can also prevent worsening of symptoms (Miravitlles, 2010).

Oxygen therapy

Controlled oxygen therapy plays an important role in optimising the delivery of oxygen to the tissues where hypoxaemia (low PaO_2) has been detected by blood gas analysis to alleviate the symptoms of dyspnoea. Hypoxaemia is a result of alveolar hypoventilation (including ventilation/perfusion mismatch) caused by airway obstruction and the increase in mucus production. Oxygen therapy is the obvious first-line treatment for Arthur. The prescribed dosage must be carefully considered to reflect his underlying respiratory disease and reflect individualised oxygen saturation target range (NICE, 2010).

Normally the respiratory stimulus to breathe, i.e. the 'respiratory drive' is a detected rise in arterial carbon dioxide levels ($PaCO_2$) but in a few patients with long-standing respiratory disease such as COPD the respiratory centre becomes desensitised to high CO_2 levels and so a low PaO_2 becomes the 'respiratory drive'. Therefore, high levels of administered oxygen therapy to an individual with COPD may depress or 'switch off' the natural respiratory drive and lead to respiratory failure. These patients are required to carry an 'alert' card, identifying the need to be prescribed low levels of oxygen.

The aim of oxygen therapy in Arthur's case is to:

1. increase the level of oxygen at the alveolar–capillary interface;
2. maintain oxygen saturations at about 90 per cent (rather than aiming for a normal SpO_2 of 99 to 100 per cent);
3. increase the arterial oxygen level without risking further carbon dioxide retention (increase in $PaCO_2$) and respiratory acidosis.

Oxygen should be administered in a controlled way (titrated) and reflect the deviation of oxygen saturation and ABGs from the expected normal (NICE, 2010). The interpretation of the oxygen saturations and ABG analysis will give an indication of the percentage of oxygen that should be given. The most effective (and accurate) method of delivery of oxygen is via a venturi mask where controlled low inspired oxygen concentrations of 24 per cent at 2–4/L minute to 28 per cent at 4/L minute (NICE, 2010). Some patients may prefer to have the oxygen delivered via nasal cannula though it can be difficult to assess the percentage of oxygen the patient is receiving, especially as they may breathe through their mouth. ABG analysis gives the most accurate picture of the effectiveness of gaseous exchange when receiving oxygen therapy. After one hour of receiving 28 per cent oxygen Arthur's oxygen saturations had decreased from 87 to 86 per cent. A worsening in respiratory failure was evidenced by a decreasing pH (respiratory acidosis) and increasing carbon dioxide. This demonstrates the sensitivity to increased $PaCO_2$ is lost and therefore hypoxaemia, not hypercapnia, is the chief respiratory stimulant. In Arthur's case the oxygen therapy appears to be reducing respiratory drive.

Normally a probe positioned on the patient's finger will provide information about the degree of oxygen saturation. Failure to correct the oxygen saturations (SpO_2) to greater than 90 per cent with an oxygen flow rate of 40 per cent may suggest the presence of additional pathophysiology that needs to be investigated. Whilst objective measurements give a good indication of the success of the oxygen therapy, monitoring Arthur's level

Figure 7.2   Non-invasive ventilation (NIV) mask
Copyright E. S. Cleave. Reproduced with permission.

of confusion and consciousness is an important indicator of worsening hypoxaemia. If, during adequate oxygenation (oxygen saturations above 90 per cent), there is a fall in pH or a rise in $PaCO_2$, this indicates worsening respiratory failure and the patient requires ventilation support (NIV or intermittent positive pressure ventilation (IPPV)).

NIV has become pivotal in the management of all patients with aeCOPD especially when the use of optimal medical therapy appears to show no improvement following initial management with bronchodilators, oxygen therapy, corticosteroids and antibiotics (NICE, 2010). An ABG pH of 7.35 or less is an indication that the patient requires NIV. NIV can reduce the intubation rate and mortality in patients presenting with aeCOPD and should be considered as a treatment option within the first 60 minutes of arrival in hospital (Popat and Jones, 2012).

NIV assists breathing by:

- augmenting tidal volume;
- decreasing the work of breathing by initiating a slower, deeper breath reflecting a more normal physiological pattern of breathing; this is achieved where inspiration and expiration parameters on the NIV machine are independently set to reflect individualised breathing pattern (Royal College of Physicians, British Thoracic Society, Intensive Care Society, 2008).

The inspiratory phase improves alveolar ventilation and as a direct result of this:

- decreases carbon dioxide;
- decreases dyspnoea;
- ultimately, decreases the use of accessory muscles.

In the expiratory phase of breathing:

- NIV forces an extra breath of air into the lung to splint the alveoli open at the end of respiration, therefore increasing the time of respiration, and this in turn increases gas exchange, decreasing carbon dioxide and increasing oxygen. This ultimately improves the ventilation/perfusion mismatch.

Arthur continued to struggle with his breathing despite being compliant with the optimum management offered. A repeat ABG analysis after one hour of management revealed a worsening of respiratory failure (Table 7.9) and therefore the decision was made to initiate NIV (Royal College of Physicians, British Thoracic Society, Intensive Care Society, 2008). NIV involves positioning a very tight-fitting mask over the mouth and/or nose to aid assisted ventilation (Figure 7.2). However, in addition to the underlying dyspnoea, the forced ventilation during expiration and the tight-fitting mask can cause feelings of claustrophobia, sweating and facial sores and anxiety, and may limit patient compliance with the device. Sensitive management is essential to promote compliance at this critical time. Initially allowing the patient to hold the mask without strap fixing may decrease the anxiety and the patient may tolerate the air delivery from the machine more readily. The selection of low initial inspiratory and expiratory pressures allows the patient to become used to the forced inspiration and expiration prior to being increased to achieve maximum NIV therapy. Simple explanation, reassurance, visibility, approachability and easy methods of communication with nurses and family may help Arthur to learn to cope with and tolerate his treatment. For any patient commenced on NIV, observations should be monitored every 30 minutes during the first four hours (see Table 7.12).

Patient compliance with the treatment is essential in determining a good outcome linked with the patient's level of consciousness and tolerance of the NIV, especially the fitting of the face mask to ensure maximum therapy.

During NIV therapy the following should be considered:

- Adequate fluid management, nutrition and communication should be planned, implemented and evaluated within the care delivery plans.

Table 7.12   NIV observations

Initial NIV observations include:

Respiratory rate
Heart rate
Level of consciousness
Chest wall movement
Ventilator synchrony

● Bed rest also necessitates careful planning of toilet and hygiene needs, especially mouth and eye care, pressure area care including facial points beneath the NIV mask and passive limb exercises to avoid deep vein thrombosis.

● Hourly ABG analysis via several arterial stab wounds will require localised manual pressure to achieve stasis and regular observation of the sites for bleeding, oozing or signs of infection such as redness and soreness. ABG analysis gives an indication as to the improvement of alveolar ventilation.

Arthur's ABGs are assessed one hour after commencing NIV (Table 7.9). The pH has increased from 7.34 to 7.41 indicating a lessening of respiratory acidosis, the arterial level of oxygen has increased from 8.0 kPa to 10.2 kPa and the arterial level of carbon dioxide has decreased from 7.4 kPa to 6.9 kPa. These results indicate a positive response to prescribed treatment.

For some patients NIV is not successful in correcting the arterial oxygen and carbon dioxide levels and the decision to proceed to full intubation and transfer to intensive care must be considered (NICE, 2010). This can be a difficult decision and the beliefs, opinions and thoughts of the patient and family must be carefully considered by the health professionals to ensure the patient is fully informed of the possible treatment options available.

As part of the management plan with NIV, inhaled bronchodilators, corticosteroids and antibiotics are seen as essential in managing aeCOPD.

Inhaled Bronchodilators: Nebulisers

Increased dyspnoea is a result of airway responsiveness to the airflow limitation and increased mucus production. The first line of management is to increase the dose and regularity of short-acting bronchodilators, where the aim is to reduce the symptoms of dyspnoea and improve airflow obstruction. Bronchodilators act to dilate the bronchioles in the lung by working on the smooth muscle cells. This results in widening the airways and should therefore improve the exchange of gases. Extensive research has revealed that bronchodilators do not produce significant improvements in FEV1, but appear to work by reducing airway smooth muscle tone, increasing airway calibre and reducing dynamic hyperinflation. Salbutamol® is the most common bronchodilator drug used in patients with aeCOPD at 2.5 to 5mg 3–4 times daily, or more frequently if symptoms dictate. Once the drug is inhaled it works quickly and the effects last up to six hours (Hennefer, 2009). This drug is normally prescribed in stable COPD but increasing the frequency of dose and strength can positively decrease any dyspnoea experienced. One potential side effect of Salbutamol® medication is tachycardia. Arthur should be made aware of this and the need to report symptoms such as palpitations as soon as possible. Four-hourly recording of heart rate should also detect signs of increasing tachycardia. Arthur was prescribed Salbutamol® 100 microgrammes (mcg) – 200 microgrammes (mcg) via a multi-dose inhaler (MDI) and was taking the drug via that route prior to being visited by the GP. As he had not experienced relief from this method of administration, he had been given the bronchodilator by nebuliser. Arthur's excess respiratory effort, often associated with a peripheral hand tremor, may have interfered with his ability to hold and use the device MDI effectively. NICE (2010) identify there is no real benefit of nebuliser over MDI but anecdotally some patients feel relief from getting the bronchodilators this way. The bronchodilator should be delivered on compressed air (NICE, 2010) rather than oxygen due to the potential effect of high alveolar oxygen tensions on ventilation/perfusion and increasing $PaCO_2$.

Ipratropium bromide (Atrovent®) (250–500mcg 3–4 times daily) is normally prescribed where the alveoli are enlarged and inflexible. The mode of action of Atrovent® differs from Salbutamol® but has the same bronchodilator effect though it takes longer to achieve the same effect. It causes smooth muscles to relax by blocking the nerve impulses which as part of the disease process are causing bronchoconstriction. The role of the nurse during oxygen/nebuliser therapy is to assist Arthur in gaining maximum effect from the oxygen/nebulised drugs by ensuring correct use of the delivery chamber and assisting him to sit in an upright position to maximise lung expansion. Theophylline® can be used as an adjunct to the management of aeCOPD, by increasing respiratory drive if there is an inadequate response to nebulised bronchodilators (NICE, 2010). Prior to Theophylline® use, care must be taken to ensure that Arthur is not taking the drug as part of routine management, as it is easy to exceed the therapeutic range and induce side effects such as nausea and cardiac arrhythmias.

Systemic Corticosteroids

Corticosteroids are given to relieve the symptoms of inflammation, reduce the length of the exacerbation and improve symptoms although the benefit of corticosteroids has remained contentious (Miravitlles, 2010). The medication is given by the oral route as opposed to the inhaled route. Corticosteroids improve lung function and reduce the risk of treatment failure (Greenstone 2010). Arthur was commenced on a dose of 30 mg of Prednisolone® for seven days as longer courses have not been found to be beneficial and increase the risk of side effects (NICE, 2010).

Antibiotics

Antibiotics are commonly prescribed for episodes of purulent sputum (NICE, 2010). The bacteria that have been isolated during exacerbations are generally sensitive to most broad-spectrum antibiotics. There has been some controversy about whether antibiotics have benefit in an exacerbation but treatment is usually based on patient symptoms and the purulence of the sputum. Little data exists on the optimum duration of the therapy. As Arthur is experiencing an increased sensation of breathlessness, increased sputum production and an observed colour change to the sputum, antibiotics have been prescribed. The antibiotic chosen may be dictated by antibiotic policies and local resistance patterns but it is generally agreed that the drug of choice (Trimethoprim®, Doxycycline®, Erythromycin®) will cover common pathogens such as *Haemophilus influenzae, Moraxella catarrhalis* and *Streptococcus pneumoniae* (Bourke and Burns, 2011). It is not considered necessary to take sputum samples prior to initiating antibiotics except where patients do not appear to be responding to treatment or to check whether the correct antibiotic has been prescribed. Safety of drug prescribing should be detailed regarding previous administration of antibiotics or to determine any drug allergies or details of drugs that may interact. It should also be noted that aeCOPDs are not always caused by infection, as air pollutants and adverse weather conditions may lead to an exacerbation.

Preventing Exacerbations

A positive partnership between the patient and the GP will enable the patient to recognise the symptoms of deterioration (Russell et al., 2012). Early treatment can be initiated and prevent further deterioration of the patient's lung function. Arthur and his GP had worked together to develop a self-management plan and this was used successfully when he began to experience symptoms away from his daily norms. Zwerink et al. (2014) demonstrated that self-management plans reduce hospital admissions and carry a cost saving in economic terms with patients reporting an improved quality of life (less shortness of breath) following their introduction to self-management plans.

Other strategies that may prevent the patient from needing hospital admission include:

1. Annual influenza vaccinations and pneumococcal vaccinations.
2. Education and health promotion related to smoking.

If patients with diagnosed COPD continue to experience exacerbations then the GP may consider the following:

1. Inhaled steroids with patients who are experiencing more than two aeCOPDs in a 12-month period and if the FEV1 is <50 per cent predicted.
2. Using combined therapy of long-acting bronchodilator (NICE, 2010) and inhaled steroids.

Summary

COPD is a complex disease and annual review is suggested for patients experiencing mild symptoms in stable COPD. For patients with more severe disease, bi-annual review is recommended. aeCOPD can be successfully managed within primary care, but due to the severity of symptoms experienced the patient may require hospital admission. aeCOPDs present a burden both to the patient in terms of quality of life and in cost implications to the health service, but successful treatment of acute exacerbations can prevent further deterioration in the patient's lung function. Thorough assessment of a patient experiencing an acute exacerbation will inform the management to optimise treatment availability. A critical aspect of the management of the patient is to recognise the physical and psychological impact the 'stable' disease can have on the activities of daily living and the anxiety and fear that often accompanies an acute exacerbation.

Further Reading

Caress, A., K. Luker and K. Chalmer. 'Promoting the Health of People with Chronic Obstructive Pulmonary Disease: Patients' and Carers' Views', *Journal of Clinical Nursing*, **19** (3–4) (2010), 564–73.

Goodridge, D., W. Duggleby, J. Gjerve and D. Rennie. 'Caring for Critically Ill Patients with Advanced COPD at the End of Life: A Qualitative Study', *Intensive & Critical Care Nursing* **24** (2008), 162–70.

Simpson, E. and M. Jones. 'An Exploration of Self-Efficacy and Self-Management in COPD Patients', *British Journal of Nursing*. **22**(19) (2013), 1105–9.

Sorensen, D., K. Frederiksen, T. Grofte and K. Lomborg. 'Practical Wisdom: A Qualitative Study of the Care and Management of Non-invasive Ventilated Patients by Experienced Intensive Care Nurses', *Intensive & Critical Care Nursing*, **29** (2013), 174–81.

References

Albert R. K., S. G. Spiro and J. R. Jett. *Clinical Respiratory Medicine* (Philadelphia: Elsevier, 2008).

Bourke, S. J. and G. P. Burns. *Respiratory Medicine*, 8th edn (Chichester: Wiley-Blackwell, 2011).

British Lung Foundation. *Self Management Plans* (2010) [Online]. Available from: http://shop.blf.org.uk/products/copd-self-management-plan-hcp (accessed 1 May 2015).

British Thoracic Society and Primary Care Respiratory Society. 'IMPRESS' (2012) [Online]. Available from: www.impressresp.com (accessed 6 May 2015).

British Thoracic Society, Royal College of Physicians, Intensive Care Society. 'The Use of Non-invasive Ventilation in the Management of Patients with Chronic Obstructive Pulmonary Disease Admitted to Hospital with Acute Type II Respiratory Failure' (2008) [Online]. Available from: www.brit-thoracic.org.uk/guidelines-and-quality-standards/non-invasive-ventilation-(niv)/ (accessed 6 May 2015).

Chitkara, R. and J. R. Hurst. 'Chronic Obstructive Pulmonary Disease: Aetiology, Pathology, Physiology and Outcome', *Medicine*, **40**(5) (2012), 257–61.

Department of Health (DH). 'Chronic Obstructive Pulmonary Disease Scheme: Statistics' (2011a) [Online]. Available from: www.gov.uk/government/statistics/chronic-obstructive-pulmonary-disease (accessed 1 May 2015).

Department of Health (DH). *An Outcomes Strategy for Chronic Obstructive Pulmonary Disease (COPD) and Asthma in England* (2011b) [Online]. Available from www.dh.gov.uk/publications (accessed 1 May 2015).

Department of Health/Medical Directorate/Respiratory Team. *An Outcomes Strategy for COPD and Asthma: NHS Companion Document* (2012). www.dh.gov.uk/publications (accessed 1 May 2015).

Fletcher, C. M., P. C. Elmes and M. B. Fairbairn. 'The Significance of Respiratory Symptoms and the Diagnosis of Chronic Bronchitis in a Working Population', *British Medical Journal*, **2** (1959), 257–66.

Global Initiative for Chronic Obstructive Lung Disease (GOLD). *Global Strategy for the Diagnosis, Management, and Prevention of Chronic Obstructive Pulmonary Disease* (2014) [Online]. Available from: www.goldcopd.org/uploads/users/files/GOLD_Report_2014_Jan23.pdf (accessed 22 May, 2015).

Greenstone, M. 'Management of Acute Exacerbations of Chronic Obstructive Pulmonary Disease: The First 23 Hours', *Clinical Medicine*, **10**(1) (2010), 65–67.

Hennefer, D. and E. Lawson. 'Pharmacology – A Systems Approach: Respiratory System', *British Journal of Healthcare Assistants*, **3**(3) (2009), 148–51.

Kvangarsnes, M., H. Torheim, T. Hole and L. S. Ohlund. 'Narratives of Breathlessness in Chronic Obstructive Pulmonary Disease', *Journal of Clinical Nursing*, **22** (2013), 3062–70.

Marieb, E. N. *Essentials of Human Anatomy and Physiology*, 11th edn (Pearson, 2015).

Miravitlles, M. 'Prevention of Exacerbations of COPD with Pharmacotherapy. *European Respiratory Review*, **19**(116) (2010).

National Centre for Smoking Cessation and Training. 'Standard Treatment Programme: One-to-one Smoking Cessation Support' (2012) [Online]. Available from: www.ncsct.co.uk (accessed 22 May 2015).

National Chronic Obstructive Pulmonary Disease (COPD). *Audit Programme* (2013) [Online]. Available from: www.rcplondon.ac.uk/COPD (accessed 22 May, 2015).

National Institute for Health and Clinical Excellence (NICE). *Chronic Obstructive Pulmonary Disease: Management of Chronic Obstructive Pulmonary Disease in Adults in Primary and Secondary Care* (2010) [Online]. Available from: http://guidance.nice.org.uk/cg101/Guidance/pdf/English (accessed 1 June 2015).

Office for National Statistics 'Chronic Obstructive Pulmonary Disease' (2013) [Online]. Available from www.ons.gov.uk/ons/publications/re-reference-tables.html?edition=tcm%3A77-327590 (accessed 14 April 2015).

Popat, B. and A. T. Jones 'Invasive and Non-invasive Mechanical Ventilation', *Medicine*, **40**(6) (2012), 298–340.

Royal College of Physicians, British Thoracic Society, Intensive Care Society. 'Chronic Obstructive Pulmonary Disease: Non-invasive Ventilation with Bi-phasic Positive Airways Pressure in the Management of Patients with Acute Type 2 Respiratory Failure', *Concise Guidance to Good Practice Series, No 11* (London: RCP, 2008) [Online]. Available from: www.rcplondon.ac.uk/pubs/brochure.aspx?e=258 (accessed 14 April 2015).

Russell, R., J. Norcliffe and M. Bafadhel. 'Chronic Obstructive Pulmonary Disease: Management of Chronic Disease. *Medicine*, **40**(5) (2012), 262–6.

Woodrow, P. *Intensive Care Nursing*, 3rd edn (Abingdon: Routledge, 2012).

Zwerink, M., M. Brusse-Keizer, P. D. L. P. M. van der Valk, G. A. Zielhuis, E. M. Monninkhof, J. van der Palen, P. A. Frith, and T. Effing. Self management for patients with chronic obstructive pulmonary disease. *Cochrane Database of Systematic Reviews* 2014, Issue 3. Art. No.: CD002990. DOI: 10.1002/14651858.CD002990.pub3.

8

Acute Kidney Injury

Mark Bevan

Introduction

Acute kidney injury (AKI) is a term that has recently gained worldwide acceptance to describe the condition formally known as acute renal failure. AKI describes a condition ranging from mild but significant impairment to outright failure of the kidney, and is a serious life-threatening condition that has been poorly understood, documented and managed (NCEPOD, 2009). AKI is marked by a rapid but potentially reversible decline of kidney function, which results in retention of nitrogen-based waste products of metabolism such as urea and creatinine and in most cases a reduction in urine output (Clarkson et al., 2008). It is worth noting that AKI is not inevitable in acute or critical illness and in many cases is preventable, and while it is commonly seen in acute care wards it can also be found in the primary care environment (Hegarty et al., 2005). The ability to estimate the incidence of AKI has been limited until fairly recently when there have been attempts to provide a more realistic picture of the problem. Much of this limitation has been associated with a lack of standard definition which has caused much variance. For example, Feest et al. (1993) estimated the incidence to be 51 people per million population (pmp) but they use a creatinine level of 500 µmol/L (normal range 60 to 125 µmol/L: Provan and Krentz, 2002). In a Scottish study Khan et al. (1997) using a creatinine level of 300 µmol/L saw the incidence rise to 620 pmp, with the elderly presenting a significant risk. Where a lower creatinine level is used as a marker of AKI, unsurprisingly the incidence increases. Ali et al. (2007) found, using creatinine levels of $\geq$ 150 µmol/L for males and $\geq$ 130 µmol/L for females, an incidence of 1,811 pmp/year with a high incidence in patients (336 pmp/year) with underlying chronic kidney disease (CKD). An influential study undertaken by Chertow et al. (2005) examined the effects of AKI on 19,982 patients and found that even a modest elevation of serum creatinine

214

26.5–35.36 µmol/L led to a 70 per cent increase in risk for death compared to those who had little or no rise in creatinine. Chertow et al. (2005) also reported that those who developed AKI tended to be older and had a higher severity of illness, and that AKI incidence was higher in those with cardio-vascular disease, infectious diseases, endocrine and nutritional conditions, respiratory disease, genitourinary disease, injuries and poisoning. What this study demonstrated was that a small elevation in serum creatinine increases the risk of death and as such the incidence and impact of AKI has been significantly underestimated. What can be seen is an inverse relation-ship between lower levels of elevated creatinine threshold and the higher incidence of AKI. This means in reality that in previous years there has been under-reporting; the apparent increase in patients diagnosed with AKI reflects a change in acceptable diagnostic threshold with greater sensitivity (Case et al., 2013), rather than an actual increase in AKI.

The study by Chertow et al. heralded the development of a standardised definition as identified by the Acute Kidney Injury Network (AKIN) and now endorsed by many bodies such as the Renal Association (UK), National Institute for Health and Care Excellence (NICE) and the Kidney Disease Improving Global Outcomes (KDIGO), though not without controversy. According to NICE (2013) which echoes the AKIN (Mehta et al., 2007) cri-teria, AKI occurs when there is:

> a rise in serum creatinine of 26 micromol/l or greater within 48 hours; a 50% or greater rise in serum creatinine known or presumed to have occurred within the past 7 days; a fall in urine output to less than 0.5 ml/kg/hour for more than 6 hours in adults and more than 8 hours in children and young people and a 25% or greater fall in eGFR in children and young people within the past 7 days (NICE, 2013: 176).

For full AKI staging criteria see Table 8.1.

Standardisation of AKI criteria means that more consistent and mean-ingful information is forthcoming, providing a more accurate picture. Case et al. (2013) identified the incidence of AKI in intensive care (ICU) patients ranging from 20 to 50 per cent. Case et al. (2013) also reported AKI as a significant risk factor for death associated with a mortality of greater than 50 per cent. In relation to urology patients, Caddeo et al. (2013) reported 587 episodes of AKI in 410 patients which correspond to 6.7 per cent of the total hospitalised urology patients. They also reported that males were four times more likely to get AKI and the mean age was 73 years. One-third of the patients developed AKI during the course of their elective admission. Mortality rates were identified at 7.8 per cent with the majority of deaths being in non-elective patients and mortality increased with the severity of

Table 8.1 Criteria for diagnosis of acute kidney injury

AKI stage	Serum creatinine criteria	Urine output criteria
1	Increase in serum creatinine of 26 µmol/litre or more within 48 hours OR 1.5 to 2-fold increase from baseline	Less than 0.5 mL/kg/hour for more than 6 hours
2	Increase in serum creatinine to more than 2 to 3-fold from baseline	Less than 0.5 mL/kg/hour for more than 12 hours
3	Increase in serum creatinine to more than 3-fold from baseline OR Serum creatinine more than 354 µmol/litre with an acute increase of at least 44 µmol/litre	Less than 0.3 mL/kg/hour for 24 hours or anuria for 12 hours

Source: Adapted from Mehta et al. (2007)

AKI. A study of ten acute medical units in England and Scotland over two 24-hour periods highlighted the prevalence of community-acquired AKI at 17.7 per cent with sepsis, hypovolaemia, CKD and diabetes mellitus identified as major risk factors (Finlay et al., 2013). Perhaps a more telling picture of AKI incidence is provided by Challiner et al. (2014) who performed a retrospective audit on 745 case records of unselected emergency admissions. What they found was an AKI incidence of 25.4 per cent, with one-third of AKI being present on admission and two-thirds developing post admission. Where baseline kidney function was known at admission AKI was reported as even higher at 38.1 per cent. Patients with AKI spent more than twice as long in hospital and severity of AKI correlated with longer stay in hospital, use of ICU and risk of mortality (Challiner et al., 2014).

What this indicates is that AKI is no longer seen as a rare organ failure but is very common in hospitals, ranging from 13 to 18 per cent (Challiner et al., 2014; NICE, 2014). In this case nearly 1 in 5 patients in hospital will have or have acquired AKI and 1 in 4 emergency admissions will have AKI. Minor changes in creatinine ($\geq$25 µmol/L) demonstrate a failing kidney and this is correlated to increase in likelihood of death. Up to 30 per cent of AKI episodes are avoidable if health care professionals do what is expected of them (NCEPOD, 2009). Therefore early detection of AKI cannot be neglected and understanding it and its effective prevention and management becomes a priority.

Aim and Learning Outcomes

Aim

The aim of this chapter is to explore the priorities of early accurate assessment and prevention of AKI and nursing and medical management of the individual presenting with AKI.

Learning Outcomes

At the end of this chapter the reader will be able to:

1. Define AKI and distinguish between the differing manifestations of AKI.
2. Identify and explain the pathophysiological basis of the presenting signs and symptoms of AKI.
3. Identify and explain the immediate nursing and medical assessment, specific monitoring and key investigations required to enable an accurate and timely diagnosis.
4. Explore the evidence basis for immediate priorities of medical and nursing management, with a particular focus upon pharmacological and invasive interventions.
5. Appreciate the role of different health professionals in acute assessment and management of AKI.
6. Recognise the common complications associated with AKI.

The Case Scenario: The Presenting Complaint

Ralph is an 80-year-old man who lives in an elderly care home. He is usually mobile and self-caring. The staff at the home report that over the past four days Ralph has become increasingly lethargic and drowsy following treatment for a chest infection (treated with oral Amoxicillin® 500 mg three times daily for seven days). He was found on the floor of his room by morning staff; they are unsure of how long he had been lying there. He has been taking no food and very little fluids and has had several episodes of vomiting over the past two days. On examination Ralph is drowsy but responsive to questioning, though a little disorientated. He is also irritable and has a headache. His skin is dry, he has a minor petechial rash on his upper chest and lower neck and has an unproductive cough. He complains of anorexia, nausea and has vomited once (100 mL bile-stained fluid). His bladder is not palpable.

The Case Scenario *continued*

His vital signs were recorded as:

Pulse: 110 beats/minute sinus tachycardia
Blood pressure (BP): lying = 90/40 mmHg; standing = 80/40 mmHg
Jugular venous pressure (JVP): unrecordable
Oxygen saturations (SpO$_2$): 92 per cent on room air
Temperature: 37.7 °C
Glasgow Coma Scale: 14 (E4, V4, M6)
Weight: 75 kg

Ralph's past medical history reveals:

Type 2 diabetes mellitus since age 65
Osteoarthritis of left hip
Hypertension since age 60
Urinary hesitancy awaiting urological investigation

Ralph's current medication is:

Metformin® 2 g divided with meals
Bendrofluazide® 5 mg daily
Ibuprofen 400 mg eight-hourly

A provisional diagnosis of AKI is made.

Consider the following:

1. With reference to the underlying pathophysiology describe what is meant by AKI.
2. What are the common signs and symptoms associated with AKI?
3. What further investigations need to be carried out to identify a definitive diagnosis?

Acute Kidney Injury

The medical review of Ralph's clinical features suggests that he has AKI. However, unless one knows how to interpret these clinical features it will not be clear how this conclusion was made. One way in which to make sense of these clinical features is to start with some indication of the causes of AKI. Initial assessment should be comprehensive to help determine the cause of AKI and to ensure appropriate treatment (Stevens et al., 2008), and should include physical assessment and investigations (Table 8.2).

AKI has many causes but is generally classified into three groups, known as pre-renal, intrinsic and post-renal. While each group is discrete in its content

Table 8.2 Summary of the assessment of the AKI patient

Assessment	Content
History	Presenting condition, symptoms, past medical history, drug history, family history, social history
Clinical examination	Vital signs (BP, P, resps)
	Level of consciousness
	Intravascular volume (skin turgor, mucous membranes, BP lying and standing, orthostatic pulse change)
	JVP
	Pulse oximetry
	CVP, pulmonary artery catheter
	Peripheral capillary return
	Weight
	Systems: cardiovascular, respiratory, gastrointestinal, neurological, dermatological eyes, nails, oedema
Urine	Output, volume
	Appearance and content (cells, crystals, blood, protein, glucose, pH, ketones, SG)
	Culture
	Biochemistry: sodium, protein, creatinine clearance
Blood	Estimated GFR: creatinine
	Biochemistry: sodium, potassium, chloride, bicarbonate, calcium, phosphate, pH, magnesium, urea
	Blood gases
	LFTs: CK, amylase, albumin
	Cholesterol
	Immunology
	Culture
ECG	LVF, dysrhythmia, MI
Imaging	Ultrasound, X-ray, CT scan, MRI, urography, nuclear medicine, angiography, cystoscopy

it is worth noting that there may be considerable overlap, especially with pre-renal and intrinsic causes. The causes of AKI are summarised in Figure 8.1.

Pre-renal AKI

The causes of pre-renal AKI can be identified from the term 'pre-renal', occurring before the kidney, whereby AKI is a secondary event, with the primary event occurring elsewhere in the body. In order to understand how an

Figure 8.1   Causes of acute kidney injury

illness or disease elsewhere in the body can affect the kidney some knowledge of renal physiology is required. The kidneys produce urine, which is made up of water, waste products of metabolism, hormones and drugs. The production of urine occurs within 1.2 million (approximately) functional units called nephrons housed within each kidney (Figure 8.2).

Figure 8.2   The nephron

The cellular activity of the kidney requires a huge amount of oxygen. In fact, while the kidney only occupies 1 per cent of total body weight it uses 10 per cent of the body's oxygen requirements (Cohen, 1986). The kidney's high oxygen consumption is proportionate to the amount of sodium reabsorption, which is a vitally important function for maintaining fluid balance. However, the cells in the nephrons function at very low oxygen saturation levels of 1.3–2.9 kPa (normal is 12–15 kPa) and therefore are very sensitive to change. The kidney requires 1200 mL of blood per minute, which is one-fifth of cardiac output, in order to produce 1 mL of urine per minute (Koeppen and Stanton, 2001). Kidney blood flow causes a filtration pressure within the glomerulus of about 60 mmHg, which in turn produces a glomerular filtration rate (GFR) of approximately 125 mL/min/1.73 m^2 (Koeppen and Stanton, 2001). The key point here is that given all these factors the kidney is susceptible to alterations in its blood supply and oxygenation and this is where pre-renal causes affect kidney function.

In order to provide 1200 mL/min of blood to the kidney certain factors need to be in place. These factors are the need for an effective pump (the heart), an effective circulating volume (the blood), appropriate volume pressure (blood pressure) and a patent vasculature (blood vessels). Any change to one or more of these factors may cause a reduction of kidney perfusion significant enough to cause injury. Major causes of pre-renal AKI cause a rapid loss of GFR and a reduction in urine output (oliguria). Typical causes of pre-renal AKI are hypotension of any cause, congestive cardiac failure, diuretic use and haemorrhage (Table 8.3).

Loss of significant volumes of fluid will lead to a low blood pressure (BP) and reduced kidney perfusion. Volume depletion is by far the major cause of pre-renal AKI and can be divided into two groups. One is total intravascular depletion, where intravascular volume is reduced, and the other is effective volume depletion due to arterial under-filling, where there is adequate volume (Faubel et al., 2005) (Table 8.4).

Table 8.3   Examples of causes of pre-renal AKI

Cause	*Examples of common problems*
Cardiac	Congestive cardiac failure, cardiac surgery, arrhythmia
Volume	Burns, bleeding, vomiting, diarrhoea, diuresis
Vascular resistance	Shock, antihypertensive treatment, NSAIDs, ACE inhibitors, hepatorenal syndrome
Vascular patency	Renal artery thrombosis, abdominal aortic aneurysm (AAA), bilateral renal artery stenosis

Table 8.4 Causes of volume depletion

Total intravascular depletion	Effective volume depletion
Haemorrhage	Reduced cardiac output: congestive cardiac failure, pulmonary embolism, cardiogenic shock
Renal fluid loss: diuretics, osmotic diuresis (such as glycosuria)	Peripheral vasodilation: sepsis, anaphylaxis, cirrhosis, antihypertension medication
Gastrointestinal loss: vomiting, diarrhoea and nasogastric aspiration	
Skin fluid loss: burns, sweating	
Third space syndrome: pancreatitis, peritonitis	

Source: Adapted from Faubel et al. (2005)

However, additional factors, including commonly used drugs such as non-steroidal anti-inflammatory drugs (NSAIDs), are known to cause vaso-constriction of the arterioles of the kidney, thus reducing GFR. Therefore it is important that a range of possible causes are considered. In Ralph's case, his clinical history reveals a number of clues that may point to pre-renal AKI as a possible cause. The clinical information indicates Ralph is hypoten-sive, his fluid intake has been low, he has vomited, though the frequency is not known, and he is taking medication (Bendrofluazide® and ibuprofen), which all carry the risk of reducing renal perfusion.

Intrinsic AKI

In contrast to pre-renal AKI, where a physiological insult occurs elsewhere in the body, intrinsic AKI points to the kidney as the source of the problem. Intrinsic simply means something specific to the kidney, whereas pre-renal AKI is extrinsic or from without the kidney. Other words used synonymously with intrinsic are intrarenal, renal or parenchymal, and each points to prob-lems with the functional parts (nephrons) of the kidney. The structures of the kidney that are affected are the microcapillaries (glomeruli, afferent and efferent arterioles), the tubular cells and the interstitium, which is the tissue that surrounds the nephrons (Figure 8.3). It is also important to note that if pre-renal AKI occurs this will have an impact upon the nephron and cause tubular cell death, also known as acute tubular necrosis (ATN). Examples of intrinsic AKI can be found in Table 8.5.

Afferent Arteriole
(supplies arterial blood
under high pressure)

Efferent Arteriole
(arterial blood leaves)

Glomerulus

Bowman's capsule

Glomerular Filtrate

Figure 8.3 The glomerulus

Table 8.5 Examples of causes of intrinsic AKI

Vascular	Glomerular	Tubular	Interstitial
Renal artery	Goodpasture's	Ischaemia	Drug-induced
thrombosis	Syndrome	Haemorrhage	antibiotics,
Surgical cross	Henoch-	Nephrotoxins, e.g.	NSAIDs, diuretics
clamping	Schoenlein	vancomycin	Infection:
Polyarteritis nodosa	Purpura	Myoglobin	bacterial, viral,
Haemolytic uraemic	Infective	(muscle damage)	tuberculosis
syndrome	endocarditis	Haemoglobin	
Malignant	Wegener's	(haemolysis)	
hypertension	granulomatosis		

The glomerulus is where filtering of the blood occurs (Figure 8.3). Filtration is driven by BP and so a fall in BP will cause a decline in the GFR. The filtration barrier is made up of three structures: the endothelial cells of the blood vessel, the basement membrane and the epithelial cells of the Bowman's capsule. The glomerulus has a size restriction (anything over 42 Å is retained) and is also negatively charged to prevent substances such as proteins from escaping into the urine (Koeppen and Stanton, 2001). Any pathological process that damages this structure alters its function by inhibiting filtration or essentially making it more permeable to larger substances, such as in protein (albumin) leakage (seen in diabetes mellitus) or red blood cell leakage (as found in glomerulonephritis). As already noted, the nephron is made up of highly active cells and it is here where wholesale and fine tuning reabsorption of essential substances such as water, sodium and potassium as well as the secretion of excess and toxic substances occurs. These cells are responsible for maintaining the chemical balance of extracellular fluid by manipulating substances such as sodium and potassium. Damage to these cells will alter the ability to maintain chemical homeostasis and the removal of toxins.

Intrinsic diseases that affect the kidney can be primary to the kidney or as part of a systemic disease. Where the disease is part of a systemic disease such as systemic lupus erythematosus (SLE) kidney function cannot be affected by manipulating external factors such as maintaining circulating volume. Diseases that affect the microcapillaries involve the blood vessels or the capillary bundle known as the glomerulus. There are inflammatory conditions of blood vessels such as polyarteritis nodosa and Wegener's granulomatosis, large vascular disease such as renal artery thrombosis, renal vein thrombosis and surgical cross-clamping as found in abdominal aortic aneurysm repair. Conditions that affect small vessels include thrombocytopaenic conditions such as pre-eclampsia, scleroderma, malignant hypertension and haemolytic uraemic syndrome (HUS), which is often caused by *Escherichia coli* H0157:H7 contamination of food. In these conditions there is damage to the endothelial cells of the blood vessels and stimulation of the clotting cascade (Salama, 2002).

Intrinsic AKI: Glomerular Disease

There are diseases of the glomerulus that alter the structure of the glomerular filtration barrier, causing haematuria and proteinuria. They are usually immunologically mediated and cause the condition known as glomerulonephritis. Proteinuria can be very severe and in some cases in excess of 3 grams in 24 hours can be lost, which is known as nephrotic, whereas less than 2 grams in 24 hours is called nephritic. Such conditions include Henoch–Schönlein purpura, Goodpasture's syndrome, infective carditis and post-infectious glomerulonephritis (often streptococcal infection). Patients with these diseases are usually very ill, with skin lesions and often a rash (Holley, 2001). Ralph has a petechial rash, which may indicate an intrinsic cause to his AKI. Alternatively his rash could have been caused by local capillary trauma due to coughing during his chest infection. The blood cells found in the urine of patients with glomerulonephritis are often misshapen and lumped together in 'casts' as they progress through the tubules. Haematuria can be non-visible and only found by urine dipstick testing, or visible. This simple test aids diagnosis of intrinsic disease of the kidney.

Intrinsic AKI: Tubular Disease

Damage to the renal tubules (acute tubular necrosis: ATN) is caused in 50 per cent of cases by a reduction in blood flow (ischaemia) to the kidney and in 35 per cent of cases by a nephrotoxic substance (Faubel et al., 2005). Ischaemic causes of ATN have already been identified in pre-renal AKI; however, nephrotoxins are multiple and in theory any substance is potentially toxic to the kidney. Due to the rich blood supply to the kidney and the ability to concentrate toxins in high levels the kidney is particularly vulnerable to toxic substances (Clarkson et al., 2008). Nephrotoxins can be drugs such as aminoglycoside antibiotics, including Gentamicin® and Vancomycin®; cancer drugs such as Cisplatin®; anaesthetic drugs such as Enflurane®; antiviral drugs such as Acyclovir® and immunosuppressive drugs such as Ciclosporin®. Nephrotoxins can also come from within the body, such as haemoglobin (from haemolysis), myoglobin (from muscle damage) and uric acid. Each of these nephrotoxins will damage the tubular cells to varying degrees, which may be sufficient to prevent function or lead to cell death. Subsequent tubule blockage leads to cellular casts or debris in the urine.

Intrinsic AKI: Interstitial Disease

Interstitial disease of the kidney occurs when an inflammatory process is initiated in the cells between nephrons. Commonly inflammation occurs as a consequence of hypersensitivity to drugs but it can also be caused by infection or systemic disease such as SLE (Baker, 2002). Infectious causes can be direct, as found in upper urinary tract infection leading to pyelonephritis, or they can be systemic, such as streptococcal, staphylococcal, HIV and hepatitis A. Drugs that induce acute interstitial nephritis (AIN) include many perceived safe drugs such as antibiotics (ampicillin, erythromycin), non-steroidal anti-inflammatory drugs, Ranitidine®, diuretics (Furosemide®, thiazides), paracetamol and aspirin (Baker, 2002). It is likely that any drug has the potential for initiating hypersensitivity in a person and causing kidney injury. Patients with AIN frequently present with pyrexia, rash, joint pain, hypertension, fluid retention and possible signs of systemic disease. It can occur at any time after exposure to the drug and is not dose dependent.

There are a number of possible causes in Ralph's case. He may have ATN due to low BP but he has also had an infection and was treated with an antibiotic. Further to this Ralph has been taking ibuprofen (a NSAID) and Bendrofluazide® (a diuretic), which may indicate interstitial nephritis. Ralph has a rash on his chest, which is a possible sign of a vasculitic disease, and protein in his urine could indicate glomerular damage. This information adds to the complexity of assessment of someone with AKI and by no means can it be assumed that the cause is pre-renal or intrinsic at this point.

Post-renal AKI

Post-renal AKI relates to conditions that interfere with the flow of urine from the tip of the papillae (renal pyramids) to the tip of the urethra. Obstruction is the usual cause, with elderly men being most at risk due to prostatic hypertrophy and/or cancer (Table 8.6).

In these conditions patients usually present with reduced (oliguria) or loss (anuria) of urine output, urinary retention, loin pain and possibly fever. Anuria usually suggests urinary tract obstruction; otherwise it is unusual in AKI (Hilton, 2006). Urinary retention and bilateral kidney obstruction will eventually cause back pressure into the kidney tubules, which counteracts the pressure across the filtration barrier of the glomerulus, thus reducing glomerular filtration rate and renal blood flow. This in turn would eventually cause an intrinsic AKI due to ischaemia of the tubular cells. This additional information adds more possibilities to the cause of Ralph's AKI. Ralph has a reduced urine output, which may be symptomatic of obstruction, especially as he has a history of urinary hesitancy, not uncommon for a man of his age. Ralph also has diabetes mellitus, which is known to cause papillary necrosis, which obstructs the ureters with necrotic tissue. Each of these potential causes requires investigation to differentiate cause and initiate appropriate management.

Risk Factors for AKI

It is important to note what factors increase the risk of AKI. NICE (2013) recently identified a range of risk factors particularly in relation to different clinical scenarios; however, a general theme can be seen and is summarised in Table 8.7.

In relation to Ralph, increased age is a risk factor for AKI. The reason for this is multifactorial, including multiple co-morbidities, but one major

Table 8.6 Examples of causes of post-renal AKI

Intraureteral obstruction	Bladder and urethral obstruction	Obstruction by external pressure
Stones	Urethral stricture	Malignancy: rectal,
Papillary debris caused by drugs, diabetes, stricture	Prostatic hypertrophy/ cancer	ovarian, uterine, cervical
Blood clots	Tuberculosis	Fibroids
Myeloma	Spinal cord injury	Crohn's disease
	Multiple sclerosis	Haemorrhage
	Diabetes mellitus	Aortic aneurysm

Table 8.7 Risk factors for AKI

- CKD (eGFR < 60 mL/min/1.73m^2)
- Heart failure
- Liver disease
- Diabetes mellitus
- History of AKI
- Oliguria
- Limited access to fluid
- Hypovolaemia
- Use of drugs with nephrotoxic potential
- Use of iodinated contrast
- Symptoms or history of urological obstruction
- Deteriorating early warning score
- Age 65 or over

Source: Adapted from NICE (2013)

reason is that kidney function of older people lacks renal reserve. This means that the kidney has an age-related reduced GFR which, when put under stress, such as dehydration, cannot compensate effectively (Pannu and Halloran, 2002). The elderly kidney is also sensitive to the effects of drugs, especially NSAIDs, which cause vasoconstriction and a decline in GFR and may be implicated in Ralph's AKI (Jefferson et al., 2010). Underlying chronic kidney disease, often identified by proteinuria or cardiovascular disease (especially hypertension and renovascular disease), is also a risk factor in that it will affect the kidney's ability to respond to injury. In addition, diabetes mellitus causes long-term vascular damage to the kidneys (see Chapter 10) and sepsis causes renal vasoconstriction (see Chapter 3). These four factors immediately place Ralph at high risk for AKI. Surgery, especially cardiac surgery, predisposes individuals to AKI and accounts for 25 per cent of hospital-acquired AKI (Lamiere et al., 2005, Thakar, 2013) and hypotension is a major risk factor that is increased with the use of diuretics. The increase in organ transplantation is contributing to more cases of AKI due to the use of immunosuppressive therapy (Lamiere et al., 2005).

In summary, an understanding of the underlying causes of AKI can inform the assessment strategy employed in Ralph's case. It is apparent that Ralph has a number of potential causes for his condition. His history of potential hypovolaemia and hypotension may suggest pre-renal AKI, whereas possible intrinsic causes such as his medication may have caused acute tubular necrosis. Finally, Ralph may also have a urinary system obstruction that may have contributed to his kidney injury.

The Case Scenario: The Immediate Assessment Priorities

Samples of blood and urine taken for analysis from Ralph revealed the following results:

Capillary blood glucose: 8.5 mmol/L
Venous blood biochemistry – urea and electrolytes (U&Es)
Urea: 40 mmol/L
Creatinine: 200 μmol/L
Na+: 133 mmol/L
K+: 6.5 mmol/L
Cl–: 107 mmol/L
HCO3: 19 mmol/L
Cholesterol: 7.5 mmol/L
CK: 180 iu/L
Calcium: 2.2 mmol/L
Pi: 1.2 mmol/L
Glucose: 10 mmol/L
Venous blood liver function tests (LFTs)
Albumin: 35 g/L
Bilirubin: 10 μmol/L
ALT: 15 iu/L
Alkaline phosphate: 123 u/L
Lactate: 2.0 iu/L
CRP: 72
Venous blood haematology
Hb: 13.2 g/dL
HCT: 0.45 L/L
WCC: 22 ¥ 109/L
Platelets: 10 ¥ 109/L
Immunology
ANA, ANCA, complement, protein electrophoresis, anti-GBM all tested normal
Virology
No HIV, hepatitis A or B
Urinalysis
Protein +
pH: 6
No other abnormality
Urine output: 150 mL in 8 hours
Sodium: 10 mmol/L
Fractional excretion Na: < 1 per cent
Urine osmolarity: 1250 mOsm/kg H_2O

The Case Scenario *continued*

Immediate Assessment
1. How does the information gleaned so far help with the next step of assessment?
2. Devise a comprehensive acute assessment plan for Ralph and explain the rationale for each measure.
3. How is AKI differentiated from chronic kidney disease?
4. How is Ralph's level of kidney function calculated?
5. Re-examine Ralph's biochemistry results then calculate his eGFR at www.renal. org/eGFRcalc/GFR.pl and consider what it means with respect to the amount of kidney function he has.

Assessment and Reaching a Diagnosis

The NCEPOD 2009 report *Adding Insult To Injury* highlighted some significant issues in relation to patient care that should not be ignored. The NCEPOD report identified that only 50 per cent of patients received good care, there was poor assessment of AKI risk factors and of patients once they had developed AKI, there was an unacceptable delay in recognising AKI post admission in 43 per cent of patients, one-fifth of cases were both predictable and preventable, and complications were missed in 13 per cent of cases, avoidable in 17 per cent of cases and managed badly in 22 per cent. Finlay et al. (2013) reported the need for continuing improvement when they found basic elements of care were still being omitted by practitioners. In view of this poor indictment of clinical practice it is essential that healthcare staff take note and improve their patient care.

Notwithstanding other aspects of assessment, namely ABCDE identified in Chapter 1, assessment will focus upon specific issues related to Ralph and AKI. However, it is important to note that assessment of airway, breathing and circulation is essential especially because AKI is potentially a life-threatening condition. There must be appropriate prioritisation in the assessment of Ralph and assessment of risk because focusing upon the wrong issues may prove fatal for someone with AKI. All patient management should be linked to a 'track and trigger' system/early warning system such as NEWS (RCP, 2012) for managing change in the patient's health status.

Airway and Breathing

While conscious, Ralph will be maintaining his own airway; however, his SpO_2 at 92 per cent suggests a degree of hypoxaemia. It is therefore important to observe and document his respiratory rate, depth and rhythm and sounds regularly and to monitor oxygen saturations using pulse oximetry continuously. Oxygen therapy should be commenced at 40 per cent via face mask in an effort to increase the SpO_2 above 95 per cent.

Circulation

Retention of electrolytes, in particular potassium, due to renal failure can lead to serious cardiac arrhythmias. Therefore Ralph requires continuous cardiac monitoring to assess his heart rate, regularity and rhythm. He is documented as having a sinus tachycardia, which may be a compensatory response to his low BP. Ralph's BP should be recorded at least every four hours as an indication of improvement or deterioration. Central venous pressure (CVP) measurement may also be useful in assessing Ralph's circulatory fluid status but will require insertion of a wide bore catheter into the jugular vein attached to a litre infusion of 0.9 per cent sodium chloride to enable regular measurement (see Chapter 2).

Disability

Assessment of Ralph's altered consciousness must be undertaken. Altered consciousness is a trigger factor for initiating urgent treatment in an attempt to prevent deterioration (NICE, 2007). Ralph's conscious level should prompt a bedside capillary blood glucose measurement, particularly as he has a history of type 2 diabetes and hasn't eaten well recently. His capillary and venous blood glucose are on the upper side of normal but not sufficiently abnormal to account for his drowsiness. Drowsiness is a common clinical feature in AKI. If other potential factors such as hyper- or hypoglycaemia, hypoxia and hypotension are excluded, altered consciousness occurs in AKI due to the accumulation of uraemic toxins. Vanholder et al. (2003) identified 90 potential uraemic toxins, including urea, creatinine, parathyroid hormone, guanidines, ammonia and peptides. These substances are poorly understood: for example, urea only has a very minor effect and is believed not to be the cause of uraemic symptoms, requiring accumulation with other substances to have an effect (Meyer and Hostetter, 2007). It is worth noting that uraemia does not mean high urea levels in the blood but literally means 'urine in the blood': that is to say, the products normally seen in the urine are retained in the blood but at abnormal levels.

Uraemia causes altered neurosensory function, presenting with cognitive impairment such as defects in memory, attention and concentration. Unrelieved uraemia will lead to coma and death. Clinical signs and symptoms of uraemia can be found in Table 8.8. Ralph's consciousness level must be monitored using the Glasgow Coma Scale (or equivalent) for deterioration (see Chapter 4) and the frequency of assessment will be determined by his condition, level of consciousness and potential for deterioration. Ralph

Table 8.8 Signs and symptoms of uraemia (some features may be dependent upon underlying cause)

Uraemic signs and symptoms
Altered consciousness, irritability, reduced concentration and memory numbness, weakness, tremor, stupor, coma, hearing disturbance
Dyspnoea, orthopnoea, haemoptysis, nose bleed, sinusitis
Palpitations, arrhythmias, pericarditis, cardiac failure, hypotension
Nausea, vomiting, diarrhoea, thirst, abdominal pain, acid reflux, bleeding, hiccup, stomatitis, fetor, gastritis, gastric/enteral ulceration, bleeding
Haematuria, proteinuria, frequency, dysuria, suprapubic pain, altered urine output, loin pain, colic
Arthralgia, muscular pain, cramp
Rash, pruritus, bruising, jaundice, hypothermia, dry skin, oedema, uraemic frost
Red eyes, oedema
Fever, malaise, insomnia, weight loss
Anaemia, thrombocytopaenia (bleeding), altered white cell function

currently has a GCS of 14 so every 15 to 30 minutes may initially be sufficient; however, there must be a nursing initiative to increase the frequency of testing should his condition deteriorate. Drowsiness in uraemia is a sign of very high accumulation of uraemic toxins. Patients with chronic kidney disease can usually tolerate high levels of uraemic toxins and are not usually drowsy in the way Ralph is; therefore his symptoms appear to point towards AKI, where drowsiness is more likely.

Specific Investigations

A range of specific investigations are required to reveal the exact cause of Ralph's apparent kidney failure and presenting signs and symptoms. Table 8.9 outlines investigations required for a general approach to the assessment of causes of AKI.

Estimating the Level of Kidney Function

Creatinine is a substance that is also thought to be of limited toxicity. Normal kidney function usually excretes all creatinine, unlike urea, of which about 60 per cent is reabsorbed. Creatinine is a by-product of muscle metabolism and reflects total muscle mass. Because of its complete removal by the kidney

Table 8.9 Investigations for assessment of AKI

Investigation	Specific test content	Reason for test
Urea and electrolytes	Urea and creatinine	Creatinine to estimate kidney function and hydration (Ur:Cr ratio)
	Sodium	Assess level and hydration
	Potassium	Assess level and cardiac risk
	Calcium	Assess level and differentiate CKD, high levels cause AKI, low in rhabdomyolysis
	Phosphate	Assess level and differentiate CKD
	Chloride	Assess level; acidosis/alkalosis
	Magnesium	Assess level (may be low)
	Bicarbonate	Acidosis/alkalosis
	Urate	Assess level pre-eclampsia (high uric acid levels are implicated in pre-eclampsia and lead to AKI)
	Lactate	Tissue ischaemia/under perfusion, assess lactic acidosis
eGFR	Estimate glomerular filtration rate	To assess level of kidney function
Liver function test	Albumin	Assess level; may be low in glomerulonephritis
	Creatine kinase	Assess level for muscle damage (myoglobin)
	Amylase	Assess level; pancreatitis may cause AKI
	Bilirubin, AST, ALT	Haemolysis, liver disease may cause AKI
Arterial blood gases	pO_2	Assess oxygen level for oxygenation
	pCO_2	Assess acidosis, CO_2 retention
Full blood count and coagulation studies	Haemoglobin	Assess for anaemia, need for transfusion
	White cell count	Indicator of infection
	Platelets	Level and coagulopathy (e.g. DIC)
	Group and save	Transfusion
	Haematocrit	Assess anaemia/hydration
	INR	Clotting screen
Inflammation and immunology	ESR	Indicator of inflammation
	CRP	Non-specific marker for inflammation and infection
	ANA, ANCA, Anti-GBM, IgA, IgM, IgG, electrophoresis, complement, antistreptolysin	Specific glomerular disease tests, e.g. SLE, vasculitis, myeloma

(Continued)

Table 8.9   (*Continued*)

Infection	Blood culture	Infection: sepsis may cause or prolong AKI
	Urine culture	Infection: may cause interstitial nephritis, prolong AKI
	Virology	Hepatitis A B, HIV
Urinalysis	Dipstick	Assessing for blood, protein, infection
	Electrophoresis	Specific test for multiple myeloma which causes AKI
	Albumin creatinine ratio	Assess glomerular damage to assess kidney function/damage
	Creatinine clearance	Assesses urine output/kidney function and prescribe volume replacement
	Volume	
Imaging	Chest X-ray	Evidence of pulmonary oedema, LVF
	Renal ultrasound	Assess kidney structure, size and signs of obstruction
	X-ray kidney ureter bladder	Obstruction, stones, abdominal masses
	CT/MRI	Assess kidney structure
	Isotopes studies	Assess renal perfusion, cortical necrosis, vascular obstruction
	Biopsy	Assess ATN, suspected intrinsic AKI
Cardiac	ECG	Assess cardiac function: LVF, dysrhythmia

it is a useful marker for glomerular function. It is used as a means for estimating kidney function. Current recommendations advise the use of the estimated glomerular filtration rate method (eGFR), which uses age, race, creatinine and sex to calculate kidney function (Lewington and Kanasundaram, 2011). Some caution is needed in AKI because eGFR is normally used for chronic kidney disease. The eGFR is requested at the same time as obtaining urea and electrolytes (U&Es) but there are many eGFR calculators available on the internet. Using the Renal Association (2011) calculator Ralph's GFR is 30 mL/min/1.73m² (normal: about 100 mL/min/1.73m² without signs of kidney disease), which means he has less than 30 per cent of his kidney function remaining. In addition to eGFR and following the results of the NCEPOD (2009) *Adding Insult to Injury* report in England there will be implementation of an AKI e-alerts system where an elevation of serum creatinine by 26μmol/L will automatically produce an alert on a patient's electronic records system. The aim is to identify patients with AKI and implement prompt treatment and consistency of practice across health services (NHS England, 2014).

The Case Scenario: Medical Management and Care Issues

Ralph is diagnosed with AKI and he does not appear to be showing any signs of improvement. A radial artery sample is taken for blood gas analysis and the following results received:

Arterial blood gases (ABGs)
  PO_2: 10 kPa
  PCO_2: 8.1 kPa
  Base excess: −1
  Anion gap: 18
  pH: 7.31

Immediate Medical Management
1. What two urgent priorities of management and care can you identify for Ralph?
2. How would these two priorities be managed?
3. What fluid replacement regime would best suit Ralph's needs?
4. What are Ralph's main care issues?
5. What are Ralph's additional management priorities?
6. Examine the blood gas results carefully and consider what might be done.

Differentiating between AKI and CKD

It is important to establish whether Ralph has AKI or CKD to ensure that he gets the appropriate treatment. Not only is Ralph a prime candidate for AKI but his increased age, diabetes and hypertension made him a prime candidate for CKD. Ralph may have underlying kidney disease and be presenting with an acute-on-chronic episode (which is a common presentation of AKI) or with end-stage renal disease (ESRD). Drowsiness is a common symptom of AKI but can also manifest in ESRD (National Collaboration for Chronic Conditions, 2008; Hsu et al., 2008). People with CKD usually have an absence of acute illness, and also present with anaemia, nocturia, long duration of symptoms, hyperphosphataemia and hypocalcaemia (Hilton, 2006). Renal ultrasound will identify the size of the kidney, as those with CKD will typically have small kidneys (<9 cm), though diabetes may preserve kidney size for some time. Ralph's clinical features and history indicate his problem is acute in nature rather than chronic.

Medical Management Strategies

AKI is a life-threatening condition and it is therefore important that priorities for management are promptly identified. Principles of AKI management can be found in Table 8.10, where some immediate concerns such as hyperkalaemia and fluid resuscitation are noted.

Hyperkalaemia

Ralph demonstrates signs that are potentially life threatening and may override the initial desire to find an underlying cause. The two immediate concerns are his high potassium level (hyperkalaemia), which is 6.5 mmol/L (normal range 3.2–5.0 mmol/L), and hypovolaemia. In the first instance causes of hyperkalaemia should exclude pseudohyperkalaemia caused by test tube haemolysis, prolonged tourniquet tightness, leucocytosis and infusion arm sampling to avoid inappropriate treatment (Table 8.11).

Table 8.10 Principles of management of AKI

- Identify and correct cause
- Optimise cardiac output and renal perfusion
- Restore urine flow
- Accurate fluid balance, daily body weight
- Review drugs: stop nephrotoxic drugs, adjust doses and monitor blood levels
- Identify, avoid and treat complications: e.g. hyperkalaemia, fluid overload, acidosis, hyper/hyponatraemia, hyperphosphataemia
- Optimise nutritional support: calories, potassium restriction, minimal nitrogen
- Vigilant monitoring for infection and treat aggressively.
- Minimise the use of indwelling lines and catheters: remove if unnecessary
- Avoid, identify and treat bleeding tendency
- Initiate dialysis before uraemic complications occur
- Expert nursing care

Source: Adapted from Lameire et al. (2005) and Hilton (2006)

Table 8.11 Drugs that can cause hyperkalaemia

Angiotensin converting enzyme inhibitors (ACEI)
Angiotensin II receptor blockers (ARB)
Non-steroidal anti-inflammatory drugs (NSAIDs)
Digoxin
Spironolactone especially in those with underlying renal insufficiency

Table 8.12 ECG changes in hyperkalaemia

- Peaking ('tenting') of T waves: K⁺ > 5.5 mmol/L
- Flattening and disappearance of P waves: K⁺ > 6.5 mmol/L
- Prolonged PR interval
- Progressive widening of QRS complex: K⁺ > 6.5 mmol/L
- Deepened S waves and merging with T waves
- Sine wave patterns
- Ventricular fibrillation and asystolic cardiac arrest: K⁺ > 12.0 mmol/L

Source: Adapted from Steddon et al. (2006)

Additional causes of hyperkalaemia include potassium supplementation, gastrointestinal bleeding and in Ralph's case potassium retention due to loss of kidney function (Renal Association, 2014). Ralph's medication must be considered and any drug that may cause hyperkalaemia – for example, ibuprofen – should be discontinued, if possible, without causing additional medical problems. Alternative medication may be required. The effects of hyperkalaemia are neuromuscular and cardiac but demonstrate few symptoms. Patients may complain of vague abdominal sensations or skeletal muscular weakness but more importantly they may develop cardiac arrest. Cardiac arrest occurs because of decreased membrane excitability, neuromuscular depression and cardiac arrhythmias (Weisberg, 2008). In view of this, Ralph must be closely monitored by continuous ECG for progressive hyperkalaemic changes, which occur in sequence with elevating hyperkalaemia, as seen in Table 8.12. The degree of hyperkalaemia requires immediate attention. Treatment must be instigated urgently, especially if the potassium is over 6.5 mmol/L or ECG changes are present. The aim is to reduce Ralph's potassium and limit his risk by the following the Five Key Steps to Treatment of Hyperkalaemia (Renal Association, 2014). The patient should never be left until all five have been completed.

1. Protect the heart
   - Cardioprotection: medical or advanced nurse practitioner administration of prescribed 10 mL 10 per cent intravenous calcium gluconate or calcium chloride, repeat if necessary. This drug does not reduce potassium level but 'protects' the heart from excess potassium excitability.
2. Shift potassium into the cells
   - Administration of a prescribed slow intravenous infusion of 50 mL of 50 per cent glucose.
   - Administer prescribed insulin (15 iu Actrapid®) and dextrose (50 mL of 50 per cent) infusion. Effects are seen within 15 minutes and last between two and four hours.

- Nebulised salbutamol® (which drives potassium into the cells) 10–20 mg may be used in conjunction with insulin and glucose providing an additive effect. Effects are seen within 15–30 minutes and last for two hours. Monitor for tachycardia, headache and palpitations.
- The process can be repeated after four hours.

3. Remove potassium from the body
- Oral calcium resonium (which binds with potassium in the gut) 15 g with lactulose®, though this is slow to work ($\geq$ 2 hours). This is not recommended for emergency severe hyperkalaemia but for mild to moderate hyperkalaemia.
- Renal replacement therapy only when first-line treatments fail to control potassium level or if severe hyperkalaemia ($\geq$7 mmol/L) is present.

4. Monitor potassium and glucose
- Monitor blood potassium 30 minutes after each administration then hourly.
- Monitor U&Es for hypokalaemia 30 minutes after each administration.
- Monitor blood glucose level with a blood glucose monitor 30 minutes after administration then hourly and treat hypoglycaemia with prescribed dose of 10 per cent glucose.

5. Prevent recurrence
- Review medication and stop any that may cause hyperkalaemia, in particular ACEi, ARBs, loop diuretics, NSAIDs and trimethoprim.
- Review dietary intake including salt substitutes.

Insulin and glucose are the most effective means for conservatively keeping the potassium low and their efficacy is improved with nebulised salbutamol® (Mahoney et al., 2005). Insulin works by increasing cellular uptake of potassium by increasing intracellular sodium. Intravenous access will be necessary for infusions and strict fluid balance monitoring of all intake and output commenced. All fluid volumes, including intravenous fluids, nasogastric feeds and oral fluids, must be entered onto the fluid balance chart. All types of fluid output, including urine, vomit, and wound drainage, should be measured and documented accurately. Urine output may need to be assessed on an hourly basis.

Volume Depletion

The next priority for Ralph is his fluid status. Ralph is displaying evidence of volume depletion, which if not treated may cause permanent damage to the kidney as well as more systemic problems such as hypovolaemic

Table 8.13   Assessing circulating volume

- Pulse
- Blood pressure
- JVP or CVP
- Peripheral perfusion
- Lung crackles
- Dyspnoea

---

shock, leading to inadequate tissue oxygenation and multiple organ failure (Ragaller et al., 2001). Volume depletion is evident in Ralph in a number of clinical features (Table 8.13). Most noticeably, Ralph's jugular venous pressure (JVP) is unrecordable, which means it is low (normal 0 to 3 cm above the sternal angle).

Ralph is also tachycardic with a heart rate of 110 beats per minute and his BP is low and falls when he is standing. This effect is known as a postural drop or orthostatic hypotension and is a classic sign of hypovolaemia. However, in a systematic review of studies of clinical signs of hypovolaemia, hypotension was frequently absent in supine patients. Orthostatic hypotension is also present in 10 per cent of normovolaemic adults under 65 years old and up to 30 per cent of normovolaemic adults over 65 years old (McGee et al., 1999). Tachycardia is a normal response to volume depletion in an attempt to ensure vital organs receive blood. A postural increase of pulse rate by 30 beats/min or more upon standing is an accurate sign of hypovolaemia (McGee et al., 1999) (Table 8.14). A reduced fluid intake, vomiting, continued use of diuretic medication and mild pyrexia all indicate

Table 8.14   Volume depletion: test results

Hypovolaemia
- Blood sodium variable dependent upon loss: low/normal/high sodium level
- Raised urea:creatinine ratio
- Increase urine specific gravity
- Increased urine osmolality
- Haematocrit variable dependent upon cause, e.g. low in blood loss

Dehydration
- High blood sodium level (> 145 mmol/L)
- Raised blood osmolality
- Elevated haematocrit
- Urine specific gravity above 1.030

---

uncontrolled fluid loss and fluid imbalance, which may be further substantiated when Ralph's test results are examined. Biochemistry results show Ralph's sodium level to be 133 mmol/L (normal range: 135–145 mmol/L), rendering him hyponatraemic.

There are many causes of hyponatraemia (Table 8.15) that need to be considered when assessing Ralph's condition. Hyponatraemia is an important sign because it indicates volume depletion rather than dehydration. Dehydration means a loss of intracellular water, which would increase plasma sodium levels. In contrast, volume depletion describes a loss of sodium (and water) from extracellular space caused by bleeding, excessive vomiting or diarrhoea. Ralph's sodium is low and points towards volume depletion, but there are other clues. Ralph's urea and creatinine levels are raised due to retention by the kidney (not urinary retention), but also in comparison to each other the urea is disproportionally high. This is caused by passive reabsorption of urea in the kidney (creatinine is not reabsorbed), which occurs in hypoperfusion of the kidney but also increased catabolism, steroid therapy, gastrointestinal bleeding and the use of tetracyclines. As a result the high urea level must be interpreted with caution (Goldberg, 2002). Analysis of Ralph's urine also reveals a low sodium content, less than 10 mmol/L (normal about 100 mmol/L), and a fractional excretion of sodium (FeNa) of less than 1 per cent (normal 1–2 per cent). This is typical of pre-renal AKI and demonstrates tubular sodium reabsorption in an effort to retain water to expand the circulating blood volume.

Conversely, intrinsic AKI has a FeNa of greater than 2 per cent, meaning the tubules are unable to reabsorb sodium which is lost in what urine there

Table 8.15 Some causes of hyponatraemia

Low plasma osmolality	Normal or raised plasma osmolality	Syndrome of inappropriate anti-diuretic hormone (SIADH)
Vomiting	Hyperglycaemia	Stress
Diarrhoea	Acute uraemia	Nausea and vomiting
Diuretic use	Alcohol	Pain
Excess fluid replacement	Mannitol infusion	Trauma/surgery
Congestive cardiac	Amino acid infusion	Infection
failure	Sickle cell syndrome	Stroke
Cirrhosis and ascites		Meningitis
		NSAIDs

Osmolality is the measure of osmoles of solutes (e.g. sodium, chloride, glucose) per kg of solvent (blood)

Source: Adapted from Crook (2006)

Table 8.16   Glossary of terms

Oliguria: a urine output of less than 1 mL/kg/hour or less than 400 mL/24 hours

Anuria: a urine output of less than 100 mL/24 hours

Non-oliguric AKI: high urine volumes but of poor quality

---

is (MacPhee, 2002). Urine osmolality is also high, indicating concentrated urine, and in Ralph's case it is in excess of 500 mOsm/kg H_2O, indicating pre-renal AKI. Ralph's urine output (oliguria) is reduced to 150 mL in eight hours (Table 8.16). Non-oliguric AKI can also occur where normal amounts of urine are passed but of poor quality, but this type has a better prognosis. Oliguria occurs when the kidney is attempting to retain water in the body, thus concentrating the urine, or when little urine is being made due to kidney damage. Oliguria is often followed by a polyuria (>3 litres/24 hr) phase due to recovery of kidney function but an initial inability to concentrate effectively, and usually resolves in a few days. All these points direct attention to the fact that Ralph is hypovolaemic, which needs to be addressed. Addressing these problems will require close and frequent monitoring of Ralph's fluid balance, which would include daily weight, hourly urine output, insensitive loss such as sweating and faecal loss (which is estimated a being ≥ 500 mL/24 hr) measurements and all fluid input. CVP monitoring provides for a more accurate assessment of blood volume (see Chapter 2).

Managing Hypovolaemia

Ralph is hypotensive, hypovolaemic and in need of urgent fluid resuscitation. Fluids are required to return normal circulating volume, elevate his BP, increase renal perfusion and reverse pre-renal AKI. The general 'rule of thumb' is to replace lost fluid with its equivalent. Ralph's BP is not low enough to warrant the need for colloid (e.g. human albumin solution) infusion for immediate improvement, and in fact evidence suggests that colloids appear to offer no survival benefit over crystalloids (e.g. 0.9 per cent sodium chloride) in critically ill patients (Perel and Roberts, 2007). Colloids are also thought to cause a hyperoncotic renal failure (Nadeau-Fredette and Bouchard, 2013) and should be used sparingly. In view of this Ralph needs a crystalloid infusion and 0.9 per cent sodium chloride is most appropriate. It is worth noting that 0.9 per cent saline has risks associated with it particularly causing hyperchloraemia which in itself reduces renal blood flow and sodium excretion (Prowle et al., 2010). Dextrose or dextrose/sodium chloride saline are inappropriate because they would quickly distribute among total body water with little vascular filling effect. Mannitol also plays no part in fluid management except when a patient has rhabdomyolysis, which causes nephrotoxicity from damaged muscle myoglobin. The amount of 0.9 per cent sodium chloride needed is dependent upon the extent of Ralph's hypovolaemia, his age and what it takes to restore his blood pressure. Given Ralph's advanced age it may be advisable to infuse 200–300 mL of 0.9 per cent sodium chloride over 10 minutes. Any improvement in BP, pulse, CVP and oliguria would prompt further infusions until Ralph is normovolaemic. Great care is needed to avoid overhydration, which would cause cardiac failure, pulmonary oedema, respiratory distress, hypertension, peripheral oedema and elevated JVP. In addition to this, overhydration by as little as 5–10 per cent of the patient's body weight is linked to worsening organ function and increased mortality (Bouchard et al., 2009, Prowle et al., 2010). Medical and nursing staff should endeavour to maintain urine output with fluid infusions by matching input with urine output plus 30 mL (for insensible loss) or maintaining a CVP of 8–12 cmH_2O. Ralph's AKI may move into the polyuric phase, which could increase the risk of further volume depletion as well as potassium depletion. Once again fluid balance becomes an essential monitoring activity for the AKI patient.

In some instances patients with AKI are commenced on diuretic infusions in an attempt to maintain a urine output. Ralph is prescribed a diuretic (Bendrofluazide®) but this kind of drug is ineffective when GFR is below 30 mL/min/1.73m^2 and should be discontinued. The diuretic drug of choice is Furosemide® and may be given as an infusion. This is controversial treatment with no evidence of its clinical benefit to AKI patients; however,

Table 8.17 Stages of AKI

Initiation: reduction in renal blood flow by 30–50% = oliguria phase

Extension: continued cell hypoxia, inflammatory response, cell death = oliguria/anuria phase

Maintenance: proximal cortical cell regeneration and proliferation = oliguria/anuria phase

Recovery: tubular cellular regeneration and proliferation = diuresis phase and development of concentration gradient and return to normal output

---

it is thought to promote diuresis but should only be used in patients with adequate circulating volume (Lamiere et al., 2005; Ho and Sheridan, 2006, Renal Association, 2014). Dopamine infusion at an alleged 'renal dose' has been shown not to improve patient outcome and has additional risks and so is not recommended for AKI patients (Kellum and Decker, 2001; Stevens et al., 2008). In some instances of deterioration such as in septic shock (but not hypovolaemic shock) it may be necessary to provide blood pressure support and thus renal perfusion with the use of inotropic drugs such as Dopexamine® or norepinephrine. However, given Ralph's health history the use of inotropic drugs is not necessary.

Managing Acidosis

Ralph's ABGs show a low oxygen level of 10.0 kPa (normal > 10.6 kPa), a high carbon dioxide level of 8.1 kPa (normal range 4.7–6 kPa) and a low but not life-threatening pH of 7.31 (normal range 7.35–7.45). The anion gap is 18 (normal range 8–16) and base excess is –1 (diagnostic range –3 to +3). These results indicate that Ralph is hypoxic and in need of oxygen. He is also retaining acid, which is demonstrated by high carbon dioxide level, low pH, high anion gap and negative base excess. The kidney is responsible for maintaining long-term acid–base balance by removal of acids from the body and reconstituting bicarbonate into the blood for buffering excess acids. Should the kidney fail then it can no longer remove acids and produce bicarbonate, which leads to metabolic acidosis. Indeed this is the case for Ralph, though his low oxygen level may be caused by his chest infection, resulting in respiratory acidosis. Ralph's acidosis is best dealt with by treating the underlying cause so fluid resuscitation is essential. Treatment with bicarbonate is not recommended unless Ralph's pH falls below 7.1 because it in fact generates more CO_2 when reacting with hydrogen ions and also delivers a large dose of sodium. Providing oxygen therapy would be beneficial in order to keep Ralph's oxygen saturation level at 95 per cent or higher with a non-rebreathe mask at 15 litres per minute until blood gas values stabilise. Then a 24 per cent venturi mask or nasal cannulae at 2 litres per minute can be used. Naturally this may change with frequent monitoring, which is determined by the patient's condition (O'Driscoll et al., 2008).

One additional point to consider is Ralph's diabetes medication. Metformin® is associated with lactic acidosis production in reduced kidney function and so would probably be discontinued. Treatment of Ralph's diabetes in the short term can be with insulin and glucose (as used in the treatment for hyperkalaemia) but will require reappraisal for long-term treatment.

Ongoing Care Issues and the Role of the Nurse

Ralph was found lying on the floor and had been there for an indeterminate period. The reason for this is unclear; however, from an AKI perspective this may be important. Long-term pressure upon muscle tissue (crush injury) leads to tissue hypoxia and tissue death. Muscle tissue breakdown is known as rhabdomyolysis and releases myoglobin, which is nephrotoxic. A common presentation of this condition in AKI is brown urine (in about 50 per cent of cases) that tests positive for blood upon urine dipstick test, limb swelling, myalgia, hypocalcaemia and hyperkalaemia. Elevations in blood levels of amylase and very high levels of creatine phosphokinase (CK) after 12 hours would indicate rhabdomyolysis. Vigilance is required in the assessment and monitoring of patients with AKI who have been involved in this kind of situation.

The Case Scenario: Ongoing Care Issues

Ralph is very ill and requires close observation. He has been commenced on an IV dextrose and insulin infusion to control his elevated plasma potassium and his diabetes. He has an intravenous infusion of 0.9 per cent sodium chloride with 10-minute bolus infusions of 200 mL until his blood pressure is within normal limits. He will then require a continuous infusion set according to hydration and urine output. He may have been given additional medication such as calcium resonium, salbutamol® nebuliser and Furosemide®. Ralph's fluid balance must be monitored closely to avoid under- or overhydration. He is also receiving oxygen therapy to treat hypoxia and acidosis. He requires bed rest and continuous cardiac monitoring for arrhythmia detection. A detailed social, family and risk factor assessment has been completed.

Nursing Care Issues
1. Consider the appropriate ongoing assessment and monitoring required for Ralph.
2. Discuss in detail Ralph's immediate care issues.
3. What is important about Ralph being found on the floor and AKI?
4. Why should the nurse be concerned with infection control in the patient with AKI?
5. What are Ralph's nutritional requirements and how can they best be provided?
6. What are the indications for initiating renal replacement therapy (RRT)?
7. What types of RRT are available to support the treatment of AKI?

The Academy of Royal Medical Colleges (2011) has developed a five-level competency framework for AKI that identifies the required competencies of roles ranging from healthcare assistants to specialist nephrology consultants. The nursing role includes that of level 1 recorder, level 2 recogniser and level 3 primary responder (for advanced practitioners). There are different requirements of knowledge, skills and behaviours for those who have different responsibilities (these are summarised in Table 8.18) but the minimum competence for a nurse is that of a recogniser. For detailed inspection the Acute Kidney Injury Competency Framework (2011) can be viewed and downloaded from the Academy of Medical Royal Colleges Guidelines pages.

Table 8.18   AKI competency framework

Knowledge, skills and behaviour	*Competency role*		
	Recorder e.g. health care assistant	**Recogniser** e.g. staff nurse	**Primary responder** e.g. advanced practitioner
Physiological obs. (BP, P, T, resps)	✓	✓	✓
Urinalysis	✓	✓	✓
Fluid balance		✓	✓
Risk factors		✓	✓
U&Es		✓	✓
Acute illness		✓	✓
Medicine management		✓	✓
Urethral catheterisation		✓	✓
Causes of AKI			✓
Clinical examination			✓
Investigations and management			✓
Complications of AKI			✓
Recovery from AKI		✓	✓

The knowledge, skills and behaviour competencies build upon each other and increase in complexity depending upon role. The minimum role for a qualified nurse is that of a recogniser.

Infection and AKI

Ralph has been treated for a chest infection but it would appear that this has not been successful. Ralph is pyrexial and has an elevated white cell count and c-reactive protein (CRP), all indicating infection. Naturally this will require treatment with an appropriate antibiotic and the collection of samples of urine, sputum and blood for culture, bacteriology and virology. Uraemia renders a person at increased risk of infection because white cells develop functional abnormalities that reduce the ability to adhere to and destroy invading organisms (Meyer and Hostetter, 2007). There is also a reduction in the number of circulating white cells and the response to microorganisms. This is an important care issue because infection will account for a mortality rate of 76 per cent in patients with AKI and sepsis (Steddon et al., 2006). Sepsis is also a major risk factor for AKI and may delay recovery. The acutely ill patient is at risk of infection from a number of sources, particularly where invasive procedures are needed. The incidence of acquired hospital infection has been reported as up to 8.8 per cent, with lung infection accounting for 26 per cent, abdominal infection at 23 per cent, vascular access at 16 per cent, urinary tract at 10 per cent and wound infections at 6 per cent (Hoste et al., 2004). It is vitally important that Ralph does not develop sepsis and to help monitor this staff should be aware of the Surviving Sepsis Campaign (Dellinger et al., 2013) and the Sepsis Six risk factors (Daniels, 2011) (see Chapter 3). Catheterisation to assess urine output is a common procedure in the AKI patient but frequently causes infection. Ralph has known urinary retention, which may make urine output assessment difficult, and so an indwelling catheter may be necessary. This will require increased awareness and caution by the nurse in the prevention of infection. Invasive procedures should be minimised and catheters removed when not needed, such as when there is anuria. Constant vigilance is needed when monitoring the AKI patient, especially around vascular access sites and urinary catheters.

Nutritional Requirements

While Ralph is unwell and may be anorexic and nauseated (a common uraemic symptom) he will require nutritional support (Table 8.19). Malnutrition with AKI will independently increase Ralph's risk for morbidity and death (Stevens et al., 2008). Fiaccadori et al. (2009) call the malnutrition

Table 8.19   Goals of nutritional support

- Prevent protein-energy wasting
- Preserve lean-body mass and nutritional status
- Avoid metabolic derangements
- Avoid complications
- Improve wound healing
- Support immune function
- Minimise inflammation
- Improve antioxidant activity
- Reduce mortality

Source: Adapted from Fiaccadori et al. (2009)

process in AKI 'protein-energy wasting' (PEW) to explain lean body mass wasting and fat depletion. This involves a number of contributing factors: inadequate nutritional support; pre-existing poor nutritional state; acidosis; blood loss; superimposed catabolic illness (e.g. sepsis, trauma); nutrient loss in RRT; and derangements in metabolic and hormonal pathways (Fiaccadori et al. 2009). Fiaccadori et al. (1999) observed severe malnutrition in approximately 40 per cent of patients with AKI on intensive care units. Ralph is at risk of protein-energy wasting, characterised by the loss of lean body mass and fat mass (Fiaccadori et al., 1999). He is also at risk of protein catabolism, hyperglycaemia due to insulin resistance, and decreases in trace elements, water-soluble vitamins (except vitamin C) and vitamins A and E. Malnutrition exacerbates the inflammatory state found in patients with AKI.

Nutritional support requires a multidisciplinary approach, including a dietician to calculate Ralph's needs, and should commence within 24 hours of admission. Enteral feeding is preferred in order to avoid complications associated with parenteral feeding. Enteral feeding has the benefit of improved outcome should the gastrointestinal tract be functional. Each person requires individual assessment, which avoids blanket approaches to nutrition. In some instances protein restriction may be necessary to prevent nitrogen build-up but is unlikely in most cases due to the frequency of catabolism. Protein intake, often given as amino acids, can vary between 0.8 and 1.7 g/kg/day. Ralph will also need a high calorific intake to attenuate catabolism and this can vary, depending upon need, from 25 to 35 non-protein kcal/kg/day (Renal Association, 2014). In Ralph's case a minimum of 1,500 kcal/day is necessary and in many instances in excess of 2000 kcal/day may be given (Stevens et al., 2008). Nutritional demand may increase in hypercatabolism or if Ralph needs renal replacement therapy and supplementation of trace elements, vitamins and electrolytes, and fluid restrictions may be necessary and should reflect Ralph's fluid status and urine output. Nutritional status is a major prognostic factor in patients with AKI and significantly and independently influences length of stay, increased complications and increased mortality (Fiaccadori et al. 2009).

Renal Replacement Therapy

Many of the conservative measures for managing Ralph's condition may be inadequate to control metabolic imbalances caused by AKI. To prevent further deterioration renal replacement therapy (RRT) may be initiated (Table 8.20). It is generally believed that early initiation of RRT is beneficial to patient outcome but precise optimal time is unclear and remains a clinical decision (Stevens et al., 2008; Lewington and Kanagasundaram, 2011; NICE, 2013).

Ralph may require RRT if he does not improve soon. There are three options: peritoneal dialysis, intermittent haemodialysis or haemofiltration and continuous haemodialysis or haemofiltration. Each method of RRT has advantages and disadvantages (Table 8.21). In each instance Ralph would need some form of access, either a peritoneal dialysis catheter or a central venous catheter. RRT brings an additional set of challenges for the AKI patient, such as the additional invasive treatment and anti-coagulation.

Table 8.20 Indications for renal replacement therapy

Clinical indications	Biochemical indications
Urine output <0.3 mL/kg/24 hr or absolute anuria for 12 hr	Refractory hyperkalaemia > 6.5 mmol/L
AKI with multiple organ failure	Serum urea > 30 mmol/L
End organ damage: encephalopathy, myopathy, neuropathy, pericarditis, bleeding	Refractory electrolyte abnormalities: hypo/hypernatraemia, hypercalcaemia
Refractory fluid overload	Refractory metabolic acidosis: pH ≤ 7.1
Poisoning and drug overdose	Tumour lysis syndrome with hyperuricaemia and hyperphosphataemia
Severe hypo/hyperthermia	Urea cycle defects and organic acidurias: hyperammonaemia, methylmalonic acidaemia
Create intravascular space for infusions: blood, plasma, nutrition	For additional information consult the Renal Association Standards (2012) on AKI

Table 8.21 Advantages and disadvantages of renal replacement therapy

Modality	Patient haemodynamic instability	Solute clearance	Volume control	Anti-coagulation
Peritoneal dialysis (PD)	Yes	Moderate	Moderate	No
Intermittent haemodialysis (HD)	No	High	Moderate	With/without
Hybrid techniques	Possible	High	Good	With/without
CVVH	Yes	Moderate/high	Good	With/without
CVVHD	Yes	Moderate/high	Good	With/without

CVVH: continuous haemofiltration, CVVHDF: continuous haemodiafiltration

Source: Adapted from Stevens et al. (2008)

There is insufficient evidence to state which is the best form of treatment though clinical circumstances will clearly dictate choice (Lewington and Kanagasundaram, 2011). However, Macedo and Mehta (2013) suggest that RRT is commenced before there is full-blown failure and the patient is symptomatic in order to support organ function and prevent complications which will influence mortality. It is important that the correct treatment is provided for Ralph at all times and if there is any doubt or concern then referral for nephrology advice is a necessity. NICE (2013) provides referral criteria to guide staff in such circumstances (see Table 8.22).

Ralph's medication must be discontinued for the immediate situation as the action and metabolism of some drugs may be affected by reduced kidney function (Table 8.23). Most drugs are eliminated from the body by the kidney, which makes it essential to consider this in AKI. In many instances problems of toxicity or accumulation can be overcome by reducing the dose; however, this requires knowledge of GFR. Many drugs will require reduced dosage due to margins of safety from toxicity. Some drugs such as Vancomycin® and Genatmicin® will require careful monitoring of therapeutic levels with repeated doses altered accordingly. Wherever possible nephrotoxic drugs should be avoided in order to minimise any further injury to the kidney.

Table 8.22 Nephrology referral

Discuss AKI management with a nephrologist as soon as possible (and within 24 hours) if one of the following is present:

Potential diagnosis requiring specialist treatment (for example, vasculitis or glomerulonephritis)	AKI with no clear cause	Inadequate treatment response
Complications associated with AKI	Stage 3 AKI	eGFR is less than < 30 mL/min/1.73 m2 after AKI episode
Patients with renal transplant and AKI	CKD stage 4 or 5	

Refer adults immediately for Renal replacement therapy if any of the following are not responding to medical management:

Hyperkalaemia	Metabolic acidosis	Symptoms or complications of uraemia such as pericarditis or encephalopathy	Fluid overload and/or pulmonary oedema

Table 8.23 Effects of reduced kidney function on drugs

- Increased drug sensitivity
- Reduced drug and/or metabolites excretion
- Decreased toleration of side effects
- Some drugs become ineffective

Ralph will need expert nursing care to help him through his illness, which will include a multidisciplinary approach. Nursing care will include essential aspects of patient comfort and safety, such as skin care, mouth care and hydration, because of the multiple effects of uraemia. Examples of essential nursing skills as applied to AKI patients can be found in Table 8.24. In addition disease-specific knowledge is needed to minimise risks from potential complications such as infection, and management of additional problems such as nausea, vomiting, pain and itching must be assessed and implemented. Psychological care remains essential, as does accurate and sensitive communication. The prognosis for AKI over the years has remained relatively unchanged at around 50 per cent. Critically ill patients

Table 8.24 Essential nursing skills for patients with AKI

Expert nursing focus	Example AKI patient problems
Comfort	Fatigue, fever, myalgia, pain, insomnia
Infection control	Risk of infection in urinary catheters, vascular access, respiratory, gastrointestinal, wounds
Mouth care	Uraemic ulcers, anorexia, vomiting, thirst, infection
Skin care	Uraemic itching, wound care, fever, oedema, pressure care, delayed wound healing, infection, ischaemia
Hydration and fluid balance	Under/overhydration, fluid restrictions, intravenous fluids
Nutrition	Anorexia, nausea, vomiting, gastritis, dietary restrictions, malnutrition, nasogastric feeding
Medications management	Drug dose alteration, side effect surveillance, prevention of nephrotoxins
Symptoms management	Headache, irritability, erratic memory, confusion, pulmonary oedema
Oxygenation	Pulmonary oedema, LVF, infection
Elimination	Urinary catheter, urinary obstruction, infection, diarrhoea, constipation
Health surveillance: safety	Hypotension, bleeding, dyspnoea, hyperkalaemia, fluid overload, infection
Psychological support and education	Anxiety, depression, metabolic cognitive changes

who develop AKI and require RRT generally have a poor prognosis, with mortality rates exceeding 60 per cent, and unsurprisingly mortality is higher in older patients (Bagshaw, 2008).

Between 8 and 22 per cent of critically ill patients will not recover renal function and will require RRT on a permanent basis. The risk of mortality does not stabilise until after one year following discharge from hospital (Morgera et al., 2008). In one study only 57 per cent attained complete recovery of kidney function, with the remaining 43 per cent attaining partial recovery (Morgera et al., 2008). If kidney function had not recovered within 6 to 12 months of AKI there was no further recovery of function. Two per cent of AKI survivors proceed to end-stage kidney disease. There is a 76 per cent chance of recovery from a single cause but multiple causes of AKI only have a 30 per cent chance of kidney function recovery (Bagshaw, 2008). More recently a large-scale Danish study of 30,762 patients, of which 4,793 had AKI, reported 30-day mortality between 35.5 per cent (AKI risk) and 44.2 per cent (renal failure) as compared to 12.8 per cent in non-AKI patients. Further to this one-year survival ranged between 20.5 per cent (AKI risk) and 23.8 per cent (renal failure) as compared to 10.7 per cent in non-AKI patients indicating the high risk for death in patients with AKI and the need for diligence in care (Gammelager et al., 2012). Therefore, should Ralph recover he will need long-term follow-up to monitor his kidney function along with his diabetes, hypertension and arthritis.

Summary

A patient presenting with AKI requires a comprehensive assessment and management strategy that utilises both general and specific knowledge. Developing knowledge of specific medical conditions can enhance a nurse's ability to care for and manage a patient. While it is acknowledged that some conditions appear more complex than others this should not prevent nurses from learning to care for such patients. Integration of nursing care and medical knowledge enables the development of nursing expertise that can only benefit the patient and enhance the nurse's confidence.

Suggested reading:

National Confidential Enquiry into Patient Outcomes and Death (NCEPOD). *Adding Insult to Injury: A Review of the Care of Patients who Died in Hospital with a Primary Diagnosis of Acute Kidney Injury (Acute Renal Failure)* (London: NCEPOD, 2009) [Online]. Available from: www.ncepod.org.uk/2009report1/Downloads/AKI_report.pdf

National Health Service (NHS). 'Think Kidneys' www.thinkkidneys.nhs.uk/

National Institute for Health and Care Excellence (NICE). *Acute Kidney Injury Prevention, Detection and Management of Acute Kidney Injury up to the Point of Renal Replacement Therapy. NICE Clinical Guideline CG:169* (2013) [Online]. Available from: www.nice.org.uk/Guidance/CG169 (accessed 30 May 2015).

References

Ali, T., I. Khan, N. Simpson, G. Prescott, J. Townend, W. Smith and A. McLeod. 'Incidence and Outcomes in Acute Kidney Injury: A Comprehensive Population-based Study', *Journal of the American Society of Nephrology*, **18** (2007), 1292–8.

The Academy of Royal Medical Colleges. 'Acute Kidney Injury: A Competency Framework Defining the Role of the Expert Clinician (London: The Academy of Royal Medical Colleges, 2011) [Online]. Available from: www.aomrc.org.uk/doc_view/9503-acute-kidney-injury-a-competency-framework (accessed 30 May 2015).

Bagshaw, S. M. 'Short and Long-term Survival after Acute Kidney Injury', *Nephrology, Dialysis and Transplantation*, 23 (2008), 2126–8.

Baker, R. 'Acute Interstitial Nephritis', in P. Glynne, A. Allen and C. Pusey (eds), *Acute Renal Failure in Practice* (London: Imperial College Press, 2002).

Bouchard, J., S. B. Soroko, G. M. Chertow et al.. 'Fluid Accumulation, Survival, and Recovery of Kidney Function in Critically Ill Patients with Acute Kidney Injury', *Kidney International*, 76 (2009), 422–7.

Caddeo, G., S. T. Williams, C. W. McIntyre and N. M. Selby. 'Acute Kidney Injury in Urology Patients: Incidence, Causes and Outcomes', *Nephrology Urology Monthly* 5(5), (2013), 955–61.

Case, J., S. Khan, R. Khalid and A. Khan (2013) 'Epidemiology of Acute Kidney Injury in the Intensive Care Unit', *Critical Care Research and Practice* (2013), Article ID 479730, http://dx.doi.org/10.1155/2013/479730

Challiner, R., J. P. Ritchie, C. Fullwood, P. Loughan and A. Hutchinson. 'Incidence and Consequence of Acute Kidney Injury in Unselected Emergency Admissions to a Large Acute UK Hospital Trust, *BMC Nephrology*, 15(84) (2014). doi: 10.1186/1471-2369-15-84.

Chertow, G. M., E. Burdick, M. Honour, J. V. Bonventre and D. W. Bates. 'Acute Kidney Injury, Mortality, Length of Stay, and Costs in Hospitalized Patients', *Journal of the American Society of Nephrology*, 16 (2005), 3365–70. doi: 10.1681/ASN.2004090740.

Clarkson, M. R., J. J. Friedewald, J. A. Eustace and H. Rabb. 'Acute Kidney Injury', in *Brenner and Rector's The Kidney*, 8th edn (Philadelphia: Saunders Elsevier, 2008).

Cohen, J. J. 'Relationships between Energy Requirements and Na^+ Reabsorption and Other Renal Functions', *Kidney International*, 29 (1986), 32–40.

Crook, M. A. *Clinical Chemistry and Metabolic Medicine*, 7th edn (London: Hodder Arnold, 2006).

Daniels, R. 'Surviving the First Hours in Sepsis: Getting the Basics Right (An Intensivist's Perspective)', *Journal of Antimicrobial Chemotherapy*, 66 (Suppl 2) (2011), ii11–ii23, doi:10.1093/jac/dkq515.

Dellinger, R. P., M. Levy, A. Rhodes et al.. 'Surviving Sepsis Campaign: International Guidelines for Management of Severe Sepsis and Septic Shock 2012', *Critical Care Medicine Journal*, 41(2) (2013), 580–637, doi: 10.1097/CCM.0b013e31827e83af.

Faubel, S., C. L. Edelstein and R. E. Cronin. 'The Patient with Acute Renal Failure', in R. W. Schrier (ed.), *Manual of Nephrology*, 6th edn (Philadelphia: Lippincott Williams and Wilkins, 2005).

Feest, T. G., A. Round and S. Hamad. 'Incidence of Severe ARF in Adults: Results of a Community Based Study', *British Journal of Medicine*, 306 (1993), 481–3.

Fiaccadori, E., M. Lombardi, S. Leonardi, C. F. Rotelli, G. Tortorella and A. Borghetti. 'Prevalence and Clinical Outcome Associated with Pre-existing Malnutrition in Acute Renal Failure: A Prospective Cohort Study', *Journal of American Society of Nephrology*, 10 (1999), 581–93.

Fiaccadori, E., G. Regolisti and A. Cabassi. 'Specific Nutritional Problems in Acute Kidney Injury, Treated with Non-dialysis and Dialytic Modalities', *Nephrology Dialysis Transplantation Plus* (2009), 1–7. doi:10.1093/ndtplus/sfp017.

Finlay, S., B. Bray, A. J. Lewington, C. T. Hunter-Rowe, A. Banerjee, J. M. Atkinson and M. C. Jones. 'Identification of Risk Factors Associated with Acute Kidney Injury in Patients Admitted to Acute Medical Units, *Clinical Medicine*, **13**(8) (2013), 233–8.

Gammelager, H., C. F. Christiansen, M. B. Johansen et al.. 'One-year Mortality among Danish Intensive Care Patients with Acute Kidney Injury: A Cohort Study', *Critical Care*, **16** (2012), R124. doi: 10.1186/cc11420.

Goldberg, L. 'Biochemical Investigations', in P. Glynne, A. Allen and C. Pusey (eds), *Acute Renal Failure in Practice* (London: Imperial College Press, 2002).

Hegarty, J., R. Middleton, M. Krebs, H. Hussain, C. Cheung, T. Ledson, A. Hutchison, P. A. Kalra, H. Rayner, P. Stevens and D. O'Donoghue. 'Severe Acute Renal Failure in Adults: Place of Care, Incidence and Outcomes', *Quarterly Journal of Medicine*, **98**(8) (2005), 661–6.

Hilton, R. 'Acute Renal Failure', *British Medical Journal*, **333** (2006), 786–90.

Ho, K. M. and D. J. Sheridan. 'Meta-analysis of Frusemide to Prevent or Treat Acute Renal Failure', *British Medical Journal*, **430** (2006), 330.

Holley, J. 'Clinical Approach to the Diagnosis of Acute Renal Failure', in A. Greenberg (ed.), *Primer on Kidney Disease*, 3rd edn (San Diego: Academic Press, 2001).

Hoste, E. A., S. I. Blot, N. H. Lameire, R. C. Vanholder, D. de Bacquer and F. A. Colardyn. 'Effect of Nonsocomial Bloodstream Infection on the Outcome of Critically Ill Patients with Acute Renal Failure Treated with Renal Replacement Therapy', *Journal of American Society of Nephrology*, **15** (2004), 454–62.

Hsu, C. Y., J. D. Ordonez, G. M. Chertow, D. Fan, C. E. McCuloch and A. S. Go. 'The Risk of Acute Renal Failure in Patients with Chronic Kidney Disease', *Kidney International*, **74** (2008), 101–7.

Jefferson, J. A., J. M. Thurman and R. W. Schrier (eds). 'Pathophysiology and Aetiology of Acute Kidney Injury, in J. Floege, R. J. Johnson and J. Feehally, *Comprehensive Nephrology*, 797–812 (St Louis: Saunders, 2010).

Kellum, J. A. and J. Decker. 'Use of Dopamine in Acute Renal Failure: A Meta-analysis', *Critical Care Medicine*, **29**(8) (2001), 1526–31.

Khan I. H., G. R. Catto, N. Edward, and A. M. MacLeod. 'Acute Renal Failure: Factors Influencing Nephrology Referral and Outcome', *Quarterly Journal of Medicine*, **90** (1997), 781–5.

Koeppen, B. M. and B. A. Stanton. *Renal Physiology*, 3rd edn (St Louis: Mosby, 2001).

Lamiere, N., W. van Biesen and R. Vanholder. 'Acute Renal Failure', *Lancet*, **365** (2005), 417–30.

Lewington, A. and N. S. Kanagasundaram. *Clinical Practice Guidelines: Acute Kidney Injury* (London: Renal Association, 2011) [Online]. Available from: www.renal. org/guidelines/modules/acute-kidney-injury#sthash.LEeva74i.dpbs (accessed 30 May 2015).

McGee, S., W. B. Abernathy and D. L. Simel. 'Is This Patient Hypovolaemic?', *Journal of the American Medical Association*, **281**(11) (1999), 1022–9.

MacPhee, I. 'Urine Output and Urinalysis', in P. Glynne, A. Allen and C. Pusey (eds), *Acute Renal Failure* (London: Imperial College Press, 2002).

Macedo, E. and R. L. Mehta. 'Timing of Dialysis Initiation in Acute Kidney Injury and Acute-on-chronic Kidney Injury', *Seminars in Dialysis*, **26**(6) (2013), 675–81, doi: 10.1111/sdi.12128.

Mahoney, B. A., W. A. D. Smith, D. S. Lo, K. Tsoi, M. Tonelli and C. M. Clase. 'Emergency Interventions for Hyperkalaemia', *Cochrane Database of Systematic Reviews*, 2 (2005), art. no. CD003235. doi: 10.1002/14651858.CD003235.pub2.

Mehta, R. L., J. A. Kellum, S. V. Shah, B. A. Molitoris, C. Ronco, D. G. Warnock, A. Levin and the Acute Kidney Injury Network. 'Acute Kidney Injury Network: Report of an Initiative to Improve Outcomes in Acute Kidney Injury', *Critical Care*, **11**(2) (2007) [Online]. Available from: http://ccforum.com/content/11/2/R31.

Meyer, T. W. and T. H. Hostetter. 'Pathophysiology of Uraemia', in *Brenner and Rector's The Kidney*, 8th edn (Philadelphia: Saunders Elsevier, 2007).

Morgera, S., M. Schneider and H. H. Neumeyer. 'Long-term Outcomes after Acute Kidney Injury', *Critical Care Medicine*, **36** (2008), S193–7.

Nadeau-Fredette, A-C and J. Bouchard. Fluid Management and Use of Diuretics in Acute Kidney Injury@, *Advances in Chronic Kidney Disease*, **20**(1) (2013), 45–55.

National Collaboration for Chronic Conditions. *Chronic Kidney Disease: National Clinical Guideline for Early Identification and Management in Adults in Primary and Secondary Care* (London: Royal College of Physicians, 2008).

National Confidential Enquiry into Patient Outcomes and Death (NCEPOD). *Adding Insult to Injury: A Review of the Care of Patients who Died in Hospital with a Primary Diagnosis of Acute Kidney Injury (Acute Renal Failure)* (London: NCEPOD, 2009) [Online]. Available from: www.ncepod.org.uk/2009report1/Downloads/AKI_report.pdf (accessed 30 May 2015).

National Health Service (NHS) England. 'Patient Safety Alert on Standardising the Early Identification of Acute Kidney Injury' (2014) [Online]. Available from: www.england.nhs.uk/2014/06/09/psa-aki/ (accessed 1 June 2015).

National Institute for Health and Care Excellence (NICE). *Acutely Ill Patients in Hospital: Recognition of and Response to Acute Illness in Adults in Hospital* (London: National Institute for Clinical Excellence, 2007).

National Institute for Health and Care Excellence (NICE). *Acute Kidney Injury: Prevention, Detection and Management up to the Point of Renal Replacement Therapy, NICE Clinical Guideline CG:169* (2013) [Online]. Available from: www.nice.org.uk/Guidance/CG169 (accessed 30 May 2015).

O'Driscoll, B. R., L. S. Howard and A. G. Davison. 'BTS Guidelines for Emergency Oxygen Use in Adults', *Thorax*, **63**(suppl. VI) (2008), vi1–vi10.

Pannu, N. and P. F. Halloran. 'The Aging Kidney', in A. Greenberg (ed.), *Primer on Kidney Disease*, 3rd edn (San Diego: Academic Press, 2002).

Perel, P. and I. G. Roberts. 'Colloids versus Crystalloids for Fluid Resuscitation in Critically Ill Patients', *Cochrane Database of Systematic Reviews*, **4** (2007), art. no. CD000567. doi: 10.1002/14651858.CD000567.pub3.

Provan, D. and A. Krentz. *Oxford Handbook of Clinical Laboratory Investigations* (Oxford: Oxford University Press, 2002).

Prowle, J. R., J. E. Echeverri, V. Ligabo, C. Ronco and R. Bellomo 'Fluid Balance and Kidney Injury', *Nature Reviews Nephrology*, **6** (2010), 107–15.

Ragaller, M. J. R., H. Theilen and T. Koch. 'Volume Replacement in Critically Ill Patients with Acute Renal Failure', *Journal of the American Association of Nephrology*, **12** (2001), S33–S39.

Renal Association. *eGFR Calculator* (2011) [Online]. Available from: http://egfrcalc. renal.org/ (accessed 01 June 2015).

Renal Association. 'Treatment of Acute Hyperkalaemia in Adults, Clinical Guidelines' (London, UK: Renal Association, 2014) [Online]. Available from: www.renal. org/docs/default-source/guidelines-resources/joint-guidelines/treatment-of-acute-hyperkalaemia-in-adults/hyperkalaemia-guideline-march2014pdf (accessed 26 January 2016).

Royal College of Physicians (RCP). 'National Early Warning Score (NEWS) – Standardising the Assessment of Acute-illness Severity in the NHS' (2012). www. rcplondon.ac.uk/resources/national-early-warning-score-news (accessed 9 April 2015).

Salama, A. 'Haemolytic Uraemic Syndrome and Thrombocytopaenic Purpura', in P. Glynne, A. Allen and C. Pusey (eds), *Acute Renal Failure in Practice* (London: Imperial College Press, 2002).

Steddon, S., N. Ashman, A. Chesser and J. Cunningham. 'Acute Renal Failure', in S. Steddon, N. Ashman, A. Chesser and J. Cunningham (eds), *Oxford Handbook of Nephrology and Hypertension* (Oxford: Oxford University Press, 2006).

Stevens, P., A. Davenport, S. Kanagasundaram and A. Lewington. *Acute Renal Failure (Acute Kidney Injury), Clinical Practice Guidelines* (London: The Renal Association, 2008).

Thakar, C. V. 'Perioperative Acute Kidney Injury', *Advances in Chronic Kidney Disease*, **20**(1) (2013), 67–75.

Vanholder, R., R. de Smet, G. Glorieux et al.. for the European Uremic Toxin Work Group (EUTOX). 'Review on Uremic Toxins: Classification, Concentration, and Interindividual Variability', *Kidney International*, **63** (2003), 1934–43.

Weisberg, L. S. 'Management of Severe Hyperkalaemia', *Critical Care Medicine*, **36**(12) (2008), 3246–51.

9

Small Bowel Obstruction

Beverley Gallacher

Introduction

Small bowel obstruction is a common reason for admission to hospital and surgical consultation, accounting for between 12 and 16 per cent of surgical admissions annually (Maung et al., 2012). In one study, 76 per cent of all patients who presented with a bowel obstruction had an obstruction in the small bowel (Markogiannakis et al., 2007). It is most common in people who have had previous surgery during which the bowel has been handled, as this predisposes the formation of adhesions. Adhesions are created when the sections of the bowel adhere or 'stick' together, a process that impairs small bowel function and its ability to transport partially digested food. A small bowel obstruction is said to occur when the normal flow of the small bowel is interrupted (Huci, 2013). The general consensus is for surgical treatment for large bowel obstruction; however, there is a difference of opinion regarding the need for surgical treatment for small bowel obstruction (Hayanga et al., 2005; Williams et al., 2005; Foster et al., 2006), particularly if the cause of the small bowel obstruction is adhesions. Cox et al. (1993) found that in 123 patients admitted with adhesive small bowel obstruction, the obstruction resolved without surgery in 85 cases (69 per cent); 75 of these resolved within 48 hours and the remaining 10 within 72 hours. Patients who did not require surgery in the study were managed medically and regularly assessed for signs of deterioration as an indication for surgical intervention. Cox et al. (1993) concluded that most adhesive small bowel obstructions resolve with medical treatment within 48 hours; however, they also state that if the patient shows no signs of resolution within 48 hours, surgical intervention should follow. In a 2012 systematic review of 184 studies published between 1991 and 2011, Maung et al. found that patients with a small bowel obstruction who demonstrated evidence of clinical deterioration and ischaemia such as generalised peritonitis, fever, leucocytosis, tachycardia and metabolic acidosis should be managed surgically, whereas patients without these symptoms could safely undergo non-operative medical management. They do state, however, that medical management has a higher rate of failure in patients with a complete intestinal obstruction. The findings of this review form the basis of the Eastern Association for the Surgery of Trauma (EAST) (2012) guidelines for the management of small bowel obstruction (Maung et al., 2012).

Accurate diagnosis and assessment is therefore the key to management of the patient. The need for surgery has traditionally been determined by a number of factors (Table 9.1). However, although the diagnosis of a strangulated obstruction can be determined by the signs of ischaemia, as noted above, and the use of Computerised Tomography (CT), the difference between a complete and partial obstruction can be more difficult to distinguish clinically and if this is the case then a different approach to diagnose the need for surgery, or not, has been suggested (Zielinski and Bannon, 2011). This approach followed the retrospective modelling of the risk factors that were most predictive of surgery. Zielinski and Bannon (2011) suggest there are three risk factors which, if all present in a patient, should determine operative surgical management rather than non-operative medical management. These are obstipation (severe constipation due to intestinal obstruction), mesenteric oedema and presence of the small bowel faeces sign (the presence of feculent material within the small bowel visible on CT scan). This approach needs further testing as to its effectiveness and is not part of the current EAST (2012) guidelines for the management of small bowel obstruction (Maung et al., 2012).

It is important to identify strangulation as this doubles the mortality associated with small bowel obstruction from 10 to 20 per cent (Hayanga et al., 2005), and is a major cause of morbidity and mortality in small bowel obstruction (Zielinski and Bannon, 2011). Strangulation occurs as a result of impaired blood flow to and from the bowel and leads to necrosis of the bowel wall. This necrotic tissue can then become gangrenous and, as a consequence, bleeding into the lumen of the bowel and peritoneal cavity

Table 9.1 Factors that determine medical or surgical intervention

Factor	Treatment
Partial obstruction	Conservative/medical
Complete obstruction	Surgical
Strangulation	Surgical

Source: Adapted from Hayanga et al. (2005)

can occur, eventually leading to perforation (Doherty and Way, 2006). The contents of the lumen will thus contain blood, necrotic tissue, bacteria and toxic bacterial products, which can enter the circulation through lymphatic vessels and the peritoneum and cause septic shock and peritonitis (Doherty and Way, 2006).

Aim and Learning Outcomes

The Aim

The aim of this chapter is to provide the knowledge required to understand the nursing assessment, care and management of a patient suspected of having a small bowel obstruction.

Learning Outcomes

At the end of this chapter the reader will be able to:

1. Identify possible causes of bowel obstruction.
2. Explain the pathophysiological basis of the presenting signs and symptoms of small bowel obstruction.
3. Recognise the immediate assessment, specific monitoring and key investigations required to enable an accurate and timely diagnosis.
4. Describe and explore the ongoing nursing assessment and monitoring required to establish whether the obstruction requires medical or surgical intervention.
5. Appreciate the role of different health professionals in acute assessment and management of small bowel obstruction.

The Case Scenario: The Presenting Complaint

Mrs Brown is an 82-year-old lady with a two-day history of intermittent, colicky, cramping abdominal pain and bloating. Mrs Brown is alert and tells you that she is in some pain, although this has been relieved somewhat by 10 mg IV morphine given in casualty. Mrs Brown has vomited twice this morning and so is now 'nil by mouth'. An intravenous infusion of 1 litre of 0.9 per cent sodium chloride has been commenced to infuse over eight hours. On arrival to the ward Mrs Brown's vital signs are recorded as follows:

Pulse: 84 beats per minute
Blood pressure: 150/80 mmHg

The Case Scenario *continued*

Respiratory rate: 18 breaths per minute
Temperature: 36° C

Mrs Brown lives alone but is accompanied by her son, who lives locally and is her next of kin. A provisional diagnosis of small bowel obstruction has been made.

Consider the following:

1. Describe the structural anatomy of the gastrointestinal tract.
2. Explain how the gastrointestinal tract functions to enable the digestion and absorption of food and drink.
3. Does Mrs Brown's presentation represent an acute and urgent situation?
4. Describe the pathophysiological basis for Mrs Brown's presenting signs and symptoms.
5. List some of the common causes of bowel obstruction.

Structure and Function of the Gastrointestinal Tract

Mrs Brown has a two-day history of abdominal pain and bloating, she has started to vomit and her pain has increased sufficiently for her to seek medical help, which may indicate an acute presentation of bowel obstruction. A large proportion of small bowel obstructions resolve with medical management alone. Resolution is defined as the absence of abdominal pain, reduced abdominal distension, the passage of flatus and/or faeces, and the successful intake of food and drink without recurrence of symptoms (Cox et al., 1993). However, although many obstructions resolve spontaneously, some will not and symptoms worsen, indicating the need for surgical removal. If a deterioration in symptoms is not acted upon swiftly, Mrs Brown could develop hypovolaemic shock and the bowel could perforate, resulting in peritonitis, which is associated with increased mortality. The situation is not urgent at the moment as Mrs Brown's vital signs are within normal limits and her pain has been relieved by morphine. However, she is seriously ill and will require close monitoring as her symptoms could worsen and her condition deteriorate. In order to appreciate the severity and impact of small bowel obstruction a basic knowledge and understanding of the normal anatomy and physiology of the gastrointestinal tract is necessary.

Brief Overview of the Gastrointestinal Tract

Figure 9.1 illustrates the gastrointestinal tract. The bowel, also known as the intestine, is divided into two sections based upon the diameter of the lumen, and includes the small bowel and large bowel. The diameter of the

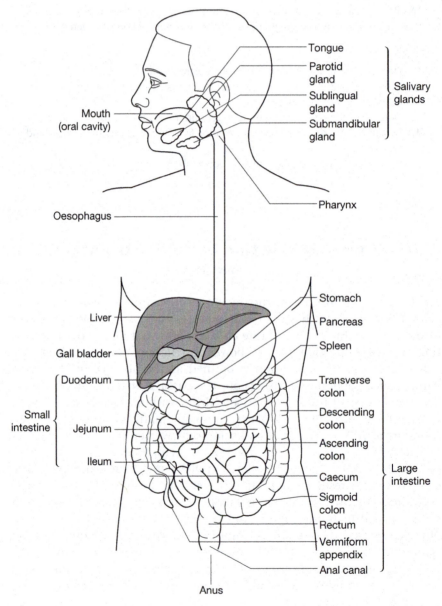

Figure 9.1 The gastrointestinal tract

small bowel varies between 4 cm at the stomach and 2.5 cm at the junction with the large intestine. The large bowel has a diameter of 7.5 cm (Martini, 2014). The purpose of the gastrointestinal tract is to transfer modified nutrients, water and electrolytes from the external environment into the body's internal environment (Martini, 2014). Modification of ingested nutrients is necessary as most food eaten is in the form of molecules that are too large to pass from the bowel into the blood or lymph (internal environment). Large molecules are 'modified' or broken down into small ones that can 'pass' or be absorbed by mechanical and chemical processes.

The Small Bowel

The small bowel achieves mechanical digestion through peristalsis and segmentation. Peristalsis is the rhythmical muscular contraction that breaks down and pushes partially digested food through the gastrointestinal tract. The muscular layer responsible for peristalsis is known as the muscularis externa (Figure 9.2). Segmentation is a similar process to peristalsis; however, muscular movement is both forwards, towards the anus, and backwards.

The large and small bowel have the same common structure as the whole of the gastrointestinal tract, which can be divided into four layers (Figure 9.2). The inner mucosal layer is the surface from which intestinal

Figure 9.2 The layers of the gastrointestinal tract

Source: https://commons.wikimedia.org/wiki/File:Layers_of_the_GI_Tract_english.svg

secretions are produced and through which absorption of essential water and nutrients into the circulation occurs. Anatomically the mucosal layer is made up of thousands of villi and microvilli, which increase the surface area over which secretion and absorption can take place. The second layer is the sub-mucosa, which contains blood and lymphatic vessels and a nervous network called the Meissner's plexus. These are all vital for transporting the absorbed products of digestion, and for stimulating the secretion of digestive juices from the mucosa, respectively. The third layer is composed of two layers of muscle (the stomach has an additional third layer) arranged in a longitudinal and circular manner. Rhythmical contractions of the muscle layers are responsible for peristalsis and segmentation. The final outer layer is the serosa, which is a serous membrane composed of epithelium and connective tissue. Below the diaphragm the serosa is called the peritoneum. The peritoneum is a double membrane, one of which forms the outer layer of the gastrointestinal tract (visceral peritoneum) and the other of which lines the abdominal cavity (parietal peritoneum).

Between the two layers of the peritoneum lies a thin layer of serous, 'peritoneal' fluid, which acts as a lubricant enabling the bowel to move within the abdominal cavity with as little friction as possible. Peristalsis moves partially digested food along the gastrointestinal tract while segmentation allows it to thoroughly mix with digestive chemicals such as bile and pancreatic and intestinal enzymes that are secreted into the small bowel (Figure 9.3). Bile is produced by the liver and secreted via the right and left hepatic ducts (Figure 9.3) for storage in the gall bladder before being released

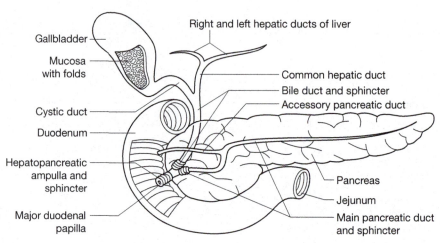

Figure 9.3   The duodenum and related organs

by the relaxation of the hepatopancreatic sphincter, in response to hormonal stimulation. Sphincter relaxation also allows the entry of pancreatic enzymes via the pancreatic duct into the small bowel.

Bile and enzymes thoroughly mix with the food via segmentation. Bile does not contain enzymes, but does contain bile salts, which emulsify lipids (fats). Normally lipid and water do not mix unless an emulsion is created. Bile converts large lipid droplets into many small droplets that are suspended in the watery contents of the intestine, creating an emulsion. This process increases the surface area of the lipid droplets over which the enzyme lipase can act, thus speeding up the chemical digestion of lipid.

Enzymes play a key role in chemical digestion and act as catalysts in the digestive process. Catalysts are compounds that accelerate chemical reactions without being permanently changed or consumed themselves (Martini, 2014). Digestive enzymes speed up the breakdown of food into absorbable molecules. There are three main classes of enzymes, determined by the food group they act upon (Table 9.2).

The approximate quantity of fluid that is ingested and secreted into the gastrointestinal tract per day is shown in Table 9.3. In addition to the daily intake of fluids by mouth, approximately 7 litres of fluid is produced by the intestine every day (Martini, 2014). Much of this liquid will be absorbed

Table 9.2 Enzyme classification

Food group	Enzyme group	Absorbable units	Example
Carbohydrate	Carbohydrase	Monosaccharides	Glucose
Protein	Protease	Amino acids	Tryptophan
Lipid	Lipase	Fatty acids + glycerol	Linoleic acid + glycerol

Table 9.3 Quantity of fluid in the gastrointestinal tract in 24 hours

Source	Daily quantity (mL)
Food and drink	2,000
Saliva	1,500
Gastric secretions	1,500
Bile	1,000
Pancreatic secretions	1,000
Intestinal secretions	2,000

from the lumen of the gut into the blood, along with the small absorbable nutrient molecules produced from the mechanical and chemical digestion of food, such as monosaccharides and amino acids. Indeed, the prime function of the small bowel is to facilitate the final stages of digestion and to absorb the nutrients generated into the blood and lymph. Ninety per cent of nutrient absorption occurs in the small intestine and the rest occurs in the large intestine (Martini, 2014). This is achieved via large circular folds, 'plicae circulares', villi and microvilli. See Martini (2014) for detailed mechanisms of digestion and absorption.

The close proximity of blood and lymphatic vessels to the absorptive mucosal surface facilitates their transport. Monosaccharides and amino acids are absorbed into the blood, and fatty acids and glycerol are largely absorbed into the lymph via lymphatic vessels (also known as lacteals).

The Large Bowel

The large bowel connects the end of the ileum to the anus. Its four main functions are absorption of water, compaction of intestinal contents into faeces, absorption of vitamins generated by the bacteria that occupy it and storage of faeces prior to defecation.

Bowel Obstruction

Definition and Classification of Bowel Obstruction

Intestinal obstruction 'is the blockage or slowing down of the normal flow of intestinal contents and may be partial or complete' (Punder, 2010: 327). Mrs Brown's presenting symptoms of a two-day history of intermittent, cramping abdominal pain, bloating and vomiting typify the halting of digestive processing associated with small bowel obstruction.

There are two broad types of bowel obstruction: mechanical and paralytic (Table 9.4). Mechanical obstruction is caused by a physical blockage of the intestinal lumen – for example, by a cancerous growth – and paralytic obstruction relates to the halting of peristalsis caused by neuromuscular disorders such as multiple sclerosis, vascular disorders such as a mesenteric thrombosis or temporary problems such as post-operative paralytic ileus.

The Causes of Bowel Obstruction

Mechanical obstruction occurs when something physically halts the progression of the contents of the gastrointestinal tract. The intestine may be blocked from the inside by the severe inflammation of inflammatory bowel

Table 9.4 Classification of bowel obstruction

	Type of obstruction	*Definition*
Causes	Mechanical	Lumen physically obstructed with mass or narrowed opening
	Paralytic	Halted peristalsis – causes build up of intestinal contents
Type of lesion	Intrinsic	Obstruction involves lumen or bowel wall
	Extrinsic	Obstruction is external to bowel
Onset	Acute	Usually single occurrence and rapid onset of symptoms
	Chronic	Repeated episodes of partial or complete obstruction due to an ongoing risk factor
Extent	Partial	Lumen partly open – some movement of bowel contents, but activity slowed
	Complete	Total occlusion of lumen – build up of intestinal contents proximal to obstruction
Location	High small bowel	Occurring in duodenum and jejunum
	Low small bowel	Occurring in jejunum and ileum
	Large bowel	Occurring in the large intestine

disease, thickened pancreatic secretions of cystic fibrosis, tumour growth into the lumen or the presence of the parasitic worm ascaris, although this is more common in children living in less developed nations (Gil et al., 2006) (Table 9.5).

Extrinsic causes that originate from outside the intestine can be a tumour and, in women, endometriosis and pregnancy, when the foetus physically presses on the bowel. Obstruction during pregnancy is uncommon, with a reported incidence of 1 in 16,709 deliveries (Hayanga et al., 2005). The bowel can also twist (volvulus), loop back on itself (intussusception Figure 9.4) or protrude through a weak spot in the muscular wall of the abdomen (hernia), which can result in obstruction. External pressure on the herniated bowel impairs its venous drainage and the resultant swelling and oedema can cause it to become permanently trapped (incarcerated). With time, this can compromise the blood supply to the gut and the herniated bowel may become strangulated, leading to ischaemia and necrosis.

Lastly, adhesions can cause bowel obstruction, and with an approximate incidence of 49–60 per cent this is by far the most common cause

Table 9.5 Causes of bowel obstruction

Congenital	Intussusception; cystic fibrosis; Meckel's diverticulum; Hirschprung's disease
Mesenteric vascular disease	Bowel ischaemia
Neuromuscular diseases	Multiple sclerosis; myasthenia gravis; paralytic ileus
Other intrinsic causes	Crohn's disease; ulcerative colitis; volvulus; foreign body in GI tract; abdominal trauma
Infectious diseases	Cytomegalovirus; ascariosis; tuberculosis
Other extrinsic causes	Adhesions (post-operative or radiation induced); endometriosis; tumours; pregnancy; abdominal hernia

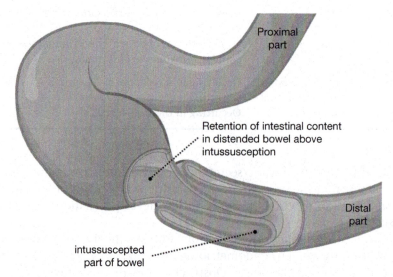

Figure 9.4 Intussusception

Source: https://commons.wikimedia.org/wiki/File:Intussusception_EN.svg (intussusception image)

of small bowel obstruction in developed nations (Zielinski and Bannon, 2011, Doherty and Way, 2006; Foster et al., 2006). Adhesions are bands of scar tissue that cause organs and tissues to stick or bind together and commonly occur following surgical operations. The trauma and inflammation associated with surgical procedures triggers the leakage of plasma and the deposition of fibrin. Fibrin is one of the key factors that cause adhesions. Fibrin is naturally broken down by the enzyme plasmin, which is itself produced in an inactive form called plasminogen. Plasminogen is converted to plasmin in the presence of plasminogen activator, produced by the peritoneum. Adhesions are associated with reduced levels of plasminogen activator, levels that are further lowered by the abrasions and drying that occur during the manual handling of the bowel during an operation (Garden et al., 2012). Ultimately the low levels of plasminogen activator mean that fibrin is not broken down and adhesions are created. Adhesions can also follow irradiation of the bowel: for example, after radiotherapy treatment. Mrs Brown's history may reveal some clues to the potential cause of obstruction in her case.

Pathophysiology Associated with Bowel Obstruction

Once the bowel has become obstructed the contents cannot move forward beyond the obstruction. As a result the contents 'build up' and 'back up' as fluid and food are ingested. The excess build-up of intestinal contents characteristically results in vomiting. Typically when the bowel is obstructed there is heightened peristalsis proximal to the obstruction in an attempt to force the contents of the bowel past the obstruction, often causing abdominal pain. Mrs Brown has experienced both vomiting and pain. Beyond or 'distal' to the obstruction peristalsis is reduced. The absence or presence of peristalsis can be assessed by listening for bowel sounds with a stethoscope, normally performed by a doctor or advanced nurse practitioner.

In addition to partially digested food, the bowel becomes distended with gastrointestinal secretions and gas, from swallowed air, which are unable to move beyond the obstruction and which create additional pressure on the gut wall (Grossman and Porth, 2014). The intestinal distension stimulates the secretion of fluid, electrolytes and succus entericus (intestinal juice) into the bowel, producing further distension, which stimulates further secretion in a positive feedback manner (Zielinski and Bannon, 2011). As this continues, the increased pressure of fluid in the lumen acts directly on the four tissue layers that make up the bowel wall (Figure 9.2), compressing the mucosal blood and lymphatic vessels of the mucosa (Grossman and Porth, 2014). Compression of the blood vessels produces an increase in blood pressure or hydrostatic pressure. As a result normal capillary fluid exchange is compromised and the increase in hydrostatic pressure forces excess leakage of fluid and electrolytes from the capillaries into the surrounding interstitial tissues. At the same time, compression of the lymphatic vessels impairs their ability to drain away excess tissue and interstitial fluid, which naturally accumulates in health, back into the bloodstream (Zielinski and Bannon, 2011). Therefore fluid accumulates in the interstitial space around the bowel and eventually leaks through the mucosa into the gut lumen. If the pressure continues to build within the bowel, fluid will eventually also move through the visceral peritoneum into the peritoneal cavity. Movement of interstitial fluid into the lumen of the bowel triggers a local inflammatory response that increases mucosal permeability, further exacerbating the movement of fluid into the lumen. The altered permeability of the mucosa also facilitates the movement of electrolytes within the interstitial fluid (which originated from the circulation) into the lumen itself, which will be detected as a loss of serum electrolytes. The large shift of fluid from the circulation to the lumen of the bowel results in further intestinal distension, hypovolaemia and dehydration and may result in hypovolaemic shock (Zielinski and Bannon, 2011).

The pressure created by the accumulation of fluid and gastric contents in an obstructed bowel, exerted upon the four tissue layers of the bowel, may result in the perforation of the visceral peritoneum. This gives rise to the serious complication of peritonitis, which carries a high risk of mortality. Clinical signs and symptoms that suggest peritonitis is imminent or has occurred are rebound tenderness, muscular rigidity and spasm, guarding of the abdomen and often the patient adopting a lying position on their side with hips and knees flexed, which reduces peritoneal irritation (Melander, 2004; Grossman and Porth, 2014). In addition, there can be a marked increase in abdominal pain, which is not relieved by analgesia, accompanied by pyrexia. Though they are not yet evident Mrs Brown requires careful observation for these signs, which should be reported immediately to senior nursing and medical staff, as it is likely that surgical intervention would need to follow as a matter of urgency. Every effort should be made to avoid this by relieving the obstruction before perforation occurs. Lastly, compression of blood vessels can lead to a compromised circulation in the bowel, which could result in necrosis and strangulation.

The Case Scenario: The Immediate Assessment Priorities

The initial assessment of signs, symptoms and observations indicates that Mrs Brown is seriously ill and could develop hypovolaemic shock and/or peritonitis and she may require surgery to relieve the obstruction. She is nursed in a bed close to the nurse's station that has piped oxygen and suction. A nurse chaperones and assists the doctor to complete a full clinical examination, making a mental note of the discourse between the doctor and Mrs Brown. During this time, Mrs Brown's past medical history is confirmed as a colectomy for cancer of

The Case Scenario *continued*

the colon five years ago and a cholecystectomy 30 years ago. She does not take any regular medication and is allergic to penicillin. Mrs Brown's pain has eased following morphine 10 mg, which was given in casualty two hours ago; however, her abdomen is quite distended. Venous blood samples are collected and a provisional diagnosis of suspected small bowel obstruction is documented. Mrs Brown is nil by mouth and requires insertion of a nasogastric tube.

Consider the following:

1. Given the large volumes of fluid constantly produced within the small bowel, what problem is Mrs Brown likely to experience at this time?
2. What are the immediate assessment priorities in Mrs Brown's case and what is the rationale for each measure?

Assessment and Reaching a Diagnosis

Mrs Brown will be anxious about her condition and will find herself in an unfamiliar environment on the ward. It is therefore important that the nurse endeavours to reduce her anxiety by introducing herself in a friendly confident manner, explaining to her where she is and what is likely to happen to her in the near future. It is recognised that most people, 58 per cent, broadly fall into one of two groups when it comes to innate coping styles. Some people, 'vigilant copers', require copious amounts of information as too little makes them more anxious, whereas 'avoidant copers' should receive small amounts of information as too much increases anxiety (Mitchell, 2005). However, not everyone falls into one of these two extremes, and two further categories have also been identified, 'flexible copers', whose information requirements adapt depending on the situation, and 'fluctuating copers', whose information requirements vary (Mitchell, 2005). In a systematic review of 11 qualitative studies of patients' experiences of preoperative communication published between 2006 and 2010, Chan et al. (2011) found patients did indeed have different needs for information, that involvement of the relatives reduced both patient and relative anxiety, that patients needed control and time to discuss the information that was given to them, and that healthcare professionalism was important to patients. Healthcare professionalism was associated with reassuring explanations from understanding healthcare professionals. Mrs Brown should be reassured that her condition will be closely monitored every 30 minutes for the next 24 hours in an effort to ensure her safety and comfort and to reduce anxiety. A reduction in pain and abdominal distension and a return of normal bowel sounds would suggest that the obstruction had resolved spontaneously and the need for surgery abated, whereas an increase in the severity of symptoms would indicate the need for surgical laparotomy to resolve the obstruction. The nurse should communicate this information to Mrs Brown and her son, ideally at the same time, as he will be able to reinforce and clarify what his mother has been told, should she require it. Involving relatives in this way will further reduce patient anxiety (Chan et al., 2011).

The Preliminary Assessment

A systematic ABCDE approach to assessment is advocated.

Airway and Breathing

As Mrs Brown is conscious, alert and verbally participating in her assessment on the ward it is obvious that her airway is patent. However, episodes of vomiting are a potential source of airway obstruction and so an ongoing assessment of airway should continue. Mrs Brown's respiratory rate is 18 breaths per minute and the depth is normal. Oxygen saturation is 97 per cent, which is within normal parameters, and therefore she does not need oxygen therapy at this stage. Mrs Brown's respiratory status should be observed and documented every 30 minutes to establish a trend and provide early indication of any deterioration until her abdominal symptoms have been relieved and her condition considered stable.

Circulation

Pulse and blood pressure (BP) will also be assessed initially at 30-minute intervals as they can provide an early indication of hypovolaemic shock (see Chapter 2). Mrs Brown's observations should be carefully compared against her admission results and normal parameters. Circulation can also be assessed indirectly by measuring Mrs Brown's urine output as the first process in urine formation, filtration, is determined by the BP. A fall in BP lowers the glomerular filtration rate (see Chapters 2 and 8), thus reducing urine output. As intestinal obstruction can result in fluid movement from the blood into the intestine and latterly the peritoneal cavity, a fall in BP and subsequent urine output may be observed. Insertion of a urinary catheter to enable accurate hourly monitoring of urine output is a priority and an hourly urine measurement of at least 0.5 to 1 mL/kg/hr is considered satisfactory (Woodrow, 2012). Strict measurement and recording of fluid balance should be maintained. Inspection of the skin and oral mucosa for dryness can also help assessment of the presence of dehydration but a more accurate measure of circulatory volume would be central venous pressure (CVP) monitoring (see Chapter 2).

Disability

Disability or altered state of consciousness should be assessed, although this is often one of the first obvious judgements nurses make when they communicate and interact with the patient. Mrs Brown is alert and communicating freely at this stage and there is no cause for concern. However, if her BP falls sufficiently and she develops hypovolaemic shock her consciousness levels may alter and prompt more specific assessment such as the AVPU (see Chapter 1) or Glasgow Coma Scale (see Chapter 4).

Exposure

Exposure is important to assess in surgical patients as skin integrity can be compromised during bed rest and while in the operating theatre itself. As a result, pressure areas should be observed on admission and an assessment undertaken to determine whether a specific pressure-relieving mattress is required. This assessment should be carried out in accordance with the NICE (2014) guidelines on the prevention and management of pressure ulcers. Four-hourly peripheral temperature is also an assessment priority, as pyrexia may indicate perforation of the bowel and acute peritonitis.

Signs, Symptoms and Immediate Nursing Care

Mrs Brown's most obvious problems are nausea, vomiting and pain. A vomit bowl, tissues and plain water mouthwash should be within easy reach as Mrs Brown's mouth is likely to feel extremely dry as a result of the restriction of oral fluids (Whiteing and Hunter, 2008). Lubricant may be applied to her lips if appropriate (Dougherty and Lister, 2015). As the small bowel is obstructed, the section distal to or beyond the obstruction will not be active in absorbing fluid and nutrients. This, coupled with the vomiting, will contribute to dehydration, electrolyte imbalances and malnutrition. Therefore assessment of the amount, colour and consistency of vomit is important and should be documented clearly on the fluid balance chart.

A nasogastric tube is passed to remove fluid and accumulated air or gas in the gastrointestinal tract and thus relieve pressure. It should also relieve vomiting and thus prevent aspiration, and limit the effect that further swallowed air would have on the abdominal distension (Doherty and Way, 2006). Once a nasogastric (NG) tube has been inserted via the oesophagus, aspirate should be checked for acidity by turning blue litmus paper red to ensure that the tip is situated in the stomach and not the lungs. In order to effectively relieve her symptoms, the tube should be aspirated every 30 to 60 minutes initially, depending on the volume of the aspirate. Between aspirations the tube can be left on 'free drainage' and attached to a drainage bag. If single-use syringes are used it is important that they are discarded into the clinical waste stream after every aspiration attempt. Aspirate from a high small bowel obstruction is likely to have a yellowish green colour and reflects a high proportion of bile. Aspirate from a patient with a low small bowel obstruction is likely to be a darker colour and is described as faeculent, as it contains faecal-like sediment that has an offensive odour. The removal of fluid and gases from the stomach will also help to relieve some pain, distension and discomfort.

Vomiting can lead to dehydration, and although intravenous fluids have been commenced, the intravenous infusion site should be inspected for patency in case it has dislodged from the vein during transit (infiltration or 'tissued') and the infusion checked against the prescription for accuracy of fluid and rate administration. Intravenous access is vital to replace plasma and fluid secreted into the intestinal lumen. IV 0.9 per cent sodium chloride infused at a litre every four to eight hours dependent upon the degree of dehydration is usually favoured; however, a dextrose/sodium chloride infusion may be indicated if blood glucose levels are below 4 mmol/L.

Pain assessment is an important means of establishing the site, character and intensity of the abdominal pain. Mrs Brown should be able to locate where the pain is and describe its character, which typically would be intermittent, colicky and cramp-like as it relates to spasm of the dysfunctional intestine. A verbal rating scale, such as 0 for no pain and 10 for the worst possible pain, allows Mrs Brown to verbalise the pain from her perspective and provides a benchmark against which the effect of pain relief can be measured. IV morphine 5 to 10 mg dependent upon Mrs Brown's body mass should relieve the pain but discomfort from abdominal distension may still be present. Regular pain assessment at 30-minute intervals or if prompted by Mrs Brown should be maintained and documented in the clinical notes. A failure to alleviate the pain at all or worsening pain should be reported to senior nursing and medical staff immediately, as it may signal perforation of the bowel.

As Mrs Brown is likely to be in bed for 48–72 hours while being managed medically, it is vital that she wear knee-length thrombo-embolus deterrent stockings (TEDs), in order to prevent the complication of a deep vein thrombosis (DVT) (NICE, 2010). The graduated compression they provide facilitates the venous return of blood in the legs, preventing stasis, which is the perfect condition for the development of a venous thrombosis. Mrs Brown's legs should be measured to ensure the correct size TEDs are fitted. Prophy-lactic subcutaneous heparin or a weight-adjusted dose of low molecular heparin such as Tinzaparin® sodium would normally be prescribed to pre-vent deep vein thrombosis (NICE, 2010). Finally, encouraging Mrs Brown to bend and flex her knees and ankles while in bed will improve venous return, reducing blood stasis and hence DVT formation.

Specific Investigations

Abdominal girth measurements are one way of assessing abdominal disten-sion. It is thus important to measure the abdomen in the same place every time and it should therefore be marked with a pen. A disposable tape measure should be used and can be left in situ to promote patient comfort. Abdomi-nal inspection by the doctor requires Mrs Brown to lie flat and she will need explanation and assistance from the nurse to achieve this position. The gen-eral shape and contours of the abdomen would be noted: a visible swelling, for example, could indicate a hernia, which could relate to the cause of the obstruction. Surgical scars are important to note as they indicate previous surgical procedures, which could suggest adhesions. Visible movement and pulsation of the abdomen is assessed, as marked visible rippling is strongly suggestive of bowel obstruction (Zielinski and Bannon 2011).

Bowel sounds are listened for by auscultation with a stethoscope. When the bowel is dilated, stretch receptors are activated, resulting in reflex peristaltic contractions (Garden et al., 2012), the effects of which can be heard with a stethoscope as bowel sounds. Peristalsis is increased proximal to the obstruction and the bowel is described as hyperactive. Hyperactive bowel sounds are 'loud, high-pitched tinkling sounds that occur frequently' (Springhouse, 2008: 431) and typically in bowel obstruction the sounds coincide with the patient experiencing abdominal cramps. The bowel distal to the obstruction collapses as fluid and gas no longer enter it and peristalsis is reduced or absent (Garden et al., 2012). The bowel is therefore hypoac-tive and sounds are heard very infrequently. Generally, people with a high small bowel obstruction have hyperactive bowel sounds in the left upper quadrant of the abdomen, and hypoactive bowel sounds elsewhere. A low small bowel obstruction is associated with hyperactive bowel sounds in the left and right upper quadrants of the abdomen, with hypoactive bowel sounds elsewhere.

Abdominal percussion and palpation, by their very nature, may alter bowel activity and can affect bowel sounds and should therefore be per-formed after auscultation. Percussion consists of listening to the sounds made by tapping the abdomen with the hand or finger. It can determine the presence of fluid and air in the abdomen which, if present, is heard as a clear, hollow, drum-like sound. Palpation involves first light and then deep touch, to assess the nature and tenderness of the abdominal organs and the presence of fluid. An abdominal mass may be identified on palpation and may signify the cause of the obstruction. Percussion and palpation may, however, be painful for Mrs Brown; therefore painful areas should be assessed last, and the procedures may be postponed as radiological investigations can provide similar information.

Diagnostic Imaging

Diagnostic imaging provides information that often cannot be obtained by patient history and assessment of clinical signs and symptoms alone. Traditionally, plain abdominal X-rays have been undertaken to assist in the diagnosis of small bowel obstruction as X-ray equipment is commonly available and the procedure is inexpensive; however, there is some debate as to their sensitivity in diagnosis and in many settings plain abdominal X-rays have been supplanted by CT scan (Dayton et al., 2012). A systematic review of patients with ischaemia and complete small bowel obstruction found that CT scan had high positive and negative predictive values for obstruction coupled with a high sensitivity and specificity (Mallo et al., 2005). CT is also extremely useful in identifying the cause of the obstruction, such as a tumour, hernia, intussusception or inflammatory bowel disease (Dayton et al., 2012), and is particularly valuable in identifying ischaemic changes associated with strangulation, and specific types of obstruction such as closed loop obstruction, both of which require urgent surgical intervention (Furukawa et al., 2003, Zielinski and Bannon, 2011). 'A closed loop obstruction is a form of mechanical intestinal obstruction where two points of the intestine along its course are obstructed at a single site' (Furukawa et al., 2003: 346).

Diagnosis of small bowel obstruction has become faster and easier since the development of multidetector CT scanners (Desser and Gross, 2008). Unlike conventional CT scanners, these are able to generate multiple slices through the abdomen simultaneously, increasing the speed at which images are generated. As a result, CT scan, and if available multidetector CT scan, is now recommended for the diagnosis of small bowel obstruction within the Eastern Association for the Surgery of Trauma (EAST) practice management guidelines for small bowel obstruction (Maung et al., 2012).

There is also evidence that diagnostic imaging can have a therapeutic role in the management of small bowel obstruction as well as a diagnostic one. Patients given a water-soluble contrast medium such as Gastrografin® via their NG tube have been shown to have a shorter time to resolution of their small bowel obstruction, shorter hospital stay and reduced operative rate (Di Saverio et al., 2008; Safamanesh et al., 2013). Water-soluble contrast is hyperosmotic, which means it causes water to move into the lumen of the bowel. This reduces the oedema in the bowel wall enabling its normal function to be resumed, and also increases the pressure gradient at the obstruction site which stimulates motility.

Medical Management

Continuous unrelieved pain of increasing severity and a distended abdominal girth suggest that Mrs Brown's obstruction has not resolved spontaneously and her observations reveal deterioration in her haemodynamic status. Movement of fluid and electrolytes from the circulation into the intestinal lumen will result in a fall in BP, which will initially be compensated for by an increase in heart rate and peripheral vasoconstriction. If the fluid loss is not reversed, compensation will fail to maintain the BP and a decrease will be observed. In turn the renal glomerular filtration rate will fall, leading to a decrease in urine output below 0.5 mL/kg/hr. Mrs Brown's increased pulse, low BP and poor urine output suggest that she may be developing hypovolaemic shock, which requires immediate resuscitation (see Chapter 2). Although sodium and potassium are lost from the circulation, toxic products of metabolism such as urea and creatinine are retained as a consequence of reduced renal blood flow, as reflected in Mrs Brown's blood results. The resultant hypoperfusion will stimulate an increase in respiratory rate in an effort to deliver more oxygen to the tissues; however, this may not be sustainable and an initial period of tachypnoea may be followed by a period of bradypnoea. Lastly, a rise in temperature and leucocyte count could indicate strangulation and/or peritonitis. Peritonitis is associated with a high mortality rate, particularly in the presence of hypovolaemic shock, and so the underlying cause requires immediate surgical intervention.

The Case Scenario: Management and Care Issues

Mrs Brown has been stable overnight. She has received two injections of morphine for abdominal pain. However, as the morning progresses Mrs Brown's condition begins to deteriorate. She has been given a further 10 mg of IV morphine to minimal effect and her pain is continuous and increasing in severity. Her observations and some blood results are compared to those taken on admission and the normal range below. Given this deterioration, Mrs Brown is planned for theatre within the hour.

The Case Scenario *continued*

	Normal range	On admission	12 hours later
Pulse (beats/min)	60–100	84	98
BP (mmHg)	100–140 systolic	150/80	115/75
Respirations (/min)	12–18	18	24
Temperature (°C)	35.6–37.8	36	37.5
SpO$_2$ (per cent)	95–99	97 on 40% oxygen	92–96 on 40% oxygen
Urine output	0.5 mL/kg/hr	Nil	100 mL
Sodium (mmol/L)	135–145	136	130
Potassium (mmol/L)	3.5–5.0	3.7	2.5
Chloride (mmol/L)	98–108	108	97
Urea (mmol/L)	2.2–7.7	7.2	12.4
Creatinine (μmol/L)	50–130	100	140
Leucocytes (¥ 109/L)	3.5–9.0	5.4	9.0

Consider the following:

1. Explain the difference in blood results received over 12 hours.
2. What are the current treatment options for an obstructed bowel?
3. What factors might inform the choice of immediate surgical management?
4. What are Mrs Brown's main care issues?

Surgical Management

Given the progression in her symptoms Mrs Brown is likely to have an abdominal laparotomy, which will be guided by the radiological findings. Any adhesions that are likely to be responsible for her obstruction will be divided to relieve the obstruction. Should an obstructing lesion also be present and be located wholly within the section of small bowel, then this would be resected and the remaining small bowel rejoined in a 'primary re-anastomosis'. If a malignant lesion was responsible for the obstruction, then the bowel proximal to the obstruction may be brought to the surface of the abdomen in a stoma. If possible the malignancy would be removed; however, this may not always be the optimal course of action if the cancer has spread to secondary areas (metastasised), as a better quality of life may be achieved by not performing this surgery.

Table 9.6 Theatre checklist

- Informed consent – gained by the surgeon and / or anaesthetist and documented in notes.
- Trend of vital signs observations clearly recorded and present.
- Medical notes, X-rays, prescription chart and supporting documentation.
- Weight (kg).
- Waterlow score (or similar pressure sore risk assessment).
- Pre-theatre oxygenation with 24% oxygen via a venturi mask to maintain oxygen saturation at more than 95%.
- Venous blood sample results received and documented clearly in the notes.
- Blood group, save and cross match ready for use in the blood bank.
- Check current drug therapy and ensure the patient has not been taking anticoagulant therapy. A clotting screen may be required.
- Intravenous access with IV 0.9% sodium chloride infusion.
- Empty urinary catheter and document on fluid balance chart.
- Pain assessment and relief.
- Pre-medication – might not be required if the patient has been receiving regular opiate pain relief.
- Prophylactic IV antibiotic cover may be administered at the surgeon's discretion.
- Nil by mouth: 4 hours is considered to be sufficient time to ensure that the stomach is emptied, Nasogastric bag emptied and contents measured and documented if appropriate.
- Name bands on both wrists stating name, date of birth and hospital ID number.
- Allergy alert bands for penicillin on both wrists.
- Skin cleansing will be determined by local hospital policy and surgeon preference.
- Operation site clearly marked by the surgeon.
- MRSA screening: nasal, axilla and groin swabs sent for MC&S.
- MRSA prophylaxis: Octenesan® body wash and hair shampoo and Bactroban® ointments.
- Measure and fit TED stockings.
- Theatre gown and cap to cover hair to reduce risk of infection.
- Remove personal items such as jewellery (or cover band rings), contact lenses, dentures, hair pieces, hearing aids, body piercing (or cover), false nails. Safely store belongings as per local policy.

Open vs. Laparoscopic Surgery

Adhesive small bowel obstruction can be relieved by laparoscopic surgery, although 'laparotomy remains the standard surgical approach to acute SBO' (O'Connor and Winter, 2012: 12). It is felt that some surgeons may be reluctant to use a laparoscopic technique, believing that the distension of the bowel reduces visibility during the operation, thus increasing the chances of bowel

injury (O'Connor and Winter, 2012). Indeed, often an additional surgical incision of up to 5 cm (laparoscopic assisted) is required to resect necrotic bowel,
and in some patients a larger incision (laparoscopic converted) is necessary. A
retrospective review of over 2000 patients who had undergone laparoscopic
surgery, however, suggested that it was associated with a lower morbidity and
shorter hospital stay (O'Connor and Winter, 2012). In addition, the review
highlighted the reduced risk of recurrence with laparoscopic surgery, as laparotomy itself is associated with bowel handling and future adhesion risk.

Mrs Brown should be aware from admission that she may ultimately need
surgery to resolve her small bowel obstruction. Nevertheless she is likely
to feel anxious, and should be reassured in a calm manner. The nurse can
help by giving information about the procedure itself, what to expect in
the anaesthetic room, details of the wound, the possibility of a stoma and/
or drains, intravenous fluid lines and the patient-controlled analgesia (PCA)
she may have on return to the ward. The nurse is responsible for completing
the theatre preparation checklist (Table 9.6) pertinent to Mrs Brown, ensuring that the safety checks in relation to patient identification and patient
preparation have been made.

Mrs Brown's son should be contacted and fully informed and Mrs Brown
should be warned that she may have a temporary or permanent stoma formed.
According to local policy, prophylactic antibiotics may be given to Mrs Brown
on her induction in the anaesthetic room. This precaution is indicated due to
the large number of bacteria present in the bowel, which could potentially move
into the bloodstream during her surgery causing septicaemia, though penicil-
lin-based drugs would be avoided due to her allergy. Surgical site infection is
also reduced by the use of prophylactic antibiotics, as indicated within the NICE
(2008) guidelines for the prevention and treatment of surgical site infection as
this type of surgery involving the bowel is classified as 'contaminated'.

Mrs Brown has had previous abdominal surgery, which predisposes her
to developing adhesions, which is one explanation for her obstruction. A
second could be that the cancer that she was treated for five years ago has
returned; this could be intrinsic or extrinsic to the bowel, but either way
could result in an obstruction. At surgery it became apparent that Mrs Brown
did in fact have adhesions that caused her small bowel obstruction, which
were successfully divided, and a small portion of her bowel was resected. She
made a good recovery and was discharged home six days after her surgery.

Summary

Small bowel obstruction is said to occur when the contents of the small
bowel fail to move forward. Causes are either mechanical or paralytic and
the most common cause in the developed world is adhesions associated

with previous surgery or radiotherapy. In 69 per cent of cases adhesive small bowel obstruction will resolve spontaneously, though some patients do need immediate surgery particularly if the blood supply to the bowel has been compromised, such as in strangulation (Maung et al., 2012). This is more often associated with a total rather than partial obstruction and thus current practice is to assess the completeness of the obstruction and whether the bowel circulation has been compromised (Williams et al., 2005). This chapter has discussed the pathophysiology of small bowel obstruction and illustrated how such changes can be identified from the signs and symptoms presented by patients such as Mrs Brown. Key aspects of patient management include nursing the patient 'nil by mouth', regular aspiration of a nasogastric tube, intravenous fluids to prevent hypovolaemia and strict fluid balance measurement. Increasing pain, further abdominal distension and signs of shock or peritonitis (suspected if increasing pain is less responsive to analgesia, there is guarding of the abdomen, raised white cell count and pyrexia) are all signs of deterioration that should prompt immediate surgical intervention. The management of a patient with small bowel obstruction is, as Williams et al. (2005: 1144) state, 'a fine balance between waiting for the obstruction to resolve with conservative therapy and rushing the patient off to the operating room'. The nurse has a crucial role in the assessment of this fine balance.

Further Reading

Martini, F. H. *Fundamentals of Anatomy and Physiology*, 9th edn (e book) (San Francisco: Pearson, Benjamin Cummings, 2014).

References

Chan, Z. C. Kan, P. Lee, I. Chan and J. Lam. 'A Systematic Review of Qualitative Studies: Patients' Experiences of Preoperative Communication', *Journal of Clinical Nursing*, **21** (2011), 812–24.

Cox, M. R., I. F. Gunn, M. C. Eastman, R. F. Hunt and A. W. Heinz. 'The Safety and Duration of Non-operative Treatment for Adhesive Small Bowel Obstruction', *Australia and New Zealand Journal of Surgery*, **63** (1993), 367–71.

Dayton, M. T. et al.. 'New Paradigms in the Treatment of Small Bowel Obstruction', *Current Problems in Surgery*, **49** (2012), 642–717.

Desser, T. S. and M. Gross. 'Multidetector Row Computed Tomography of Small Bowel Obstruction', *Seminars in Ultrasound CT and MRI*, **29** (2008), 308–21.

Di Saverio, S., F. Catena, L. Ansaloni, M. Gavioli, M. Valentino and A. D. Pinna. 'Water-Soluble Contrast Medium (Gastrografin) Value in Adhesive Small Intestine Obstruction (ASIO): A Prospective, Randomised, Controlled Clinical Trial', *World Journal of Surgery*, **32** (2008) 2293–2304.

Doherty, G. M. and L. W. Way (eds). *Current Surgical Diagnosis and Treatment*, 12th edn (New York: McGraw-Hill, 2006).

Dougherty, L. and S. Lister (eds). *The Royal Marsden Manual of Clinical Nursing Procedures*, 9th edn (Chichester: John Wiley & Sons Inc. 2015)

Foster, N. M., M. McGory, D. Zingmond and C. Y. Ko. 'Small Bowel Obstruction: A Population Based Appraisal', *Journal of the American College of Surgeons*, **203** (2006), 170–6.

Furukawa, A., M. Yamasaki, M. Takahashi, N. Nitta, T. Tanaka, S. Kanasaki, K. Yokoyama, K. Murata and T. Sakamoto. 'CT Diagnosis of Small Bowel Obstruction: Scanning Technique, Interpretation and Role in the Diagnosis', *Seminars in Ultrasound, CT and MRI*, **24**(5) (2003), 336–52.

Garden, O. J., A. W. Bradbury, J. R. L. Forsythe and R. W. Parks. *Principles and Practice of Surgery*, 6th edn (Edinburgh: Churchill Livingstone, 2012).

Gil, J. M. G., C. M. L. Esturo and R. P. Ayala. 'Intestinal Obstruction due to Ascaris', *The Internet Journal of Surgery*, **8**(2) (2006).

Grossman, S. C. and C. M. Porth. *Porth's Pathophysiology: Concepts of Altered Health States*, 9th edn (Philadelphia, Wolters Kluwer Health/Lippincott Williams & Wilkins, 2014).

Hayanga, A. J., K. Bass-Wilkins and G. B. Bulkley. 'Current Management of Small Bowel Obstruction', *Advances in Surgery*, **39** (2005), 1–33.

Huci, T. 'Acute GI obstruction', *Best Practice & Research in Clinical Gastroenterology*, **27** (2013) 691–707.

Mallo, R. D., L. Salem, T. Lalani, 'Computed Tomography Diagnosis of Ischaemia and Complete Obstruction in Small Bowel Obstruction: a Systematic Review', *Journal of Gastrointestinal Surgery*. **9** (5) (2005) 690–4.

Markogiannakis, H., E. Messaris, D. Dardamanis, N. Pararas, D. Tzertzemelis, P. Giannopoulos, A. Larentzakis, E. Lagoudianakis, A. Manouras and I. Bramis. 'Acute Mechanical Bowel Obstruction: Clinical Presentation, Etiology, Management and Outcome', *World Journal of Gastroenterology*, **13** (3) (2007) 432–7.

Martini, F. H. *Fundamentals of Anatomy and Physiology*, 9th edn (e book) (San Francisco: Pearson, Benjamin Cummings, 2014).

Maung, A. A., D. C. Johnson, G. L. Piper, R. R. Barbosa, S. E. Rowell, F. Bokhari, J. N. Collins, J. R. Gordon, J. H. Ra and A. J. Kerwin. 'Evaluation and Management of Small-Bowel Obstruction: An Eastern Association for the Surgery of Trauma Practice Management Guideline', *The Journal of Trauma and Acute Care Surgery*, **73**(5), Suppl 4 (2012), S362–9.

Melander, S. D. *Case Studies in Critical Care Nursing. A Guide for Application and Review*, 3rd edn (Philadelphia: Saunders, 2004).

Mitchell, M. *Anxiety Management in Adult Day Surgery: A Nursing Perspective*. (London: Whurr, 2005).

National Institute for Health and Clinical Excellence (NICE). *Surgical Site Infection: Prevention and Treatment of Surgical Site Infection Guideline CG:74* (2008) [Online]. Available from: www.nice.org.uk/guidance/cg74/chapter/1-recommendations#preoperative-phase (accessed 30 April 2015).

National Institute for Health and Clinical Excellence (NICE). *Venous Thromboembolism: Reducing the Risk: Reducing the Risk of Venous Thromboembolism (Deep Vein Thrombosis and Pulmonary Embolism) in Patients Admitted to Hospital)* (2010) [Online]. Available from: www.nice.org.uk/guidance/cg92 (accessed 30 April 2015).

National Institute for Health and Clinical Excellence (NICE). *Pressure Ulcers: Prevention and Management of Pressure Ulcers Guideline CG:179*. (2014) [Online]. Available from:

www.nice.org.uk/guidance/cg179/chapter/1-recommendations#prevention-adults (accessed 30 April 2015).

O'Connor, D. B. and D. C. Winter. 'The Role of Laparoscopy in the Management of Acute Small Bowel Obstruction: A Review of over 2000 Cases', *Surgical Endoscopy,* **26** (2012) 12–17.

Punder, R. *Nursing the Surgical Patient,* 3rd edn (Edinburgh: Bailliere Tindall, 2010).

Safamanesh, S., A. Pazouki, Z. Tamannaie, B. Mohammadalipour, K. Ramezani, E. Hajnasrollah and S. Chaichian. 'Evaluation of Gastrografin Therapeutic Role in the Management of Small Bowel Obstruction', *Journal of Minimally Invasive Surgical Sciences,* **2**(1) (2013) 90–3.

Springhouse, Inc. (ed.). *Critical Care Nursing Made Incredibly Easy* (Philadelphia: Lippincott, Williams and Wilkins, 2008).

Whiteing, N. and J. Hunter. 'Nursing Management of Patients Who Are Nil by Mouth', *Nursing Standard,* **22**(26) (2008), 40–5.

Williams, S. B., J. Greenspon, H. Young and B. Orkin. 'Small Bowel Obstruction: Conservative vs. Surgical Management', *Diseases of the Colon and Rectum,* **48** (2005), 1140–6.

Woodrow, P. *Intensive Care Nursing: A Framework for Practice,* 3rd edn (Abingdon: Routledge, 2012).

Zielinski, M. and M. Bannon. 'Current Management of Small Bowel Obstruction', *Advances in Surgery,* **45** (2011) 1–29.

10

Diabetic Ketoacidosis

Paula Mayo and David Clarke

Introduction

Diabetes mellitus is a metabolic disorder that has multiple causes and is identified by the continued presence of a fasting plasma glucose level above 7 mmol/L with associated disturbances of carbohydrate, fat and protein metabolism. There are two distinct types of diabetes mellitus.

- Type 1 diabetes: reduced or absent insulin secretion caused by the auto-immune destruction of the pancreatic beta cells.
- Type 2: the action of the circulating insulin is reduced due to the presence of insulin resistance, which occurs with increased weight gain and inactivity.

Chronic absence of or insufficient active circulating insulin causes blood glucose levels to rise, which over time will lead to the development of diabetes-related complications which result in human and financial burden to primary care, acute hospitals and community services. However, with appropriate management and control many of the diabetes-related complications can be avoided.

Diabetes is an increasingly common, costly, serious, potentially debilitating and life-threatening condition which affects people across the globe in both developed and developing countries (Ginter and Simko, 2012). At present it affects approximately 6 per cent of the UK population with 3.9 million people now known to have been diagnosed with the condition; of these approximately 250,000 have type 1 diabetes and the remainder have type 2 (Diabetes, UK, 2015). However, due to the insidious and hidden nature of diabetes it is estimated that there are a further 630,000 people living with type 2 diabetes in the UK who have not been diagnosed, and if current trends continue it is estimated that by 2025, five million people in the

UK will have diabetes (Diabetes UK, 2015). Indeed, the incidence of both type 1 and type 2 diabetes is rising so rapidly that it is considered to have reached epidemic proportions. While the rise in type 2 diabetes worldwide is largely attributed to increasing levels of obesity as a result of sedentary lifestyles and high calorie, fat-laden diets, the rapid rise of type 1 diabetes is less easy to explain (Shaw et al., 2010; Ginter and Simko, 2012). The burden of diabetes to both individuals and the economy is substantial. In 2012, it was estimated that the total direct and indirect costs associated with diabetes in the UK currently stand at £23.7 billion; this figure is predicted to rise to £39.8 billion by 2035–6 (Hex et al., 2012). These authors noted that a very high percentage (79 per cent) of NHS diabetes spending is incurred in treating complications, many of which are preventable.

The long-term complications of diabetes resulting from poor blood glucose control are well recognised; these include impairments resulting from vascular complications such as renal failure, neuropathy, stroke, retinopathy and amputation. However, suboptimal blood glucose control in people with diabetes can also cause the acute complications of hypoglycaemia and hyperglycaemia. The seriousness of both conditions should not be underestimated as they can both be life threatening if not treated quickly and appropriately. A rapid escalation of blood glucose levels causing hyperglycaemia is responsible for the acute presentation of diabetic ketoacidosis (DKA). DKA is a life-threatening complication that affects a significant number of people, leading to hospital admission each year. It is due to a relative or absolute deficiency of insulin and is the most common hyperglycaemic emergency in patients with diabetes (Umpierrez et al., 2004; Savage et al., 2011), with the person often requiring high level monitoring and management in an intensive care unit (Savage and Kilvert, 2006). DKA occurs predominantly in people who have type 1 diabetes but it can occur with type 2 diabetes, particularly in the presence of severe infection or episodes of metabolic stress. Therefore the focus of this chapter is the acute assessment and management of a young person presenting with DKA. The management strategies are based upon recommendations from the Joint British Diabetes Societies Guidelines (JBDS) (2013) and Clinical Guidelines (NG:18) from the National Institute for Health and Care Excellence (2015).

Aim and Learning Outcomes

The Aim

The aim of this chapter is to provide the reader with a logical and comprehensive approach to the assessment and first line management of a person with DKA.

Learning Outcomes

At the end of this chapter the reader will be able to:

1. Identify and discuss the normal and altered pathophysiology of blood glucose control.
2. Differentiate between type 1 and type 2 diabetes.
3. Define and explain the pathophysiological changes that occur in the body as a result of hyperglycaemia.
4. Outline and describe the main causes of DKA.
5. Consider the assessment process and the investigations required to enable an accurate and timely diagnosis.
6. Using evidence-based practice, consider the immediate care and management that a person admitted to hospital with acute DKA will require.

The Case Scenario: The Presenting Complaint

Lucy is an 18 year old who was diagnosed with type 1 diabetes when she was six years old. Her diabetes is currently controlled with a basal/bolus insulin regimen. Lucy's insulin regimen comprises Lantus® (ultra long-acting peakless insulin) 22units at bedtime to provide Lucy with her basal insulin requirements, supplemented by bolus administration of Novorapid® (rapid-acting insulin) prior to each main meal to control the expected rise in post-prandial blood glucose level. The dose of Novorapid® is determined by Lucy and is based upon the type and amount of food she is about to eat and her current blood glucose levels. On the day of admission Lucy had been shopping with her mother and friend. At lunchtime, having ordered a meal, Lucy realised that she did not have her Novorapid® insulin but, as she was hungry and her lunch had been served, she decided to eat and administer her insulin as soon as she returned home. Lucy was aware that this was not ideal but felt confident that her post-meal blood glucose levels would be partially maintained by the amount of walking around the shops she had done. Approximately two hours after lunch, Lucy complained of abdominal pain, leg cramps and nausea. She subsequently vomited, and appeared pale, sweaty and clammy and less alert than usual. Her mother and friend escorted her to the nearest accident and emergency unit. On admission Lucy is semi-conscious, her abdomen is tender and distended and she continues to vomit bile-stained fluid. A provisional diagnosis of DKA is made.

Consider the following:

1. Describe the normal physiology of the pancreas, the production of insulin and the normal homeostatic control of blood glucose levels to maintain them between 4 and 7 mmol/L.
2. Note the distinct features of type 1 and type 2 diabetes mellitus.
3. Consider the physiological changes in the body caused by diabetes that result in the development of hyperglycaemia.
4. What are the common predisposing factors, signs and symptoms of DKA?

Normal Blood Glucose Regulation

A good working knowledge of the normal physiological mechanism of blood glucose control is essential if healthcare practitioners are to fully understand, recognise and manage the implications of disordered blood glucose control.

Anatomy and Physiology in the Absence of Diabetes

The pancreas, a major organ in the body with endocrine and exocrine functions, plays a significant role in the normal homeostatic control of blood glucose. The endocrine pancreas consists of small clusters of cells called the islets of Langerhans, which are scattered among the exocrine cells and named after the German anatomist Paul Langerhans. There are approximately one million individual clusters of islet cells within the pancreas and each islet contains approximately 1,000 endocrine cells (Rorsman, 2005; Marieb, 2015).

Within each islet of Langerhans there are four main types of cells. The alpha and beta cells are predominantly responsible for the regulation of blood glucose levels.

1. Alpha (α) cells make up approximately 20 per cent of all the cells in each islet. These secrete glucagon, which raises blood glucose levels.
2. Beta (β) cells account for approximately 75 per cent of all of the islet cells. These secrete insulin, which lowers blood glucose levels.
3. Delta (δ) cells are the majority of the remaining cells and they secrete somatostatin, which is a growth hormone-inhibiting hormone.
4. F cells, also known as PP cells, are limited in number and are scattered sparsely throughout each islet of Langerhans. They secrete pancreatic polypeptide, which has a part to play in the exocrine function of the pancreas and is therefore not relevant to diabetes.

Normal Blood Glucose Homeostasis

At a cellular level, the availability of glucose is essential for normal energy production and cell function and the presence of insulin is required for the uptake of glucose into the cell. A range of mechanisms exist to control blood glucose levels and ensure adequate availability for the cells. The commonest source of glucose is from the ingestion of dietary simple sugars and/or complex carbohydrate foods such as pasta, potatoes, cakes and bread. The glucose from these foods is absorbed from the stomach and small intestine into the bloodstream, causing a direct rise in blood glucose levels. The detection

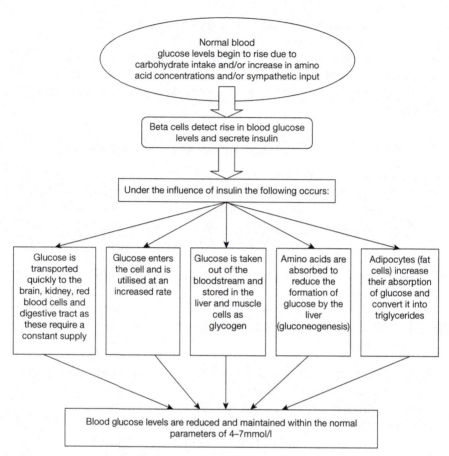

Figure 10.1   Action of insulin on target cells

of a rise in glucose levels stimulates beta cells to secrete insulin and facilitate the uptake of glucose into the cell (Figure 10.1).

Glucagon Secretion

The secretion of glucagon from the pancreatic alpha cells is equally important as insulin in the maintenance of optimal blood glucose levels. In response to falling blood glucose levels glucagon is released, causing the conversion of glycogen into glucose within the liver. This process serves to raise blood glucose levels and prevent the person from experiencing hypoglycaemia (Figure 10.2). These homeostatic mechanisms are designed to maintain blood glucose levels within the normal range of 4 to 7 mmol/L. Amino acids, found in dietary protein as well as being synthesised by the

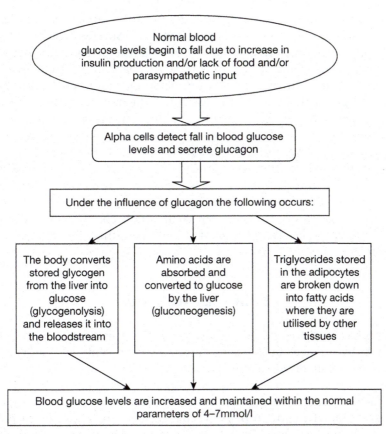

Figure 10.2   Action of glucagon on target cells

body, also play a part in blood glucose control. In between meals or during a fast as blood glucose levels decrease amino acids are released from muscle cells into the bloodstream and transported to the liver. The liver converts amino acids into glucose via a process called 'gluconeogenesis'. This 'new' glucose is then transported back into the bloodstream, causing blood glucose levels to rise (Figure 10.2). This process is part of the body's compensatory mechanism to ensure that vital organs such as the kidneys and brain, which cannot store glucose, have a continuous supply regardless of whether the person has eaten or not.

The 'fight or flight' sympathetic nervous system mechanism, which is triggered when faced with a dangerous, difficult or frightening situation, can also enable an increase in blood glucose. Sympathetic stimulation of the anterior pituitary gland releases adreno-cortico-trophic hormone (ACTH), which stimulates the adrenal gland to release growth hormone, cortisol and adrenaline, which promote hepatic glucose release via the processes of gluconeogenesis and glycogenolysis. Simultaneously the pancreatic alpha cells secrete glucagon to provide the person with the extra energy that may be required to escape the dangerous situation. Each mechanism causes further increases in blood glucose levels (Figure 10.2). Once the fight or flight situation has abated, the parasympathetic nervous system triggers the release of insulin to reduce the elevated blood glucose levels back to within normal limits. Once insulin has been secreted it is degraded and removed from the circulation by the liver and kidneys. This occurs quite rapidly after secretion, giving insulin an active biological half-life of only 6 to 10 minutes. It is expected that all insulin produced will be broken down within 12 to 20 minutes of secretion, thus preventing an abundance of circulating insulin, which could cause a decrease in blood glucose levels to below 4 mmol/L, leading to hypoglycaemia (Marieb, 2015).

Diabetes Mellitus

Diabetes has been recognised as a disease since ancient times and was first described by Aretaeus of Cappadocia in the second century AD as a serious condition that involved the 'melting down of flesh and limbs into urine.' With greater insight into the causes and pathophysiology of diabetes it is now known that Aretaeus' description was not strictly accurate but it does illustrate some of the main physical changes that are witnessed in poorly controlled diabetes, such as weight loss and polyuria. It was not until 1889 that scientists discovered the link between the pancreas and the development of diabetes, and insulin as a treatment for diabetes was not developed until 1921 (Williams and Pickup, 2004).

Type 1 Diabetes

Type 1 diabetes is a chronic autoimmune disease in which the T lymphocytes progressively destroy the insulin-producing beta cells of the pancreas (Faideau et al., 2005), resulting in little or no production of insulin (Pozzilli and Mario, 2001). The rate of beta cell destruction varies quite considerably between people, but there is a tendency for it to be more rapid in infants and children and slower in adults. By the time Lucy exhibited classical signs and symptoms of diabetes (Table 10.1) when first diagnosed it is thought that over 90 per cent of her beta cells would have been destroyed, causing a marked insulin deficiency, which is the hallmark of type 1 diabetes. Lucy was diagnosed as having type 1 diabetes when she was just six years old.

Table 10.1 Signs and symptoms of diabetes

Type 1 diabetes	*Type 2 diabetes*
• Sudden/quick onset	• Gradual onset
	• May be no symptoms
• Polyuria	• Polyuria
• Thirst	• Thirst
• Glycosuria	• Glycosuria
• Weight loss	• Often no weight loss
	• Usually obese
• Tiredness and weakness	• Tiredness and weakness
• Ketosis	• No ketosis
• Blurring of vision	• Blurring of vision
• Skin infections	• Skin infections
• Genital soreness	• Genital soreness
• Absent C peptide	• C peptide detectable
• Islet cell antibodies present	• No markers of autoimmunity

Table 10.2 Predisposing factors for the development of diabetes

Type 1 diabetes	*Type 2 diabetes*
1. Familial or genetic link (Bonifacio et al., 2004)	1. Ethnic group particularly Afro-Caribbean and South Asian people (Diabetes UK, 2015)
2. Viral infections such as measles, mumps, rubella	2. Obesity
3. Early exposure to cow's milk (Akerblom, 2002)	3. Reduced physical activity
	4. Advancing age
4. Deficiency of vitamin D	5. Smoking (Will et al., 2001)
5. Rapid growth and obesity in childhood	6. Thrifty phenotype hypothesis (Hales et al., 2001)
6. Toxins such as Vacor and bafilomycins (Hettiarachichi et al., 2004)	7. Psychological stress
	8. Exposure to pesticides (Kuehn, 2008)
	9. Drinking fruit juice (Bazzano et al., 2008)
	10. IRS1 gene identified (Rung et al., 2009)

There are a number of factors that can increase the risk of developing diabetes (Table 10.2). Although Lucy does not report a history of diabetes in her family it is recognised that type 1 diabetes can be hereditary and there is a 23.3 per cent risk of developing multiple islet auto-antibodies if both parents have type 1 diabetes (Bonifacio et al., 2004).

Lucy will have developed auto-antibodies that will have progressively destroyed her beta cells. As she was quite young when this happened the onset of symptoms would have been rapid, probably spanning from a few days up to about a month in duration, when she would have presented at her general practitioner or accident and emergency unit. She would probably have been very unwell, with the typical signs and symptoms of ketoacidosis (Table 10.1). A diagnosis of type 1 diabetes means that Lucy would no longer have the beta cell capacity to produce insulin naturally and she would therefore rely upon artificially administered insulin, usually via the subcutaneous route, to control blood glucose levels for the rest of her life.

Type 2 Diabetes

The aetiology of type 2 diabetes is quite different from type 1 – so much so that they can almost be considered to be two different conditions. Type 2 diabetes accounts for 85–90 per cent of the total UK population with diabetes (Diabetes UK, 2015). Unlike type 1 diabetes, type 2 diabetes is an insidious disease that can be present for up to 12 years before symptoms appear and a diagnosis is made. As a consequence, up to 50 per cent of people may have developed one or more of the complications of diabetes at the time of diagnosis (Table 10.3).

Type 2 diabetes is now a major healthcare concern and the association between obesity, sedentary lifestyles and diabetes is so close that in the 1970s the term 'diabesity' was coined (Haslam and James, 2005). The development of visceral abdominal fat found typically in 'apple shaped' people is the main link between obesity and diabetes. Visceral fat cells decrease the action of the circulating insulin, causing insulin resistance (Williams and Pickup, 2004). It is thought that currently up to 25–30 per cent of the population of the UK have a level of insulin resistance similar to that of people who have type 2 diabetes. This condition is commonly referred to as prediabetes, a situation where blood glucose levels are higher than normal but not high enough for a diagnosis of diabetes. A person with prediabetes is at increased risk for developing type 2 diabetes, as well as for heart disease and stroke.

Table 10.3　Long-term complications of poorly controlled diabetes

- Diabetic retinopathy leading to blindness
- Peripheral neuropathy leading to loss of peripheral sensation and predisposing to the development of diabetic foot ulcer, which may necessitate limb amputation
- Ineffective immunity leading to poor healing and the potential for devastating infections requiring limb amputation
- Renal nephropathy leading to end stage renal disease (Happich et al., 2008)
- Peripheral and cardiovascular disease and stroke

Many people with prediabetes develop type 2 diabetes within ten years (National Institute of Diabetes and Digestive and Kidney Disorders, 2015).

In type 2 diabetes insulin is secreted but the presence of insulin resistance adversely affects the action and efficiency of the secreted insulin and therefore its ability to reduce blood glucose levels is impaired. The presence of insulin resistance also actively increases blood glucose levels further by stimulating the liver to form and release more glucose. This results in further rises in blood glucose levels and the development of symptoms of type 2 diabetes (Table 10.1). As a result, blood glucose levels continue to rise, signalling a need for further insulin to be secreted. The beta cells respond by producing more insulin, but over time they become exhausted and eventually the numbers of beta cells diminish. A state of hyperinsulinaemia exacerbates the insulin resistance further, creating other metabolic risk factors such as raised blood pressure and hyperlipidaemia (Broom, 2006). In turn, these metabolic risk factors increase the risk of developing cardiovascular disease, peripheral vascular disease and stroke (Table 10.3). In comparison to people without diabetes, those with diabetes are estimated to have a 138 per cent increased risk of angina, a 94 per cent risk increase of myocardial infarction, 126 per cent risk of heart failure and 62 per cent risk of stroke (Haffner et al., 1998; Diabetes UK, 2015; Centers for Disease Control, 2014). The link between chronic elevated blood glucose levels and the development of diabetes-related complications is evident in both type 1 and type 2 diabetes (Diabetes Control and Complications Trial (DCCT), 1993). In type 2 diabetes careful dietary control may be sufficient to control blood glucose levels, but in many cases anti-diabetic agents such as Glicazide® or Metformin® may be required. Careful blood glucose control in persons with type 1 and type 2 diabetes is the key ingredient to preventing acute hypoglycaemia and hyperglycaemia and delaying the progression of serious and life-threatening complications of diabetes (DCCT, 1993; UK Prospective Diabetes Study, 1998; Hayes et al., 2013). Further to this the NICE (2004, 2009) published optimal target blood glucose levels that a person with diabetes is expected to achieve in order to significantly reduce their risk of complications. NICE also recommends close blood pressure and cholesterol monitoring and maintenance within set limits, given the strong link between diabetes and heart disease. Medical management strategies and patient education aimed at achieving these targets are also offered by NICE (2004, 2009).

Hyperglycaemia and DKA

In normal circumstances if Lucy is carefully monitoring and appropriately managing her diabetes with routine blood glucose monitoring and administering the required background and rapid-acting bolus doses of insulin then this would normally compensate for the absence of insulin production seen in type 1 diabetes. However, given the clinical picture outlined in the case scenario (see page 294), Lucy's self-managed diabetes control has not been effective; the physiological consequences will now be considered. In Lucy's case the absence of insulin means that the normal homeostatic control of blood glucose does not occur: serum glucose levels rise yet cells are deprived of glucose for normal energy production and cellular function. Hyperglycaemia is the term used to describe a blood glucose level >10 mmol/L. In response to the low intracellular glucose, accelerated hepatic glucose production is mediated by a range of compensatory mechanisms in a futile effort to enable cellular glucose uptake (Figure 10.3). Counter-regulatory hormones such as catecholamines, glucagon, growth hormone and cortisol are released to further increase the high blood glucose levels.

Figure 10.3 Compensatory mechanisms in response to hyperglycaemia and low intracellular glucose

The lack of cellular glucose uptake leads to energy depletion and would lead to Lucy feeling tired and lethargic. In response to the lack of cellular glucose there will be an increase in the breakdown of proteins into constituent amino acids, which are subsequently converted by the body to energy. The liver will also increase absorption of the circulating amino acids and convert them to glucose, leading to a further increase in hyperglycaemia. The increased secretion of glucagon stimulates the liver to release stores of glycogen, which are also converted into glucose in a further misguided effort to increase blood glucose and intracellular levels of glucose. Once the liver's glycogen stores have been utilised, the breakdown of triglycerides into their constituent fatty acids will begin. These are converted by the liver into ketones in an attempt by the body to obtain further energy supplies. Ketones are then excreted via the kidneys and can be detected in the urine; however, when the production of ketone bodies exceeds the rate of excretion this can cause significant, life-threatening acidosis (Kettyle and Arky, 1998; JBDS, 2013). Circulating ketones are acidic and may lower the serum pH sufficiently to cause metabolic ketoacidosis. Hyperglycaemia leads to excessive diuresis and subsequent dehydration, and facilitates the movement of water and potassium out of the cells, which leads to intracellular dehydration, hypokalaemia, expansion of extracellular fluid and a loss of sodium (Kitabchi and Wall, 1999). Thus, these mechanisms merely serve to increase blood glucose further; however, they do not facilitate cellular uptake and they do instigate a number of undesirable, life-threatening side effects such as ketone production. Typically the signs and symptoms of hyperglycaemia such as polyuria, thirst and lethargy become evident when the blood glucose level rises to above 15 mmol/L.

Assessment and Reaching a Diagnosis

The serious nature of DKA should not be underestimated because if there is underlying serious illness or if the DKA is misdiagnosed, left untreated or not treated sufficiently it can be life threatening (Ilag et al., 2003; Umpierrez et al., 2004; JBDS, 2013). Lucy is acutely unwell and therefore requires a systematic and comprehensive assessment to provide a rapid, accurate diagnosis to inform immediate appropriate management and care. The Joint British Diabetes Societies Guidelines (JBDS, 2013) include an Adult Diabetic Ketoacidosis Emergency Care Pathway; the majority of hospitals in the UK have now adopted this pathway. As Lucy is 18 years of age, her care should follow this pathway. As Lucy presented in a semi-conscious state this would prompt an ABC approach (see Chapter 1). Monitoring by the nurse will be based on the use of the NEWS tool discussed in Chapter 1.

The Case Scenario: The Immediate Assessment Priorities

Lucy is currently studying full time at school for her examinations, which she is finding quite stressful. She does not smoke, drink alcohol or take drugs and is of a slim build. She is an active member of the school swimming and netball teams. Both of her parents are alive and well and she has an older brother who is fit with no health concerns. There is no other history of diabetes in her immediate family. Further information gleaned from Lucy's mother confirms the omission of insulin with her lunch prior to admission. Lucy's mother also shares concerns regarding her daughter's general health and diabetes control recently and reports a three-to-four week history of increasing tiredness, lethargy, thirst, frequency of micturition (passing urine) and weight loss.

An immediate physiological assessment revealed the following:

Temperature: 36.8 °C
Pulse: 128 beats/min, regular
Respirations: 24/minute
Blood pressure: 104/64 mmHg
Capillary blood glucose level: 22.6 mmol/L
Potassium: 4.0 mmol/L
Venous blood ketones: 7.0 mmol/L
HbA1c: 75 mmol/mol

Consider the following:

1. Explain the pathophysiological basis for Lucy's presenting signs and symptoms.
2. What are the common causes of DKA?
3. What are the immediate assessment priorities in this case and why?
4. Identify further clues in the information given by Lucy's mother that might be a cause for concern.

Airway

Dehydration and metabolic acidosis can lead to altered conscious levels. Depending upon the stage of development of DKA, Lucy's level of consciousness may be anywhere along the conscious–unconscious continuum; however, true coma at admission is rare, being present in fewer than 10 per cent of patients. Therefore airway assessment will be based upon individual circumstances. As Lucy is semi-conscious she will need to have her airway assessed at very regular intervals using the 'look, listen and feel' method of airway assessment (see Chapter 1) and the findings must be clearly reported and documented. It is good practice to include this assessment as part of the Glasgow Coma Score (GCS), which must be performed every 30 minutes initially due to Lucy's decreased level of consciousness (see Chapter 4). Altered consciousness levels should prompt an early assessment of capillary blood glucose and ketones via the finger prick method, particularly when a history of diabetes is known. Lucy's capillary blood glucose was grossly raised above the normal levels of 4 to 7 mmol/L at 22.6 mmol/L and the presence of ketones as a consequence of this abnormally high level of blood glucose may explain her semi-conscious state.

Lucy presented with a history of nausea and vomiting, which presents a potential threat to airway patency. Nausea and vomiting may result from the compensatory breakdown of fats (lipolysis), initiated in an effort to release energy stores, leading to increased circulating fatty acids. Liver cells degrade fatty acids into fatty acyl-CoA, which can be converted by cell mitochondria into acetoacetate (ketone bodies). Excessive accumulation of ketones will increase blood acidity, lower the pH and lead to metabolic acidosis, which can present as nausea and vomiting. In some cases of decreased consciousness a nasogastric tube may be inserted as a precautionary measure to avoid the potential aspiration of gastric contents and therefore protect the airway. As Lucy's condition improves and she becomes fully alert and conscious and able to maintain her own airway, the frequency of assessment of her airway and GCS can be reduced.

Breathing

Lucy is tachypnoeic with a respiratory rate of 24 breaths per minute. She may begin to hyperventilate and develop Kussmaul respirations (Savage et al., 2011) in a compensatory effort to correct the metabolic acidosis. Chemoreceptors sense a fall in blood pH, which will activate the respiratory centre housed within the medulla, leading to an increased respiratory stimulus to 'blow off' carbon dioxide (CO_2). Carbon dioxide forms carbonic acid when dissolved in the bloodstream, further exacerbating acidity. Therefore increased excretion of CO_2 helps to reduce the acidity and increase the blood pH to a more normal level, which is slightly alkaline at 7.35 to 7.45. The abnormally high level of ketones evident in the venous blood and urine may result in the smell of ketones on Lucy's breath. This gives rise to a distinctive smell of acetone or pear drops on the breath which may be noticed by the nurse caring for Lucy, although it should be noted that not everyone can smell or detect this. With appropriate intervention (see below) the acidosis should be corrected; a decrease in her respiratory rate back to within the normal parameters of 12 to 16 noiseless and effortless breaths per minute should then be noted. The characteristic ketotic acetone smell on Lucy's breath should then no longer be evident. Until this time Lucy will require her respiratory rate, depth, regularity, pattern and smell to be observed and recorded by the nurse for a minimum of one minute every 30 minutes, and any negative changes reported to a senior nurse and the doctors responsible for her treatment. Lucy's oxygen saturation levels should be recorded via continuous non-invasive oxygen saturation monitoring and be maintained at > 95 per cent. A fall in oxygen saturation levels below 95 per cent will necessitate administration of 100 per cent oxygen via a mask.

Circulation

Compensatory increased secretion of adrenaline and stress hormones such as cortisol leads to increased blood glucose levels. Increased circulating adrenaline also has a direct effect upon the cardiovascular system, leading to increased heart rate, contractility and peripheral vasoconstriction. Lucy's heart rate may reflect this effect as it is above normal at 128 beats per minute, which is considered to be a tachycardia. As abnormal serum potassium levels (see below) can lead to potentially fatal cardiac arrhythmias, Lucy should be commenced on three- or five-lead cardiac monitoring to provide a continuous analysis of heart rate and rhythm, which should be documented every 30 minutes.

Currently Lucy's blood pressure (BP) is 104/64 mmHg, which may be normotensive for Lucy or could be lower than anticipated due to dehydration, but this will need to be monitored and charted every 30 minutes. A rising blood glucose level >15 mmol/L causes osmotic diuresis and polyuria, with consequent thirst and lethargy. The subsequent loss of fluids and electrolytes leads to dehydration. Hyperglycaemia facilitates water and potassium movement out of the cells, leading to intracellular dehydration and hypokalaemia and extracellular fluid accumulation. Strict monitoring of fluid input and output is essential to assess the degree of dehydration and rehydration. Lucy will also require observation for other signs of dehydration, such as skin turgor, thirst, dry mouth, muscle cramps and a decreased urine output (<30 mL/hour), and a baseline measurement of these must be ascertained, from which improvement or deterioration can be determined. Low circulating volume results in a fall in stroke volume, cardiac output and consequent low BP, which will also initiate a range of compensatory mechanisms. A fall in BP causing less vessel wall stretch will be sensed by baroreceptors situated within the carotid sinus and aortic arch, which in turn stimulate the cardiac acceleratory centre housed within the medulla. Subsequent sympathetic nervous activation will lead to a further increase in heart rate and myocardial contraction in an effort to increase cardiac output and BP.

Excessive diuresis can lead to further depletion of potassium (K^+) levels and hypokalaemia. Lucy's potassium level is within normal limits but the serum level does not give an accurate representation of the total body potassium levels, which will always be markedly depleted, with a deficit ranging from 3 to 12 mmol/kg (Savage et al., 2011; JBDS, 2013). This has the potential of causing fatal cardiac arrhythmias and consequently needs to be corrected immediately and carefully monitored. A 12-lead electrocardiograph should be performed, as T wave changes may indicate hypokalaemia. The JBDS (2013) emergency care pathway for adults with DKA provide specific guidance on medical management based on the level of serum potassium; the guidelines indicate that the medical team should anticipate a fall in potassium and should replace lost potassium in accordance with the guideline once the first serum potassium level is obtained. Lucy's serum potassium levels will be determined on admission and at one and two hours from commencement of treatment and then every two hours (JBDS, 2013).

On admission venous blood will be tested for ketones using a hand-held blood ketone meter. This detects the presence of 3-beta-hydroxybutyrate, which is the dominating ketone body produced in the liver during periods of insulin deprivation and rising blood glucose levels. The measurement of blood ketones now represents best practice in monitoring the suppression of ketonaeamia compared to urinalysis and arterial blood measurements (JBDS, 2013).

Lucy's medical and nursing assessment has revealed poor control of her blood glucose. This can be further substantiated from serum measurement of haemoglobin A1c (HbA1c) levels taken on admission. The HbA1c measures the amount of glucose in the blood that has bound irreversibly to a specific part of haemoglobin in red blood cells. HbA1c increases proportionately with increasing blood glucose concentration over prolonged periods. HbA1c circulates for the lifespan of the red blood cell, and so gives an indication of average blood glucose levels over the preceding two to three months. An unusually high blood glucose level for one or two days is unlikely to alter the HbA1c, but high blood glucose levels for longer periods of time will be reflected in a high HbA1c. The HbA1c target to be achieved in order to reduce the risk of long-term complications of diabetes is 48 mmol/mol. Lucy's most recent HbA1c result of 75mmol/mol indicates that she has had poor blood glucose control for at least the past two to three months. This result suggests that her blood glucose levels have been higher than the normal limits of 4 to 7 mmol/L and as a consequence she is putting herself at an increased risk of developing serious acute and chronic diabetes-related complications. Previous HbA1c levels will help to identify a trend in Lucy's blood glucose control.

Specific questions may also reveal a more detailed history of Lucy's diabetes control. She has experienced increased levels of stress associated with examinations, which may have caused increased sympathetic-mediated adrenaline release, leading to a physiological increase in blood glucose levels. In this situation Lucy should have been monitoring her blood glucose levels a minimum of four times per day, before breakfast and two hours after each of her main meals. The insulin regimen that Lucy is currently prescribed allows her the flexibility to give extra rapid-acting insulin as a 'correction dose' to correct a high blood glucose level. In addition, if her pre-prandial blood glucose level is raised consistently in the morning then an increase in her basal insulin, Lantus®, may be required. Lucy and her family may require extra help and support from their healthcare team in managing fluctuating blood glucose levels during this stressful period.

On admission to the accident and emergency department Lucy's temperature is within normal limits, which at this stage of the assessment allows infection and/or sepsis to be ruled out as the potential cause of the DKA; however, it would be prudent for the doctor treating Lucy to take a blood sample for microscopy, culture and sensitivity (MC&S). In the immediate situation, if treatment for DKA is delayed or not sufficient the levels of acidosis will continue to rise and the body will eventually decompensate, causing the person to develop warm dry skin, hypothermia, hypoxia, a decreasing consciousness state and decreased renal, cardiac and respiratory output.

Reaching a Diagnosis: Specific Investigations

Rapid treatment of DKA is crucial and will impact on the potential survival of the patient (Savage et al., 2011; JBDS, 2013). Therefore specific investigations need to be arranged immediately DKA is suspected in order to be able to confirm the diagnosis, determine a possible cause and commence treatment promptly.

Investigations will include:

- capillary blood glucose (tested at the bedside);
- venous blood glucose (laboratory test);

- blood 3-beta-hydroxybutyrate (blood ketones);
- venous pH (tested at the bedside);
- urea and electrolytes;
- arterial blood gases;
- full blood count;
- electrocardiograph;
- chest X-ray if clinically indicated;
- urinalysis;
- urine specimen for microscopy, culture and sensitivity;
- blood cultures;
- continuous cardiac monitoring;
- continuous pulse oximetry;
- consider precipitating causes and treat appropriately;
- establish usual medication for diabetes;
- pregnancy test in women of child-bearing age.

Causes of Hyperglycaemia and DKA

In Lucy's case, the main cause of DKA was having had lunch without a prior injection of insulin to counteract the expected rise in blood glucose levels. Other causes include:

- Insulin leaking out of the injection site.
- Lipohypertrophy caused by insulin being injected repeatedly into the same site, causing delayed and erratic absorption and action of insulin.
- The dose of insulin not being enough for the amount and type of food eaten.
- In the event of planned exercise, the insulin dose being reduced to prevent possible hypoglycaemia, but the exercise then being cancelled or reduced in duration and/or intensity.
- Infection, injury, emotional stress and myocardial infarction causing the production of stress-responding hormones such as adrenaline and cortisol, which antagonise the effects of insulin and can result in hyperglycaemia and DKA (Kettyle and Arky, 1998).
- Menstruation causing a rise in blood glucose levels a few days before a menstrual period is due (Tamas et al., 1996).
- Steroids, thiazide diuretics and tricyclic antidepressants which have been shown to increase blood glucose levels; this can lead to the development of DKA.

The Case Scenario: Medical Management and Care Issues

Within 15 minutes of arriving in the accident and emergency department, Lucy has undergone a series of investigations and has given a detailed medical and social history.

The results of the specific investigations are as follows:

Capillary blood glucose level: 22.6 mmol/L
Venous blood glucose level: 29.8 mmol/L
Blood 3-beta-hydroxybutyrate: 3.0 mmol/L
Sodium: 129 mmol/L
Potassium: 3.5 mmol/L
Bicarbonate: 11.0 mmol/L
pH: 7.28
Electrocardiograph: sinus tachycardia, 132 beats/min
Chest X-ray: no abnormalities detected
Urinalysis: ++++ glucose and ketones

A definitive diagnosis of DKA is reached and treatment is commenced immediately.

Consider the following:

1. With reference to the rationale consider what the immediate medical treatment would be.
2. What are Lucy's main care issues?

Management Strategies and the Role of the Nurse

DKA is a medical emergency with a significant morbidity and mortality. It should be diagnosed quickly and managed intensively by the diabetes specialist team (JBDS, 2013). Diagnosing DKA is not generally difficult but the combination of hyperglycaemia, acidosis and ketosis must be found. A thorough and careful assessment is required, however, to rule out the possibility of other conditions that can cause acidosis, such as salicylate overdose, sepsis or lactic acidosis.

The criteria to diagnose DKA are:

- raised blood glucose level > 11.1 mmol/L;
- blood ketones (ketonaeamia) 3.0 mmol/L and over;
- significant metabolic acidosis measured as a serum venous bicarbonate level of < 15 mmol/L and/or venous pH < 7.3.

(JBDS, 2013)

The aim of treatment for DKA is threefold and may require slight modifications to suit the individual patient, so frequent reassessment is essential:

1. To correct the fluid and electrolyte disturbances.
2. To raise intracellular and lower extracellular levels of glucose.
3. To increase the blood pH.

Correct Fluid and Electrolyte Disturbances

Lucy will require good intravenous access via a large bore cannula into a peripheral vein. If this is not possible, or too difficult, then a central line will be inserted. Patients with DKA can typically have a 100 mL/kg of body weight water deficit and will require substantial amounts of intravenous fluids to reach an acceptable level of rehydration. Fluid replacement will normally be rapid initially and then be slowed down as Lucy's condition improves.

The JBDS Inpatient Care Group (2013) suggests giving a previously well 70 kg adult:

- 1 L 0.9 per cent sodium chloride solution over the first hour;
- 1 L 0.9 per cent sodium chloride solution with potassium chloride over the next two hours and repeat (x1);
- 1 L 0.9 per cent sodium chloride solution with potassium chloride over the next four hours and repeat (x1);
- 1 L 0.9 per cent sodium chloride solution with potassium chloride over the next six hours.

The JBDS (2013) guidelines note that a slower rate of infusion with more frequent monitoring in a high-dependency unit should be considered, with central venous pressure monitoring used if required (see Chapter 3). Reassessment of cardiovascular status is mandatory at 12 hours and further fluid may be required.

Potassium chloride (KCl) will be added to the intravenous fluids to correct hypokalaemia. The serum potassium level should be checked at 60 minutes and two hours and two-hourly thereafter. If the potassium level is outside the normal reference range, the appropriateness of potassium replacement should be reassessed hourly. If the abnormal potassium level does not resolve quickly then senior medical advice should be sought (JBDS, 2013). Once the ketoacidosis has resolved and the blood glucose and potassium levels are returned to within normal limits, the addition of KCl to the intravenous fluids can be discontinued.

Lucy also has a low sodium level, which is characteristic in DKA. Decreased levels of sodium in the gastrointestinal system may also exacerbate feelings of nausea and vomiting. The low sodium levels are compensated for with the infusion of 0.9 per cent sodium chloride, which is the recommended fluid of choice, and it is not usually necessary to give extra sodium as the blood sodium levels will correct themselves as the blood glucose levels return to normal.

An accurate fluid balance record should be kept to ensure that Lucy does not develop circulatory overload. Signs of circulatory overload include a rise in BP, rapid pulse rate, rapid breathing, shortness of breath, an abnormal crackling or rattling sound heard upon chest auscultation (termed rales), and dilation of veins with neck veins sometimes visibly engorged. The date and time of all intravenous and oral fluid intake and the amount of urine and other fluid losses such as vomit should be carefully recorded. A nasogastric tube may be considered if vomiting persists. If Lucy fails to pass a minimum urine output of 0.5 mL/kg/hr she will require a urinary catheter to be inserted using a strict aseptic technique (Savage et al., 2011). This will allow her renal function to be monitored more closely and hourly urine measurements to be taken and recorded.

Raised Intracellular and Lower Extracellular Levels of Glucose

It is crucial that insulin therapy is instigated at the same time as the fluid replacement to prevent gluconeogenesis by the liver, which if allowed to develop and continue will serve to worsen the DKA and put Lucy's life in jeopardy. JBDS (2013) recommendations are to commence a continuous fixed rate intravenous insulin infusion (FRIII) via an infusion pump. This should be made up of 50 units of human soluble insulin (Actrapid® or Novorapid®) made up to 50 mL with 0.9 per cent sodium chloride (which should be available pre-prepared). This should be infused at a fixed rate of at least 0.1 unit/kg/hour (Kitabchi et al., 2009; JBDS, 2013). This is preferred over a sliding scale regimen as it is able to accommodate obese or other insulin-resistant states such as pregnancy more effectively. However, the fixed rate may need to be adjusted in insulin-resistant people if the ketone concentration does not fall quickly enough (JBDS, 2013). A stat dose of intramuscular insulin (0.1 unit/kg) should be given *only* if there is a delay in setting up the fixed rate intravenous insulin infusion. As Lucy normally takes Lantus® subcutaneously this should continue at the usual dose and usual time. The same principle applies if the patient is taking Levemir® or Trebisa®.

Lucy's capillary blood glucose and blood ketone levels will need to be recorded hourly until the ketoacidosis has subsided and be carefully entered on the appropriate chart. It is anticipated that the blood glucose should fall by 3 mmol/L/hour. If the blood glucose levels do not begin to fall with the administration of insulin the nurse should check that the syringe driver is turned on and working and the intravenous connections are connected and patent. Any problems found should be rectified and the insulin infusion recommenced at the set dose. While administering intravenous insulin it is important not to allow Lucy to become hypoglycaemic. Once the glucose level falls below 14 mmol/L a 10 per cent glucose infusion should be commenced at 125 mL/hour alongside the 0.9 per cent sodium chloride infusion. The fixed rate insulin infusion should be continued until Lucy has less than 0.3mmol/L of serum ketones and a venous pH over 7.3. It is important not to rely on the absence of urinary ketones in determining when to discontinue the insulin infusion, as urinary ketones will still be present for some time after the DKA has resolved.

To Increase the Blood pH

The administration of intravenous insulin is usually sufficient to increase the blood pH level and the level of ketones is a good indicator of the adequacy of the insulin regimen. The administration of bicarbonate has been associated with the development of potentially fatal cerebral oedema and hypokalaemia (Williams and Pickup, 2004; JBDS, 2013) and should therefore be avoided as a treatment modality in DKA.

If Lucy's condition requires bed rest with limited mobility for three or more days she will be prescribed twice-daily, weight-adjusted subcutaneous injections of low molecular weight heparin as prophylaxis against the development of venous thromboembolism, as per NICE (2010) guidance. Once Lucy is rehydrated and her blood glucose levels have returned to within normal limits she should resume a normal diet and fluid intake and the insulin infusion can be discontinued. Once the intravenous insulin has been disconnected, within 10 to 15 minutes Lucy will no longer have any circulating active short-acting insulin. The Lantus® insulin injections should have been continued while she was receiving intravenous short-acting insulin, which means that when the insulin infusion is discontinued Lucy will not be completely insulin depleted and will have the required basal insulin still circulating in an effective form. She will therefore need to recommence her rapid-acting Novorapid® insulin, which should be given immediately prior to each of her meals or within 15 minutes of eating to avoid a recurrence of hyperglycaemia and potential ketoacidosis.

Following recovery from the acute event, care must focus upon returning Lucy to a well-informed, healthy lifestyle. The Department of Health (DH, 2001) and the National Audit Office (NAO) Report (NAO, 2012) recognise that diabetes is a condition in which, with the right education, support and motivation, the individual can have almost total control. This requires healthcare professionals to ensure that all people with diabetes are

encouraged and assisted to take an active role in their diabetes management. They also need to facilitate the patient's learning to enable them to
develop the appropriate knowledge, skills and confidence to be able to make
sometimes complex decisions regarding their blood glucose control. It is
crucial that Lucy's lifestyle choices are incorporated into her blood glucose
control regime. Although she altered her insulin dosage to suit her dietary
intake she must also learn to be more vigilant with blood glucose monitoring and be prepared to alter her insulin regime to accommodate activities
such as increased exercise or extreme changes to her normal pattern of
daily activity. Diabetes UK has made available a smartphone application
(app) which can be used to enter and track a range of levels including blood
glucose, insulin, carbohydrates, calories, weight and ketones. The app allows
the users' data to be viewed in day and week graphs to spot trends such as
recurring episodes of blood glucose levels exceeding 11mmols/L. (Other
apps with these functions also exist.) This approach, together with support from the specialist diabetes team in Lucy's local primary care centre,
may ensure Lucy feels more confident in the ongoing management of her
diabetes.

Summary

This chapter has considered DKA, which is a potentially life-threatening
complication of diabetes. Following a brief outline of the anatomy and
physiology of diabetes and the ways in which insulin and glucagon are
secreted and broken down, the differences between type 1 and type 2 diabetes were highlighted. This information was then used to underpin the
immediate assessment priorities and medical management of Lucy, a young
person with diabetes, who presents at an accident and emergency unit with
DKA. Within this, the physiology of hyperglycaemia and ensuing ketoacidosis is given, as well as the causes of high blood glucose levels. Information
is given regarding the immediate assessment of Lucy and how her medical
management and nursing care should be prioritised. Finally, the severity of
ketoacidosis should not be underestimated. The high level of monitoring
required during the acute event may necessitate transfer to an intensive care
unit or high dependency unit for care by a specialist diabetes team until the
condition becomes more stable.

Further reading

Joint British Diabetes Societies (JBDS) Inpatient Care Group. *The Management of
    Diabetic Ketoacidosis in Adults. Second Edition Update: 2013* (London: NHS Diabetes,
    2013) [Online]. Available from: www.diabetes.org.uk/Documents/About%20Us/
    What%20we%20say/Management-of-DKA-241013.pdf (accessed 1 May 2015).

Holt, P. *Diabetes in Hospital: A Practical Approach for Healthcare Professionals* (Oxford: Wiley Blackwell, 2009).

Levy, D. *Practical Diabetes*, 2nd edn (Hertfordshire: Altman, 2006).

Whettem, E. *Nursing & Health Survival Guide: Diabetes* (London: Pearson Education, 2012).

The British Society for Paediatic Endocrinology and Diabetes (BSPED) 'Diabetic Ketoacidosis Guidelines' (2015) [Online]. Available from: http://bsped.org.uk/ clinical/docs/DKAguideline.pdf (accessed 26 January 2016).

References

Akerblom, H. K., O. Vaarala, H. Hyoty, J Ilanen and M. Knip. 'Environmental factors in the etiology of type 1 diabetes', *American Journal of Medical Genetics*, **115** (2002) (1), 18–29.

Bassano, L. A., T. Y. Li, K. J. Joshipura and F. B. Hu. 'Intake of fruit, vegetables and fruit juices and risks of diabetes in women', *Diabetes Care*, **31** (2008), 1311– 7.

Bonifacio, E., M. Hummel, M. Walter, S. Schmid and A. G. Ziegler. 'IDDM and Multiple Family History of Type 1 Diabetes Combine to Identify Neonates at High Risk for Type 1 Diabetes', *Diabetes Care*, **27** (2004), 2695–700.

Broom, I. 'Thinking about Abdominal Obesity and Cardiovascular Risk', *British Journal of Diabetes and Vascular Disease*, 6(2) (2006), 58–61.

Centers for Disease Control. *National Diabetes Statistics Report* (Atlanta: National Center for Chronic Disease Prevention and Health Promotion, 2014).

Department of Health (DH). *National Service Framework for Diabetes*, (London: Department of Health, 2001).

Diabetes Control and Complications Trial (DCCT) Research Group. 'The Effect of Intensive Treatment of Diabetes on the Development and Progression of Long-term Complications in Insulin-dependent Diabetes Mellitus', *New England Journal of Medicine*, **326** (1993), 683–9.

Diabetes UK. 'Diabetes Facts and Stats' (2015) [Online]. Available from: www. diabetes.org.uk/Documents/About%20Us/Statistics/Diabetes-key-stats-guidelines-April2014.pdf (accessed 26 January 2016).

Faideau, B., E. Larger, F. Lepault, J. C. Carel and C. Boitard. 'Role of β-cells in Type 1 Diabetes Pathogenesis', *Diabetes*, **54** (2005), S87–S96.

Ginter, E. and V. Simko. 'Type 2 Diabetes Mellitus, Pandemic in the 21st Century', *Advances in Experimental Medicine and Biology*, **771** (2012), 42–50.

Haffner, S. M., S. Lehto, T. Ronnemaa et al.. 'Mortality from Coronary Heart Disease in Subjects with Type 2 Diabetes and in Nondiabetic Subjects with and without Prior Myocardial Infarction', *New England Journal of Medicine*, **339** (1998), 229–34.

Hales, C. N. and D. J. P. Barker. 'The thrifty phenotype hypothesis', *British Medical Bulletin*, 60(1) (2001), 5–20.

Happich, M., R Landfraf, W. Piehlmeier, P. Falkenstein and S. Stamentis. 'The economic burden of nephropathy in diabetic patients in Germany 2002', *Diabetes Research in Clinical Practice* (2008). doi:10.1016/j.diabres.2007.11.012.

Haslam, D. W. and W. P. T. James. 'Obesity', *Lancet*, **366**(9492) (2005), 1197–209.

Hayes, A. J., J. Leal, A. M. Gray, R. R. Holman and P. M. Clarke. 'UKPDS Outcomes Model 2: A New Version of a Model to Simulate Lifetime Health Outcomes of

Patients with Type 2 Diabetes Mellitus Using Data from the 30 year United Kingdom Prospective Diabetes Study: UKPDS 82', *Diabetologia*, 56 (2013),1925–33.

Hettiarachchi, K. D., P. Z. Zimmet and M. A. Myers. 'Transplacental exposure to bafilomycin disrupts pancreatic islet oranogenesis and accelerates diabetes onset in NOD mice', *Journal of Autoimmunity*, 22 (4) (2004), 287–96.

Hex, N., C. Bartlett, D. L. Wright, M. J. Taylor and D. Varley. 'Estimating the Current and Future Costs of Type 1 and Type 2 Diabetes in the UK, Including Direct Health Costs and Indirect Societal and Productivity Costs', *Diabetic Medicine*, 29(7) (2012), 855–62.

Ilag, L. L., S. Kronick, R. D. Ernst, L. Grondin, C. Alaniz, L. Liu and W. H. Herman. 'Impact of a Critical Pathway on Inpatient Management of Diabetic Ketoacidosis', *Diabetes Research and Clinical Practice*, 62(1) (2003), 23–32.

Joint British Diabetes Societies (JBDS) Inpatient Care Group. *The Management of Diabetic Ketoacidosis in Adults. Second Edition Update: 2013*. (London: NHS Diabetes, 2013) [Online]. Available from: www.diabetes.org.uk/Documents/About%20Us/What%20we%20say/Management-of-DKA-241013.pdf (accessed 1 May 2015).

Kettyle, W. M. and R. A. Arky. *Endocrine Pathophysiology* (Philadelphia: Lippincott Raven, 1998).

Kitabchi, A. E. and B. M. Wall. 'Management of Diabetic Ketoacidosis', *American Family Physician*, 60 (1999), 455–64.

Kitabchi A. E., G. E. Umpierrez, J. M. Miles and J. N. Fisher. 'Hyperglycaemic Crises in Adult Patients with Diabetes: A Consensus Statement from the American Diabetes Association', *Diabetes Care*, 32 (2009), 1335.

Kuehn, B. M. 'Pesticides–Diabetes Link', *Journal of the American Medical Association*, 300(4) (2008), 386.

Marieb, E. N. *Essentials of Human Anatomy and Physiology*, 11th edn (Harlow: Pearson Education, 2015).

National Audit Office (NAO). *The Management of Adult Diabetes Services in the NHS* (London: The Stationery Office, 2012).

National Institute of Diabetes and Digestive and Kidney Disorders. *Causes of Diabetes*. (2015) [Online]. Available from: www.niddk.nih.gov/health-information/health-topics/Diabetes/causes-diabetes/Pages/index.aspx#type2 (accessed 1 June 2015).

National Institute for Health and Care Excellence (NICE). *Type 2 Diabetes. The Management of Type 2 Diabetes. Clinical Guideline 87* (London: National Institute for Health and Clinical Excellence, 2009) [Online]. Available from: www.nice.org.uk/guidance/cg87 (accessed 30 May 2015).

National Institute for Health and Care Excellence (NICE). *Venous Thromboembolism: Reducing the Risk. Clinical Guidance 92* (London: National Institute for Health and Clinical Excellence, 2010) [Online]. Available from: www.nice.org.uk/Guidance/CG92 (accessed 1 May 2015).

National Institute for Health and Care Excellence (NICE). *Diabetes in Adults: NICE Quality Standard QS6*. (London: NICE, 2011) [Online]. Available from: www.nice.org.uk/guidance/qs6 (accessed 30 May 2015).

National Institute for Health and Care Excellence. (NICE) *Diabetes (type 1 and type 2) in children and young people: diagnosis and management*. (NICE Guideline 18) (2015). www.nice.org.uk/guidance/ng18 (accessed 26 January 2016).

Pozzilli, P. and U. D. Mario. 'Autoimmune Diabetes not Requiring Insulin at Diagnosis (Latent Autoimmune Diabetes of the Adult)', *Diabetes Care*, **24** (2001), 1460–7.

Rorsman, P. 'Insulin Secretion: Function and Therapy of Pancreatic Beta-cells in Diabetes', *British Journal of Diabetes and Vascular Disease*, **5** (2005), 187–91.

Rung, J., S. Cauchi, A. Albrechtsen., L. Shen, G. Rocheleau, C. Cavalcanti-Proenca, F. Bacot, B. Balkau, A. Belisle, K. Borch-Johnsen et al.. 'Genetic variant near IRS1 is associated with type 2 diabetes, insulin resistance and hyperinsulinaemia', *Nature Genetics*, **41** (2009), 1110–15.

Savage, M. W., K. K. Dhatariya, A. Kilvert, G. Rayman, J. A. E. Rees, C. H. Courtney, L. Hilton, P. H. Dyer and M. S. Hamersley for the Joint British Diabetes Societies 1. 'Diabetes UK Position Statements and Care Recommendations: Joint British Diabetes Societies Guideline for the Management of Diabetic Ketoacidosis', *Diabetic Medicine*, **28** (2011), 508–15.

Shaw, J. E., R. A. Sicree and P. Z. Zimmet. 'Global Estimates of the Prevalence of Diabetes for 2010 and 2030', *Diabetes Research and Clinical Practice*, **87** (2010), 4–14.

Tamas, G., A. G. Tabak, P. Vargha and Z. Kerenyi. 'Effect of Menstrual Cycle on Insulin Demand in IDDM Women', *Diabetologia*, **39**(suppl. 1) (1996), A52 (abstract 188).

UK Prospective Diabetes Study (UKPDS) Group. 'Intensive Blood Glucose Control with Sulphonylureas or Insulin Compared with Conventional Treatment and Risk of Complications in Patients with Type 2 Diabetes (UKPDS 33)', *Lancet*, **352** (1998), 837–53.

Umpierrez, G. E., R. Cuervo, A. Karabell, K. Latif, A. X. Freire and A. E. Kitabchi. 'Treatment of Diabetic Ketoacidosis with Subcutaneous Insulin Aspart', *Diabetes Care*, **27** (2004), 1873–8.

Will, J. C., D. A. Galuska, E. S. Ford, A. Mokdad and E. E. Calle. 'Cigarette smoking and diabetes mellitus: evidence of a positive association from a large prospective cohort study', *International Journal of Epidemiology*, **30** (3) (2001), 540–6.

Williams, G. and J. C. Pickup. *Handbook of Diabetes*, 3rd edn (Oxford: Blackwell, 2004).

11

Care and Management in Liver Disorder following Drug Misuse

Michelle Clayton

Introduction

Drug misuse, whether deliberate or accidental, for recreational or self-harm purposes, is a growing concern for health services. The real and potential harms caused by drug misuse appear to be largely underestimated and to be misunderstood by many. This chapter seeks to address the challenges faced by healthcare professionals in assessing and managing the effects of misuse of paracetamol, one of the most widely available over-the-counter drugs. The chapter will also explore the devastating impact that misuse of paracetamol can have on individuals and their families.

Paracetamol

Paracetamol is a simple yet effective analgesic that until 1998 could be bought in large quantities from many retail outlets in the UK. It is the most commonly used substance for deliberate self-poisoning, with over 42 per cent of individuals using pure paracetamol or paracetamol compound combinations (Hawton et al., 2007). Hawton et al. (1995) reported that individuals who had taken an overdose knew that paracetamol was dangerous but there was a lack of knowledge about the specific effects that occurred and the timing of these side effects. Many individuals who have ingested excess paracetamol do not generally feel unwell in the first 24 to 48 hours despite the potential catastrophic harm to their liver that may occur during this period. Acute liver failure is a serious and life-threatening event that may result from the toxic effects of excess paracetamol.

The British National Formulary (BNF) (2015) recommends between 0.5 and 1 g of paracetamol every four to six hours up to a maximum of 4 g in a 24-hour period for normal analgesic use in adults. This relatively narrow therapeutic range means that accidental as well as deliberate overdose is not difficult. A range of other over-the-counter medications also contain paracetamol, which may only be apparent on reading the product information. It is therefore important that individuals are cognisant of this to prevent an accidental overdose occurring. Due to its popularity as a drug of choice for deliberate self-poisoning the Medicines Control Agency (MCA) introduced legislation in 1998 to reduce the availability of paracetamol to 16 tablets (8 g) for non-pharmacy outlets and 32 (16 g) from pharmacies. Following the MCA legislation, the use of paracetamol products in suicide deaths has decreased by 43 per cent, or 765 fewer deaths over 11¼ years (Hawton et al., 2013).

Aim and Learning Outcomes

The Aim

This chapter aims to illustrate the physiological effects of poisoning and discuss the key issues in the assessment, care and management of a patient presenting with acute liver failure following self-poisoning.

Learning Outcomes

At the end of this chapter the reader will be able to:

1. Appreciate the normal physiological effects of paracetamol use.
2. With reference to the pathophysiological effect upon different organs, describe the common symptom presentation associated with paracetamol misuse.
3. Identify the assessment and monitoring needs of the patient following paracetamol overdose.
4. Consider the available treatment options following paracetamol overdose.

Liver Function

The liver is a complex organ with a multitude of important functions that exist to help maintain normal homeostasis (Table 11.1).

Many factors affect liver function, including congestion due to congestive cardiac failure, cirrhosis due to infections such as hepatitis or alcohol misuse, obesity and diabetes and some drug toxicity, to name a few. Disruption to normal liver function will affect several homeostatic mechanisms and a number of different organs, which will manifest in a wide variety of clinical features. Many patients with acute liver failure display signs of multiple organ dysfunction or failure.

Table 11.1   Functions of the liver

The liver has more than 500 functions. Here are a few of the common ones.

1. Carbohydrate metabolism
   - conversion of glucose to glycogen (glycogenesis)
   - conversion of glycogen to glucose (glycogenolysis)
   - conversion of amino acids to glucose (gluconeogenesis)
2. Fat metabolism
   - break down of fatty acid from acetyl coenzyme A (beta oxidation)
   - break down of acetyl coenzyme A to ketones (ketogenesis)
   - cholesterol and phospholipid synthesis
   - synthesises lipoproteins to transport fatty acids, fats and cholesterol to and from cells
   - cholesterol breakdown to bile salts
   - fat storage
3. Protein metabolism
   - deaminates amino acids for use as energy or conversion to carbohydrate or fats
   - converts ammonia to less toxic urea for excretion
   - synthesis of plasma proteins eg globulin, albumin, clotting factors – prothrombin and fibrinogen, anticlotting agents: heparin
4. Removal and detoxification of drugs and hormones from blood stream
   - detoxification and excretion of drugs in bile salts, e.g. penicillin, steroid hormones: oestrogen, aldosterone, thyroxine
5. Excretion of bilirubin from red blood cell break down as bile
6. Synthesis of bile salts to aid emulsification and absorption of fats, cholesterol, phopholipid and lipoproteins
7. Storage for glucogen, vitamins A, B12, D, E, K, and minerals: iron, copper
8. Phagocytosis: Kupffer cells phagocytose old red and white blood cells and some bacteria from the gut
9. Activation of vitamin D
10. Manufacture, break down and regulation of numerous hormones including sex hormones
11. Manufacture of enzymes and proteins which are responsible for most chemical reactions in the body, e.g. blood clotting and repair of damaged tissues

The Case Scenario: Paracetamol Overdose

Lucy is 19 years old and has been admitted to the accident and emergency department at 20.00 hours. She reports having taken 42 tablets of 500 mg paracetamol, which she found in the bathroom cupboard at home at 23.00 hours the previous evening following an argument with her boyfriend. She had cried herself to sleep and woke the next morning feeling a little nauseated and miserable but with no other symptoms. She regretted that she had taken the overdose of paracetamol and felt embarrassed by her actions and decided to forget about it. The nausea was sufficient to cause Lucy to phone in sick for work and return to bed for much of the day. At 17.00 hours her boyfriend phoned to apologise and agreed to meet Lucy. During the evening Lucy started to feel unwell, complaining of abdominal pain in her right upper quadrant, and so she confided in her boyfriend about the overdose of paracetamol. He escorted her to the accident and emergency department of their local hospital. Lucy is now 21 hours post ingestion of excess paracetamol. On admission her observations are:

Conscious, alert and orientated: GCS = 15
Pulse: 98 beats/minute
BP: 140/92 mmHg
SpO_2: 98 per cent on air
Temperature: 37 °C

Consider the following:

1. What functions does the liver undertake?
2. What effects does paracetamol have on the body?
3. What assessment and investigations would be required? Consider the rationale for these investigations and relate them to the pathophysiology.

Paracetamol Metabolism

A normal dose of paracetamol tablets taken for a headache would be metabolised via two pathways within the liver. One pathway involves the conjugation of approximately 90 to 95 per cent of the drug into inactive soluble metabolites, which are then excreted via the kidney. Conjugation is the combining of one substance with another substance to produce a different molecule. The remaining paracetamol is oxidised and converted into an unstable and toxic metabolite called N-acetyl-p-benzoquinonimine (NAPQI). This oxidation takes place in the cytochrome P-450 within the hepatocytes (liver cells). NAPQI is then normally rapidly combined with reduced glutathione S-transferases to render it harmless for excretion by the kidneys. Excess ingestion of paracetamol (commonly termed an overdose) quickly saturates the first pathway involving conjugation to non-toxic metabolites. Therefore more residual paracetamol relies upon the second pathway producing large quantities of NAPQI, which quickly depletes the available glutathione. Excess toxic NAPQI is therefore left to bind to liver cell membranes, causing necrosis. Intracellular glutathione is also an important mediator against oxygen free radicals, which are produced as a result of oxidative stress and are also toxic to normal cells; therefore, glutathione depletion leads to increased levels of oxygen free radicals (Aitio, 2006). At a cellular level the toxic metabolite NAPQI and oxygen free radicals bombard liver cells, causing substantial cell injury and death. Liver cell necrosis can occur with as little as 10 g (20 tablets) and death with 15 g, which is less than that taken by Lucy.

Within the first 12 to 24 hours post paracetamol overdose there may be no apparent clinical manifestations of liver damage or there may be non-specific signs of nausea, vomiting, diarrhoea or abdominal cramps. At this point, although individuals may regret their actions, the lack of severe symptoms may lull them into a false sense of security and deter them from seeking help. Some individuals will recover without intervention; however, by 48 hours some will develop liver cell injury and necrosis and between 72 and 96 hours acute liver failure and abnormal liver function will become apparent.

Assessment and Reaching a Diagnosis

On admission to the emergency department Lucy would be assessed using the ABCDE approach (see Chapter 1).

Airway and Breathing

It is quickly established that Lucy is self-ventilating on air with a SpO_2 of 98 per cent. Lucy's respiratory rate, depth and skin colour should be recorded every four hours unless there is an evident deterioration in her condition. Pulse oximetry provides continuous monitoring of her respiratory status.

Circulation

Lucy's pulse at 98 beats/minute and blood pressure (BP) (140/92 mmHg) were slightly elevated, though this may reflect some anxiety regarding her situation. Cardiac and BP monitoring will provide a continuous trace of rate, regularity, rhythm and changes in cardiac output.

Disability

Lucy is currently alert and orientated. However, her level of consciousness should be assessed using APVU (see Chapter 1) or Glasgow Coma Score (see Chapter 4) every 30 minutes and any changes noted. Pupillary reaction should be checked hourly for size and reactiveness. Drowsiness, irritability or confusion from hepatic encephalopathy may signal liver failure.

Exposure

Additional four-hourly observations include temperature for pyrexia, capillary blood glucose for hypoglycaemia and signs of bleeding from puncture sites, as all could suggest deteriorating liver function. Assessment of renal function may reveal a decreasing urine output and a raised serum creatinine, and pain is not uncommon, either in the abdomen, particularly in the right upper quadrant, or in the back due to inflammation of the liver.

A careful history is taken from Lucy of the type, quantity and time since ingestion of the drugs. It is important to establish whether alcohol was also taken as it may potentiate the effects and contribute to altered behaviour. Vomiting since ingestion is noted, as this may reduce the amount of toxic metabolites entering the bloodstream. Lucy will be asked for any history of previous deliberate self-harm episodes, and her intentions in taking the poison. A previous history of deliberate self-harm and suicidal ideation now would indicate a high risk for further attempts at suicide and referral for early mental health assessment and close observation would be required (Dolan and Holt, 2013). Lucy recounts her history as an impulsive deliberate self-harm act with no suicidal intent, and therefore the focus moves to investigating and treating her overdose.

Specific Investigations

A detailed clinical history and review of Lucy's past medical history, drug use (prescribed and recreational) and social and family history, and routine venous blood sampling for a range of further investigations, would be collected (Table 11.2). These would be repeated potentially with a frequency to be determined by the medical team to allow for trends to be monitored.

Assessment of the liver enzymes alanine aminotransferase (ALT) or aspartate aminotransferase (AST) can be a useful indictor of the severity of liver cell damage but must be viewed with caution (Table 11.3). ALT is more liver specific than AST, which is expressed by a number of other tissues when damaged (Imperial and Keeffe, 2006). ALT levels can rise into

Table 11.2   Routine venous blood sampling

- Full blood count (FBC): low Hb (anaemia), raised WBC (infection)
- Clotting screen: prothrombin time (PT) and international normalised ratio (INR) can provide a good guide to severity of disease
- Urea and electrolytes (U&E): electrolyte and renal function
- Serum paracetamol levels
- Liver function tests: particularly for ALT, AST, ALP, albumin, bilirubin, lactate
- Capillary blood glucose: for signs of hyperglycaemia (raised blood glucose) or hypoglycaemia (low blood glucose)

Table 11.3   Liver function tests (LFTs): normal values

Test	Normal value
Alanine aminotransferase (ALT) – enzyme (also known as SGPT)	5–40 IU/L
Aspartate aminotransferase (AST) – enzyme (also known as SGOT)	5–60 IU/L
Alkaline phosphatase (ALP) – enzyme	30–130 IU/L
Gamma-glutamyl transferase (GGT or gamma GT) – enzyme	5–80 IU/L
Albumin – protein	3.9–5.0 g/dL
Globulin	20–30 g/L
Bilirubin – breakdown product of red cells	3–17 μmol/L
Lactate	0.5–2.2 mmol/L
Prothrombin time (PT)	12–16 seconds
International normalised ratio (INR)	1

the thousands following a paracetamol overdose. As ALT leaks out of damaged liver cells, serum levels rise and therefore offer some indication of the degree of liver cell damage. Once all liver cells are damaged ALT levels will start to fall. Therefore it is imperative that the ALT level is correlated with an indicator of synthetic function. Prothrombin time (PT) and international normalised ratio (INR) are measures of clotting time that rely upon the availability of clotting factors. An increase in PT and INR may suggest insufficient production of clotting factors and could therefore reflect acute cellular damage. It is not unusual for a PT to be in excess of 100 to 150 seconds and the INR to be between 8 and 12. This coagulopathy is an excellent indicator of the severity of liver cellular damage, and a continued increase in clotting time despite a falling ALT is a poor prognostic sign. Other important blood tests include urea and electrolytes (U&Es) as a measure of renal function because excess paracetamol is toxic to kidney cells. Increased serum creatinine may indicate acute tubular necrosis. Blood glucose levels may reveal hypoglycaemia due to the liver's inability to convert stored glycogen to available glucose due to liver cell damage. Acid–base balance should be assessed by ABGs and may reveal a metabolic acidosis due to hyperlactatemia. Damaged liver cells lose the ability to metabolise lactate, leading to raised levels, which can influence acid–base balance and precipitate metabolic acidosis (Table 11.3).

Immediate Management

Lucy should be admitted to an observation ward for continued monitoring of vital signs, evaluation of venous blood samples and administration of the antidote to paracetamol. Lucy's condition could be potentially life threatening and so she should be encouraged to inform her parents. They and her boyfriend will need clear, honest communication and a high level of emotional support during the next few hours.

Administration of the antidote acetylcysteine (Parvolex®) is currently dependent upon serum paracetamol levels, which are evaluated against a new nomogram produced in 2012. This is a graph that correlates the serum level of paracetamol against time since ingestion.

The Medicines & Healthcare Products Regulatory Agency (MHRA) issued the following advice in 2012:

> All patients with a timed plasma paracetamol level on or above a single treatment line joining points of 100mg/L at 4 hours and 15mg/L at 15 hours after ingestion should receive acetylcysteine (Parvolex or generics) based on a new treatment nomogram, regardless of risk factors.

> Where there is doubt over the timing of paracetamol ingestion including when ingestion has occurred over a period of one hour or more – 'staggered overdose' – acetylcysteine should be given without delay (the nomogram should not be used). (MHRA, 2012)

The dose of acetylcysteine should be calculated on the basis of Lucy's weight and administered to a set regimen (Table 11.4). Acetylcysteine assists in the production of cysteine, which acts as a glutathione donor to detoxify NAPQI. It also provides substances that bind directly to the reactive oxygen free radicals released (Jones, 2000). Side effects of acetylcysteine that should be watched for include rash, flushing and bronchospasm, which are more frequent in asthmatics (Schmidt and Dalhoff, 2001). The MHRA (2012) suggests that these will manifest themselves within the first hour.

Table 11.4 Acetylcysteine (Parvolex®) administration regime – adult loading regime

150 mg/kg body weight infused in 200 mL over 1 hour

50 mg/kg in 500 mL over the next 4 hours

100 mg/kg in 1 litre over the next 16 hours

Dosage should be calculated to patient's weight

A ceiling weight of 110 kg should be used for obese patients

Source: Adapted from MHRA (2012)

Serum paracetamol levels are only effective in determining the overall risk of organ failure when measured four hours or longer after the initial overdose. Interpretation of serum paracetamol levels requires some caution in chronic alcohol misuse and in individuals taking enzyme inducing medication such as phenytoin, carbamazepine, rifampicin and isoniazid, as chronic alcohol consumption and some drugs induce the cytochrome P-450 pathway. Careful monitoring is especially required in individuals who are malnourished, as their intracellular levels of glutathione may be diminished, those who have ingested other substances and people with mental illness, who may not recount accurate information on the timing and amount of the overdose.

Medical Management Strategies

Late presentation following paracetamol overdose as in Lucy's case is not uncommon but can often present additional healthcare challenges. Intravenous administration of acetylcysteine is recommended despite late presentation, as studies have shown that mortality was lower in groups that received acetylcysteine (Harrison et al., 1990). The improvement in survival is thought to relate to increases in cardiac output, oxygen extraction ratio and oxygen consumption (Harrison et al., 1991). Prompt treatment will resolve the insult to the liver in the majority of cases; however, between 2 and 5 per cent will develop acute liver failure (O'Grady, 2006). Signs and symptoms of acute liver failure tend to develop over time post overdose (Table 11.5).

Acute Liver Failure

Acute liver failure presents with a number of physiological manifestations that will require intensive care support. Hepatic encephalopathy is an altered neuropsychiatric state caused by failure of the liver to process

Table 11.5 Time frame and symptom presentation post paracetamol overdose

Stage	Time frame	Symptoms
1	12 to 24 hours	• Gastrointestinal cramping, nausea, vomiting or no clinical manifestations
2	24 to 48 hours	• Symptoms reduce but hepatoxocity and renal tubular necrosis developing • Increased blood level of ALT/AST • Decreased production of clotting factors – increased bleeding risk • Decreased ability to mobilise glucose – hypoglycaemia • Decreased urine output – oliguria
3	Days 3 to 5	• Peak hepatotoxic crisis. • Jaundice • Oliguria or anuria • Bruising and bleeding • Profound hypoglycaemia • Metabolic acidosis
4	Untreated or unsuccessful treatment	• Liver failure • Acute kidney injury (see Chapter 8) • Cerebral encephalopathy and oedema • Coma and death

toxins that have a deleterious effect upon cerebral function and may lead to cerebral oedema. Scales such as the West Haven Scale (Table 11.6) or the Glasgow Coma Score (See Chapter 4) or a narrative description of Lucy's temperament and manner may be used to assess the degree of hepatic encephalopathy. She is drowsy but must be observed for signs of deterioration such as irritability, confusion or coma.

The size of reaction to light of both pupils should be recorded hourly as increasing dilation and sluggish reaction may indicate an increasing intracranial pressure. The mechanism for cerebral oedema leading to raised intracranial pressure is poorly understood but it is thought to be due to raised levels of glutamine leading to an uptake of water in the astrocytes within the brain (Sargent and Fullwood, 2006). Suspected raised intracranial pressure may require invasive pressure monitoring and treatment with an intravenous infusion of mannitol (an intravascular osmotic agent that can draw fluid from brain) (Lee et al., 2011), elective ventilation and expedient transfer to a supraregional liver centre. Failure to manage cerebral

Table 11.6 West Haven criteria for semi-quantitative grading of mental state

Grade	Symptoms
1	• Trivial lack of awareness • Euphoria or anxiety • Shortened attention span • Impaired performance of addition
2	• Lethargy or apathy • Minimal disorientation for time or place • Subtle personality change • Inappropriate behaviour • Impaired performance of subtraction
3	• Somnolence to semi-stupor, but responsive to verbal stimuli • Confusion • Gross disorientation
4	• Coma (unresponsive to verbal or noxious stimuli

Source: Adapted from Ferenci et al. (2002)

The Case Scenario: Medical Management and Care Issues

Lucy is admitted to the medical assessment unit where her condition continues to deteriorate. Despite commencing an intravenous infusion of Parvolex® Lucy is becoming more drowsy and difficult to rouse, her pupils are slightly dilated at 4 mm in diameter and their reaction to light remains brisk. Lucy's capillary blood glucose levels are recorded hourly, as they were 3.2 to 3.6 mmol/L despite an intravenous infusion of 10 per cent dextrose and she has not passed urine since admission.

Specific venous blood results revealed the following:
ALT levels: 2,592 IU/L (normal 5 to 35 IU/L)
PT: 59 seconds (normal 12 to 16 seconds)
INR: > 3.0
Blood glucose: 3.2 mmol/L (normal 4 to 7 mmol/L)
Creatinine: 340 μmol/L (normal 60 to 110 μmol/L)
Paracetamol levels: 0.3 mmol/L (or 45 mg/L) 24 hours post overdose
Arterial pH: 7.28

The Case Scenario *continued*

The nearest supraregional liver unit was contacted for advice and Lucy's parents and family were informed of her deteriorating condition and referral for specialist treatment.

Immediate Medical Management
1. What are the current treatment options for Lucy?
2. What factors might inform the choice of immediate management?
3. What are Lucy's main care issues?

---

oedema and lower the intracranial pressure will lead to brain stem herniation and death.

Hypoglycaemia is a common manifestation in acute liver failure due to the liver's inability to convert stored glycogen to available glucose. Blood glucose monitoring should be undertaken at least one- to two-hourly as profound hypoglycaemia may occur. Hypoglycaemia requires support with a range of intravenous dextrose products between 10 to 50 per cent to achieve normoglycaemia in the individual. Blood glucose monitoring should continue to occur until reliance on dextrose therapy is negated by restoration of native liver function. Some degree of coagulopathy will occur and should not be prophylactically supported or corrected with blood products because PT and INR provide an excellent indictor of the liver's ability to make certain products, including clotting factors. Circulating levels of fibrinogen, prothrombin and factors V, VII, IX and X are reduced in acute liver failure (O'Grady, 2006). Administration of blood products such as fresh frozen plasma will mask the clotting results and hinder assessment of further liver deterioration. Management of risk is an important factor to ensure that Lucy remains safe and does not injure herself. Absorbent or alginate dressings should be applied to bleeding sites such as cannulae or wounds.

Hepatic lactic acid uptake and metabolism are directly affected by paracetamol overdose and will lead to a transient metabolic acidosis within 15 hours of overdose. Metabolic acidosis occurring after 15 hours is a poor prognostic indicator as it suggests a decrease in hepatic lactic acid clearance due to deteriorating liver function and an increase in peripheral lactic acid from profound tissue hypoxia (Makin and Williams, 1997). Metabolic acidosis of pH < 7.25 after fluid resuscitation and 24 hours after the overdose can be an indicator for admission onto the NHS Blood and Transplant (NHSBT) supra urgent liver transplant waiting scheme (NHSBT, 2015).

Acute liver failure creates a hyperdynamic circulation of high cardiac output, low mean arterial pressure (MAP) and low systemic vascular resistance (SVR) due to generalised vasodilation in the body from the release of cytokines and other vasoactive substances (Ellis and Wendon, 1996). Effective circulating volume is reduced and may need aggressive fluid resuscitation and vasopressors such as norepinephrine to support and improve the MAP and SVR (Bernal and Wendon 2013). Hypovolaemia is also a potential side effect of IV mannitol administration; therefore accurate monitoring of Lucy's heart rate, BP, central venous pressure, urine output and fluid intake every 30 minutes is imperative. Invasive cardiac output monitoring including arterial BP measurement may be necessary. Lucy's renal function has also shown signs of deterioration, which is either due to the toxic effect of the excess paracetamol causing acute tubular necrosis or due to hypotension and volume depletion. Oliguria or anuria may follow, along with rises in serum creatinine and urea that may be severe enough to require haemodiafiltration.

The development of these symptoms should prompt immediate referral to a specialist supraregional liver centre that offers a liver transplantation service (Table 11.7). Early transfer of Lucy is important, as her condition can deteriorate rapidly (Lee et al., 2011).

Acute liver failure has three possible treatment outcomes:

- restoration of native liver function with intensive therapy, including ventilation, monitoring of cerebral oedema, dialysis and care of the patient with multi-organ failure;
- liver transplantation due to the inability of the native liver to regenerate functional capacity;
- death.

Table 11.7   UK and Irish supraregional specialist liver centres

England
Addenbrookes Hospital, Cambridge
Freeman Hospital, Newcastle upon Tyne
King's College Hospital, London
Queen Elizabeth Hospital, Birmingham
Royal Free Hospital, London
St James's University Hospital, Leeds
Scotland
The Royal Infirmary of Edinburgh
Republic of Ireland
St Vincent's Hospital, Dublin

Due to the immense physiological changes and rapid deterioration that occurs, Lucy and her family may not be aware of the seriousness of the situation. Clear information and explanation of the cause and speed of deterioration and the intensive therapy for multi-organ failure required is necessary. The possibility of liver transplantation, its potential risks and the lifestyle adaptation, including daily immunosuppressant medication and dietary restrictions in relation to unpasteurised products and shellfish, should be discussed with Lucy and her family by members of the medical and transplant teams. Liver transplantation is an effective treatment modality for patients with acute liver failure but a poor consent rate to donate organs by families continues to impact upon organ availability. Family refusal to donate organs is 43 per cent in the UK (NHSBT, 2013). The Organ Donation Taskforce (Department of Health, 2008) set a goal to increase organ donation by 50 per cent by 2013, which it achieved; however the increase in donation is from expansion of the donation after circulatory death (DCD) programme rather than a reduction in family refusal rates (NHSBT, 2013).

Summary

Acute liver failure can have devastating effects on both individuals and their families due to the rapid deterioration that often occurs. The insult to the liver from excess paracetamol has consequences for all body systems and multi-organ failure is a common occurrence. Unfortunately individuals may be lulled into a false sense of security regarding the non-specific symptoms that present in the first instance after taking a paracetamol overdose; however, during this time major liver damage may develop. Lucy may have had a more uneventful recovery had she attended the emergency department earlier than 24 hours post ingestion. Her treatment would have commenced sooner and may have helped to prevent further liver damage and support liver function. Lucy, like many others, may have felt embarrassed that she had on impulse taken a significant amount of paracetamol in response to an argument with her boyfriend. The liver has a marvellous capacity to regenerate in some cases, but if native liver function cannot be supported and restored then liver transplantation is the only hope for survival. Early treatment and subsequent proactive referral to supraregional centres are key to survival. However, due to the shortage of donor organs, allocation of this scarce resource is required and patients must fulfil set criteria that grade the severity of their symptoms. Liver transplantation for acute liver failure has comparable survival results with other liver transplant categories and is a recognised treatment modality.

References

Aitio, M. L. 'N-Acetylcysteine: Passe-Partout or Much Ado about Nothing?', *British Journal of Clinical Pharmacology*, **61**(1) (2006), 5–15.

Bernal W., Wendon J. 'Acute Liver Failure', *New England Journal of Medicine* **369**(26) (2013).

British National Formulary. *BNF 69* (2015) [Online]. Available from: www .medicinescomplete.com/mc/bnf/current/PHP195-acetylcysteine.htm?q=acetylcy steine&t=search&ss=text&p=4#_hit (accessed 18 May 2015).

Department of Health (DH). *Organs for Transplant: A Report from the Organ Donation Taskforce* (London: Department of Health, 2008).

Dolan, B. and L. Holt. *Accident and Emergency: From Theory to Practice*, 3rd edn (London: Bailliere Tindall, 2013).

Ellis, A. and J. Wendon. 'Circulatory, Respiratory, Cerebral and Renal Derangements in Acute Liver Failure: Pathophysiology and Management', *Seminars in Liver Diseases*, **16** (1996), 379–88.

Ferenci, P., A. Lockwood, K. Mullen, R. Tarter, K. Weissenborn, A. T. Blei and Members of the Working Party. 'Hepatic Encephalopathy – Definition, Nomenclature, Diagnosis, and Quantification: Final Report of the Working Party at the 11th World Congresses of Gastroenterology, Vienna, 1998', *Hepatology*, **35** (2002), 716–21.

Harrison, P., R. Keays, G. Bray et al.. 'Improved Outcome of Paracetamol-induced Fulminant Hepatic Failure by Late Administration of Acetylcysteine', *Lancet*, **30** (1990), 1572–3.

Harrison, P., J. Wendon, A. Gimson et al.. 'Improvement by Acetylcysteine of Hemodynamics and Oxygen Transport in Fulminant Hepatic Failure', *New England Journal of Medicine*, **324** (1991), 1852–7.

Hawton K., H. Bergen, D. Casey et al.. 'Self-harm in England: A Tale of Three Cities', *Social Psychiatry and Psychiatric Epidemiology*, **42** (2007), 513–21. Available from: http://link.springer.com/article/10.1007%2Fs00127-007-0199-7 (accessed 9 June 2015).

Hawton K., H. Bergen, S. Dodd et al.. 'Long Term Effect of Reduced Pack Sizes of Paracetamol on Poisoning Deaths and Liver Transplant Activity in England and Wales: Interrupted Time Series Analyses', *BMJ* (2013). Available from: www.bmj. com/content/bmj/346/bmj.f403.full.pdf (accessed 12 May 2015).

Hawton, K., C. Ware, H. Mistry et al.. 'Why Patients Choose Paracetamol for Self Poisoning and Their Knowledge of its Dangers', *British Medical Journal*, **310** (1995), 164.

Imperial, J. and E. Keeffe. 'Laboratory Tests', in B. Bacon, J. O'Grady, A. Di Biscelgie and J. Lake (eds), *Comprehensive Clinical Hepatology*, 2nd edn (St Louis: Mosby, 2006).

Jones, A. 'Recent Advances in the Management of Late Paracetamol Poisoning', *Emergency Medicine*, **12** (2000), 14–21.

Lee, W., A. Larson, R. Stravitz. 'AASLD Position Paper: The Management of Acute Liver Failure: Update 2011' [Online]. Available from: www.aasld.org/sites/default/files/guideline_documents/alfenhanced.pdf (accessed 12 May 2015).

Makin, A. and R. Williams. 'Acetaminophen-induced Acute Liver Failure', in W. Lee and R. Williams (eds), *Acute Liver Failure* (Cambridge: Cambridge University Press, 1997).

Medicines & Healthcare Products Regulatory Agency (MHRA). 'Paracetamol Overdose: New Guidance on the Use of Intravenous Acetylcysteine' (2012) [Online]. Available from: www.gov.uk/drug-safety-update/treating-paracetamol-overdose-with-intravenous-acetylcysteine-new-guidance (accessed 5 May 2015).

NHS Blood and Transplant (NHSBT) 'Taking Organ Transplantation to 2020: A Detailed Strategy. NHS Blood and Transplant' (2013) [Online]. Available from: www.nhsbt.nhs.uk/to2020/resources/nhsbt_organ_donor_strategy_long.pdf (accessed 5 May 2015).

NHS Blood and Transplant (NHSBT). Liver Transplantation: Selection Criteria and Recipient Registration (2015) [Online]. Available at: http://www.odt.nhs.uk/pdf/liver_selection_policy.pdf (accessed 12 May 2015).

O'Grady, J. 'Acute Liver Failure', in B. Bacon, J. O'Grady, A. Di Biscelgie and J. Lake (eds), *Comprehensive Clinical Hepatology*, 2nd edn (St Louis: Mosby, 2006).

Sargent, S. and D. Fullwood. 'The Management of Hepatic Encephalopathy and Cerebral Oedema in Acute Liver Failure', *British Journal of Neuroscience Nursing*, **2**(9) (2006), 448–53.

Schmidt, L. E. and K. Dalhoff. 'Risk Factors in the Development of Adverse Reactions to N-acetylcysteine in Patients with Paracetamol Poisoning', *British Journal of Clinical Pharmacology*, **51** (2001), 87–91.

12

Musculoskeletal Trauma

Julia Maz

Introduction

There is a wide spectrum of trauma and injuries that affect the musculo-skeletal system in terms of cause, structural damage and outcome. In 2015 there were 1,700 reported road fatalities, down by 2 per cent from 1,742 in the previous year, although motor vehicle traffic increased by 2.3 per cent over the same period (Department for Transport, 2015). However, of note is the 7 per cent increase in motorcycle accidents between 2006 and 2014. Musculoskeletal problems account for an estimated 3.5 million emergency department attendances each year and are a significant cause of disability (Spinks et al., 2009). Traumatic injury is a public health concern and the World Health Organization (2013) estimates that road traffic accidents are the eighth leading cause of death worldwide among individuals between the ages of 15 and 44 years. Acute trauma is caused by a single, clear event and demonstrates a wide variety of injury patterns ranging from minor self-limiting sprains to fractures and/or dislocations of joints. Bone, soft tissue and associated neurovascular injuries are rarely emergencies unless accompanied by a life-threatening haemorrhage as in certain amputations, pelvic and femoral fractures.

Trauma-associated deaths are known to occur in three so-called 'peaks' (Committee American College of Surgeons (ACoS), 2014). The first peak of death occurs at the time of injury. It may be instantaneous or within a few minutes and is due to overwhelming primary injury to major organs or structures such as the brain, heart or great vessels. In most situations these injuries are irrecoverable, although rapid treatment and transfer may save some patients. Primary prevention, in the form of seat belts, speed limits, motorcycle helmet legislation and road traffic law enforcement, for example, has a major role in reducing the incidence of these injuries (Davis et al., 2011; Committee ACoS, 2014), though total elimination of such events is rarely possible. The second peak lasts from the end of the first period to several hours after the injury has taken place. It is during this time that many causes of morbidity and mortality are preventable by avoidance of secondary injury due to hypoxia, haemorrhage or any process that leads to inadequate tissue perfusion. Reversible life-threatening conditions may include major haemorrhage from viscera, bone and vessels or pneumothoraces. Most definitive care is directed at this period, as skilled assessment and management should reduce mortality and disability (Committee ACoS, 2014). The third peak of death occurs days or weeks after the injury and usually happens in a high-dependency or intensive therapy area where sepsis and multiple organ failure ensue (Mikhail, 1999), see Chapter 3. Advances in intensive care therapy may reduce these deaths but improvements in initial management on admission will also reduce morbidity and mortality during this period.

Trauma patients represent the highest challenges to the healthcare system because assessment and management require a multidisciplinary team effort. Treatment of an injured patient in the pre-hospital arena should consist of assessment, extrication, initiation of resuscitation and stabilisation and safe and timely transport to the closest trauma hospital or acute care facility whose capabilities match the patients' needs (Sasser et al., 2011). For musculoskeletal injuries, the essential components of resuscitation should be limited to the establishment of airway, provision of ventilation, haemorrhage control, stabilisation of fractures, and if indicated, immobilisation of the entire spine. The focus of this chapter is on the management of an individual presenting with a traumatic long bone fracture (femur) and the management strategies offered take into account current evidence-based recommendations. Successful management of musculoskeletal injury is dependent upon the efficacy of early resuscitation, followed by detailed physical examination and diagnostic studies to establish the priorities for life-saving management, further treatment and rehabilitative care. Management generally occurs in four distinct phases:

1. Acute or resuscitation period (0 to 3 hours).
2. Primary or stabilisation period (3 to 72 hours).
3. Secondary or regeneration period (3 to 8 days).
4. Tertiary or rehabilitation period (beyond day 8).

This chapter is primarily concerned with phases 1 and 2. Further reading is indicated for phases 3 and 4 at the end of the chapter.

Aim and Learning Outcomes

The Aim

The aim of this chapter is to explore the assessment and management of an individual presenting with a compound fracture of a major long bone with significant associated injury potential. A case scenario illustrates the key principles that underpin the assessment and management of such a fracture.

Learning Outcomes

At the end of this chapter the reader will be able to:

1. Discuss the normal anatomy of the musculoskeletal system.
2. Define and explain the resultant pathophysiological processes that occur following trauma.
3. Consider the initial assessment process and the immediate prioritisation of care following musculoskeletal trauma.
4. Explore the rationale for the management and care of a person with a long bone fracture.
5. Recognise the common complications associated with a long bone fracture.
6. Appreciate the value of multidisciplinary teamwork in the management of musculoskeletal trauma.

The Musculoskeletal System

The musculoskeletal system and related neurovascular structures consist of bones, joints, tendons, ligaments, muscles, blood vessels and nerves. The skeletal system contains 206 bones, which provide support, strength, movement and protection to the body and organs. Bones also store calcium and are involved in blood cell production.

Bones are characterised by shape as long (Figure 12.1), short, flat or irregular, with the shape of a particular bone suited for a unique function or purpose. The skeleton is composed of two types of bones: cancellous and cortical. Cancellous (spongy) bone is found in the skull, vertebrae, pelvis and end of long bones. Cortical (dense) bone is found in the long bones. Bones are supplied by blood vessels, nerves and lymphatic vessels that nourish bone tissue and allow the bone to repair injuries. The periosteum covers the bones and provides an additional blood supply. Bone is connected to other bone by stabilising bands of elastic, fibrous connective tissue called

The Case Scenario: The Presenting Complaint

Paul is a fit, healthy 28-year-old salesman who normally drives to work by car, but today he decided to travel on his motorbike. He left home at 8.00 a.m. wearing full protective clothing, including a helmet. Five minutes later a van pulled out of a junction without stopping and as Paul was travelling at 40 miles per hour he was unable to avoid the impact. An ambulance arrived at the scene 12 minutes later and made the following observations.

Paul is alert and orientated to time and place with no reported loss of consciousness and no apparent neurological deficit:

GCS score: 15 and both pupils are equal and react to light.
Respiratory rate: 18 breaths per minute and SpO_2 is 99 per cent on air.
Temperature: 36.3 °C.
Pulse: 80 beats per minute.
BP: 140/80 mmHg.

The paramedic crew apply a hard cervical collar and position Paul on a spinal board. An intravenous infusion of Haemaccel® 500 mL is commenced and IV morphine 2.5 mg administered for pain with PO Cyclizine 50 mgs (anti-emetic). A single wound to the right middle thigh shows a bony protrusion, which is oozing blood. Paul denies any other injury and has no ongoing health problems, his lungs are clear and his abdomen is soft. He is haemodynamically stable en route to hospital according to the ambulance report.

Consider the following:

1. Review the normal anatomy and physiology of the musculoskeletal system.
2. Understand the importance of mechanisms of injury.
3. Consider the physiological changes in the body caused by bony trauma.
4. What are the common clinical features of a fracture?

ligaments. Non-elastic fibrous cords that connect muscle to bone are tendons. Dense connective tissue found between the ribs, in the nasal septum, ear, larynx, trachea, bronchi, between vertebrae and on articulating surfaces is known as cartilage. Cartilage has a limited vascular supply, whereas bone tissue contains abundant blood vessels (Figure 12.2).

Joints are classified as non-synovial (such as the sacro-iliac) and synovial (for example, the shoulder). Synovial joints have two articulating surfaces covered with cartilage and surrounded by a two-layered synovial membrane sac to facilitate movement. The entire joint is then encapsulated by dense, ligamentous material. Joints provide mobility and stability, flexion and extension, medial and lateral rotation, and abduction and adduction. Joint movement is enhanced by muscles and ligaments that overlie the joint.

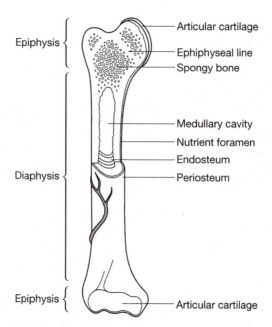

Epiphysis {
Articular cartilage
Ephiphyseal line
Spongy bone

Medullary cavity
Nutrient foramen
Endosteum

Diaphysis {
Periosteum

Epiphysis {
Articular cartilage

Figure 12.1 A long bone

Superficial epigastric
Superficial circumflex iliac
Common femoral
External circumflex
Descending ramus of
external circumflex

Superficial external pubic
Deep external pubic
Internal circumflex
Femoral profunda
First perforating

Superficial femoral
Second perforating

Third perforating
Anastomotica magna

Superior external articular
branch of popliteal

Superior internal articular
branch of popliteal

Figure 12.2 The vascular supply to the femur

Table 12.1 Key requirements of bone

Respiration
The cells of bone require oxygen for metabolism and release carbon dioxide which must be removed from their environment. If either process ceases the cells of the bone tissue will die in the same way as any other living tissue.

Assimilation
Nutrition is necessary for growth and replacement of damaged cells; therefore protein, fat, carbohydrate, water, mineral salts and vitamins must reach the cells of bone in a steady consistent supply.

Excretion
Products of metabolism are produced continually and must be excreted from bone cells and tissues. These include such products as excess water, lactic acid and urea.

Reproduction
During the skeletal growth phase (16–18 years in most people), the bones are increasing in length and diameter. After growth has ceased new cells must still be produced to replace damaged or old ones. This requires a steady process of cell division and the production of new, fresh cells.

Response to stimulation
All tissues react to chemical, mechanical or nervous irritation and bone is no exception. It must repair itself when broken or damaged, respond to increased stresses by improving its strength in given areas, provide protrusions to which muscles are attached and react in general to the need for increased size and length.

Nerves and arteries lie in close proximity to bones and muscle groups, with arterioles distributed throughout the periosteum to provide nutrients, and nerves to provide sensation and movement. Close proximity of arteries and nerves to bone structures increases the risk for injury with trauma to soft tissue, muscle, bone or joint. Bone is a living tissue with the same requirements as all living material, including respiration, assimilation, excretion, reproduction and response to stimulation (Table 12.1). The reader is referred to Marieb (2015) and Humbyrd et al. (2012) for further detail.

The Femur

The femur is the longest, strongest, largest and heaviest tubular bone in the human body (Bulstrode, 2015). It is capable of absorbing a huge amount of energy and resisting all but the greatest amount of trauma without damage. The femur can be divided into regions consisting of the head, neck, intertrochanteric, subtrochanteric (proximal), shaft and supracondylar and condylar regions (distal). In spite of the femur's strengths it is not immune to injury and when the femur is injured the situation may become life threatening. (See Dandy and Edwards (2009) for a detailed account of the anatomy of the femur.)

Long Bone Trauma: Mechanism of Injury

Musculoskeletal trauma is caused by either blunt or penetrating forces (Eckes-Roper, 2003). Blunt trauma to a femur is primarily associated with forces such as acceleration, deceleration, shearing and compression, which may result in injuries to other solid and hollow organs as well. Common causes of such injury are road traffic accidents, seat belt injuries, falls, sports injuries and explosions. Penetrating trauma is caused by an object penetrating the body, such as a gunshot wound, injuring skin, tissue, underlying organs, viscera and bone.

The mechanism of injury can be described as the effect of energy on human tissue. A clear history of the mechanism of injury is essential to make an accurate diagnosis in musculoskeletal trauma. Kinetic, thermal, electrical and radiation are examples of sources of energy that may cause injury. Paul has sustained injury (blunt trauma) resulting from kinetic energy, and it is imperative to determine how this energy was transmitted through the body and which organ systems were most likely to be affected. The most important concepts to consider when assessing the mechanism of injury are:

1. The anatomy of the area affected by trauma.
2. Newton's first law of motion, which states that an 'object at rest will remain at rest, and an object in motion will remain in motion until acted upon by an external force'.

Paul was travelling at approximately 40 miles per hour (mph) when his motorbike collided with the van. Paul's body would continue to move at 40 mph until it was acted upon by the 'external force' of the van, causing rapid deceleration to 0 mph. Deceleration forces are transferred to the body at three different points of collision. The first collision occurs when the motorbike and vehicle strike and Paul continues to move forward. The second collision occurs when Paul hits the van and his body stops. The third collision point occurs when internal organs continue to move until they impact upon another organ, cavity wall or structure, or they are restrained suddenly by vasculature, muscles, ligaments or fascia. It is important to obtain information regarding potential patterns of injury relating to the energy and force of the accident as different damage occurs with each collision point and so each point must be considered separately to avoid missed injuries.

A fracture is defined as a disruption in the integrity of living bone, involving injury to the bone marrow, periosteum and adjacent soft tissue. The fracturing force can be direct or indirect (rotation, axial compression and bending without a direct impact). Fractures are divided into two general categories (Figure 12.3). Closed or simple fractures occur when the bone is broken but the skin is intact. Open or compound fractures, as in Paul's case, are characterised by bone protrusion puncture wounds where the bone punctures the skin or a foreign object penetrates the skin and bone, causing a fracture. Examples of long bone fracture include fractures of the clavicle, the humerus, the radius and ulna, the metacarpals and phalanges, femoral shaft fractures, tibial fractures and metatarsal and phalangeal fractures. Fracture types are divided into oblique, transverse, spiral and comminuted (Figure 12.3). The clinical features of Paul's fracture include those outlined in Table 12.2.

An appreciation of high-energy mechanisms of injury and an understanding of closed or open fractures can inform appropriate and timely management of pain control, swelling or possible contamination that could require multiple trips to operating theatres for wound irrigations and surgical debridement.

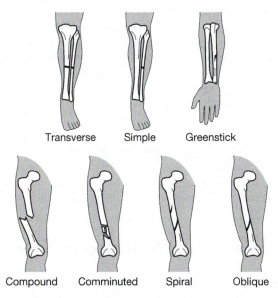

Transverse   Simple   Greenstick

Compound   Comminuted   Spiral   Oblique

Figure 12.3 Long bone fractures

Table 12.2 Classic clinical features suggestive of a bone fracture

---

Pain throbbing and localised; often aggravated by active or passive movement

Swelling at the fracture site caused by oedema and/or haematoma formation which usually increases in the first 12 to 24 hours following injury

Deformity seen and felt, loss of function due to pain and the nature of the fracture

Bony tenderness and/or bruising at the fracture site

Crepitus (grating) heard or felt when the ends of the broken bone rub together

---

The Case Scenario: The Immediate Assessment Priorities

Paul arrives at the nearest accident and emergency department with the paramedic crew at 8.40 a.m. An immediate physiological assessment reveals the following:

> Temperature: 36.2 °C
> Pulse: 110 beats/min, regular
> Respirations: 14 breaths per minute and SpO_2 = 99 per cent
> Blood pressure: 100/60 mmHg
> GCS: 15 and no apparent neurological deficits

Paul is assessed by a triage nurse, who notes that he continues to complain of severe pain, which he scores as 8 out of 10. Paul's right thigh is swollen, bruised and deformed and a compound comminuted fracture of the shaft of femur is suspected, with a 12 cm bony protrusion of the right mid thigh. He has a 2 litre intravenous infusion of 0.9 per cent sodium chloride and has received a further dose of IV morphine 2.5 mg for continued pain. He is receiving 15 litres of high-flow oxygen via a non-rebreathe face mask.

Consider the following:

1. Explain the pathophysiology of trauma on the body.
2. What are the immediate assessment priorities in Paul's case and why?
3. Consider how you would carry out a more detailed assessment of Paul's condition. In particular, how would you check for any limb-threatening conditions?

Assessment and Reaching a Diagnosis

Paul requires a systematic and comprehensive assessment to provide a rapid, accurate diagnosis to inform immediate appropriate management and care. The initial assessment and evaluation of Paul should always follow the principles of Advanced Trauma Life Support System (ATLS) (Committee ACoS,

2014), and includes the identification and treatment of life-threatening injuries. The primary efforts in the initial phase are focused on life-saving procedures within the 'golden hour', which is known to be the time period in which life-threatening conditions following major trauma may be resolved by immediate therapeutic intervention (Magee, 2005; Stahal et al., 2005). The first step is evaluation of Paul's airway, breathing and circulation while maintaining spinal precautions until injury to the complete spine can be excluded clinically and radiographically (with X-rays or computed tomography (CT) scans). In practice these activities occur simultaneously but for the sake of narrative fluency each aspect will be discussed in turn. Rapid assessment identifies major injuries of head, cervical spine, chest and abdomen, and prioritises essential interventions.

Preliminary Assessment

Airway with Cervical Spine Protection

It is imperative that a clear and unobstructed airway is present. As Paul is speaking freely it is unlikely that there is any immediate threat to his airway. He is receiving high-flow oxygen at 15 litres per minute via a non-rebreathe trauma mask with a reservoir bag so that a high concentration of oxygen can be delivered accurately. A vital nursing role is to ensure that the mask fits snugly over mouth and nose and that the flow rate is sufficient to keep the bag from collapsing during inspiration.

Given the high-velocity injury Paul has sustained, a possible spinal injury should be considered. Careful removal of Paul's helmet is imperative for protection of the cervical spine (Lui et al., 2008) (Table 12.3). Any patient with a possible cervical spine injury should have their neck immobilised in a neutral alignment to prevent further damage. Cervical spine damage is likely with deceleration injury as in Paul's case, hyperflexion or extension injury or any blunt injury above the clavicles. A fracture of the first rib seen on chest X-ray indicates high-energy transfer and should always raise suspicion of cervical injury as well as intrathoracic damage. When available a closely fitting firm cervical collar should be applied and secured with adhesive tape and sand bags placed on either side of the head to ensure immobility. Flexion of the cervical spine must be avoided to prevent airway compromise or aggravation of an existing spinal cord injury (National Association of Emergency Medicine and Surgery Physicians and ACoS, 2013).

This action has already been established by the paramedics on arrival at the accident scene. The front of the cervical collar is opened, to inspect the neck for jugular vein distension and tracheal deviation and to palpate the carotid pulse, and then securely closed. The cervical collar must fit properly

Table 12.3   Helmet removal procedure

- An adequate airway can often be achieved with helmet in place especially when the potential exists for a complicating injury during a difficult helmet removal.
- Two people are needed to remove it – one person applies in-line immobilisation by placing hands on each side of helmet with fingers on the mandible, pulling carefully. N.B. cut or remove chin strap.
- A second person concurrently receives the weight of the patient's head by placing fingers of both hands on occipital region and thumbs at the angles of the mandible. The second person is now in control of the head and neck.
- The first person then removes the helmet by pulling laterally and carefully sliding it off.

---

to prevent flexion and extension of the cervical spine. A properly fitting collar has the following features:

1. The chin rests securely in the chin holder.
2. The collar does not cover the ears.
3. The bottom of the collar rests on the upper sternum (Licina and Nowitzke, 2005).

Clinical features of spinal cord injury (Table 12.4) can be quickly ascertained, such as numbness, tingling and inability to wriggle the toes and fingers. Full spinal immobilisation with the rigid cervical collar, a cervical immobilisation device (CID) and an immobilisation board should be maintained throughout Paul's initial treatment. Should Paul vomit, he should be log rolled as a unit with the equipment remaining intact, and then suctioning should be performed. Cervical spine X-rays from C1 to T1 may be obtained to determine the presence of spinal fractures (Rodrigues and

Table 12.4   Clinical features of spinal cord trauma

Neck (cervical) and/or thoracic (chest)
Breathing difficulties (from paralysis of the breathing muscles) **and all** of list below

Lumbar and/or sacral (lower back)
- Loss of normal bowel and bladder control (may include constipation, incontinence, bladder spasms)
- Sensory changes: numbness, tingling sensation
- Motor changes: spasticity (increased muscle tone)
- Pain
- Weakness, paralysis

Qureshi, 2014). Blunt trauma, particularly when significant deceleration is involved (as in Paul's case), can affect any part of the body and imaging is used liberally. Previously X-rays or Computerised Tomography (CT) of the neck, chest and pelvis were routinely undertaken in cases of blunt trauma. However, most trauma centres now undertake imaging studies only when indicated by the mechanism of injury and clinical findings on examination (Anderson et al., 2010). Providing Paul does not have radiological evidence of bony spine abnormalities, no abnormal neurological findings and no pain on palpation, the spinal immobilisation devices can be removed. Normal neurological findings include the absence of pain with a full range of cervical motion, though this is often difficult to assess in the presence of distracting injuries or head trauma. A Magnetic Resonance Imaging (MRI) scan may be needed to evaluate the spine further.

Breathing

Respiration is assessed for rate, depth, pattern and noise every 30 minutes initially. Paul's deceleration injury may have caused rib fractures, which could affect his breathing. Signs of respiratory distress include rapid, shallow breaths, retraction of the intercostal muscles, nasal flaring and diminished or absent breath sounds. Paul's chest should be exposed and inspected for any surface trauma, penetrating wounds, paradoxical movements and flail segments. The rib cage and sternum are gently palpated for tenderness, crepitus and flail segments. A flail chest is defined as fractures in two or more adjacent ribs in two or more places or bilateral detachment of the sternum from the costal cartilage. The injury that Paul has sustained may have created a free-floating, unstable segment that moves in opposition to normal chest wall movement. Hence, a flail segment would move in when Paul breathes in and out with exhalation. A flail chest can cause hypoventilation of both lungs followed by atelectasis (alveolar collapse) and eventual hypoxia (Duggan and Kavanagh, 2005). Fortunately, Paul is not displaying these clinical features on initial assessment. Chest auscultation with a stethoscope may reveal normal air entry into both lungs, whereas unequal breath sounds on either side may indicate a collapsed lung due to a pneumothorax (air in pleural cavity) or a haemothorax (blood in pleural cavity).

Continuous pulse oximetry detects the percentage of arterial oxygen saturation in the blood and is a useful adjunct for determining adequacy of oxygenation; however, it must be remembered that the reading may not be accurate in a shocked trauma patient (Woodrow, 2012). Arterial blood gas analysis should be performed in all patients with a potential chest injury since apparently minor chest wall injuries may cause significant hypoxaemia. The mechanics of breathing may be compromised by a disruption of the bony chest wall or diaphragm, accumulation of blood or air in the pleural cavities or haemorrhage and oedema in the lung itself, which reduces compliance. A neurological injury may alter the respiratory drive or pattern of breathing.

Circulation

Untreated fractures of the limbs can lead to significant blood loss, which may be external and obvious, or covert. The estimated blood loss for a closed fracture of the femur is 1,000 to 1,500 mL and this figure can be doubled if the fracture is compound, as in Paul's scenario, and should therefore be considered a potential cause of hypovolaemic shock (see Chapter 2). Paul's pulse rate, regularity, volume and blood pressure (BP) should be assessed and recorded initially every 30 minutes until a stable trend is established. His regular heart rate of 110 beats per minute suggests a sinus tachycardia, which may be caused by pain, anxiety or both, or may signal a compensatory sympathetic response to low BP caused by a fall in stroke volume and cardiac output (see Chapter 2). Paul's BP is initially within the normal range despite potential blood loss. This may be maintained by a series of compensatory mechanisms triggered in response to a fall in circulatory volume. A fall in stroke volume (SV), cardiac output (CO) and subsequent BP will trigger baroreceptors in the carotid sinus and aortic arch to stimulate the cardiac acceleratory centre within the medulla oblongata. This will excite sympathetic nervous activity, resulting in an increased heart rate, myocardial contractility, generalised vasoconstriction and arterial redistribution of blood flow to the vital organs. A subsequent fall in renal perfusion simultaneously stimulates the renin–angiotensin–aldosterone–ADH system to retain sodium (Na^+) and water (H_2O) and conserve circulating volume to maintain SV and CO and increase the BP (see Chapter 2). Blood pressure alone can therefore be extremely misleading and should be considered in conjunction with other parameters of circulatory assessment, including pulse rate, capillary refill, respiratory rate, conscious level and urine output.

Paul should have two large bore intravenous venflons (14 or 16 gauge) inserted into large veins, such as the antecubital fossa, to administer intravenous fluid such as 0.9 per cent sodium chloride, Haemaccel®, 4 per cent albumin in 0.9 per cent saline or blood (see Chapter 2). Using National Institute of Health and Care Excellence (NICE) (2013, CG:174) guidelines would determine the best course of action. Careful monitoring of Paul's fluid input and output is essential to ensure that fluid resuscitation is optimised and that he is not volume overloaded.

A simple and important technique in reducing blood loss in Paul's situation involves immobilising the fracture with a long rigid splint such as an

Table 12.5 SHOCK mnemonic

S **Solutions** to add volume which will increase venous return. A combination of fluids, blood and plasma expanders (dextran, plasma and albumin are commonly used)

H **Haemodynamics** is a way to measure potential hypovolaemic shock and evaluate interventions. Note the normal CVP= 5–15 cm/H_2O

O **Oxygen** will saturate RBCs and decrease tissue starvation

C **Check** the skin (cold and clammy indicate the early stages of hypovolaemic shock)

K **Kick** up the feet and legs (elevate if possible) and let gravity increase venous return

---

air splint. This helps to obviate bleeding and pain. In the case of untreated femoral shaft fractures, bony overlap and large open venous channels in muscle potentiate bleeding. Paul is not displaying any signs of arterial blood loss externally (bright red and pulsating), and oozing indicates that Paul is bleeding from the capillaries adjacent to the wound site (bright red). Direct pressure in the form of firm application of a sterile gauze pad for 10 to 15 minutes and elevation (if possible) should stop the bleeding. In the presence of compressible controllable bleeding (as in Paul's case) fluid resuscitation is designed to maintain normal pulse and blood pressure. However, in the presence of non-compressible or non-controllable bleeding (pelvic fractures and bilateral limb fractures) or major bleeding elsewhere (abdomen and retroperitoneal bleeding), the object of resuscitation should be to maintain essential organ perfusion by maintaining a systolic blood pressure greater than 80 mmHg or restoring the radial pulse. The SHOCK mnemonic (Table 12.5) provides a simple but useful reminder of immediate considerations if hypovolaemic shock is suspected.

Disability

Paul may have sustained a head injury during the accident and therefore his neurological status should continue to be monitored every 30 minutes using APVU and the Glasgow Coma Scale (GCS) until a stable trend is established (see Chapters 2 and 4). The trauma score (revised) (Table 12.6) is an objective method for determining injury severity that can be used as an adjunct to vital signs observation. Ideally trauma scores are calculated during three phases: in the pre-hospital setting; on arrival at the emergency department; and one hour later. Paul's trauma score is 12 so there is no need for immediate airway intervention, high flow oxygen via a face mask can be continued and a full clinical examination can be performed.

Table 12.6 Revised trauma score

Respiratory rate		Systolic BP		GCS	
10–29	4	>89	4	13–15	4
>29	3	76–89	3	9–12	3
6–9	2	50–75	2	6–8	2
1–5	1	1–49	1	4–5	1
0	0	0	0	<4	0

Source: trauma.org; Available: http://www.trauma.org/archive/scores/rts.html

Exposure

While ensuring dignity and privacy, Paul's protective motorcycle garments must be carefully cut off using a pair of scissors to expose his entire body and allow inspection for ecchymosis (bruising), deformities, haemorrhage and skin colour. The nurse must listen for any abnormal sounds and carefully feel the movement of each bone, noting any movement that is unusual or provokes pain. Inspection, palpation, percussion and auscultation of the chest and abdomen will also be necessary to detect potential internal injuries. (See Epstein et al. (2008) for detailed clinical examination.) A warm environment should be maintained and prudent use of warmed blankets expedited.

Distal Limb Neurovascular Assessment

Once assured that no life-threatening injury has been left unattended, the nurse needs to assess the femoral injury with particular emphasis upon neurovascular function of the distal limb and the open wound. Paul has a 'golden period' of six hours before potential ischaemia and myonecrosis (death of muscle tissue) are deemed irreversible. Assessment of the distal neurovascular function (nerve and circulatory status) of the affected limb should be checked initially every 5 to 15 minutes, documented and compared with the other limb and previous assessments throughout (Table 12.7).

Table 12.7 Neurovascular limb assessment

- Pulses distal to the injury and capillary refill distal to the injury
- Colour and temperature of the limb
- Pain and tenderness
- Soft tissue swelling or discolouration
- Limitation in range of movement
- Altered sensory perception
- Loss of function

Vascular Assessment

Pulses

The femoral, popliteal, posterior tibial and dorsalis pedis (pedal) pulses all require assessment for their presence and quality. To aid in future assessments, the location of the pulse may be marked with a magic marker. If a weak pulse or no pulse is found, the fracture may be putting pressure on the femoral artery or indeed the comminuted bone fragments may have damaged the artery and the orthopaedic team should be notified immediately. A weak pulse can be determined by comparing the pulse felt below the fracture with that of Paul's uninjured extremity. If there is any uncertainty as to the nature of the peripheral pulses below the fracture site, a Doppler ultrasound probe should be used to detect blood flow and, if located, the site marked on the skin. It is important to document the quality of the pulses and words such as weak, normal quality and bounding may be used. Paul's pulses appear present and of normal quality. Capillary refill time should also be assessed by depressing Paul's right toenail until blanching occurs. The nail is then released and the speed of colour refill is observed. Refill should occur in less than two seconds. The injured extremity should be compared with the unaffected limb.

Colour

The skin colour of Paul's leg gives a good indication of the adequacy of circulation and any potential problems (Table 12.8).

The skin distal to Paul's injury site should be palpated with the whole hand to assess temperature. The dorsum of the hand is more sensitive to temperature changes (Lumley, 2008). Paul's lower right extremity is warm to touch and pink in colour but should still be observed every 15 minutes. A cool or cold right foot indicates diminished arterial blood supply and may indicate the development of circulatory compromise, termed acute compartment syndrome. This develops when pressure in a fascial compartment increases and venous return is occluded (Brown and Sayers, 2007).

Table 12.8 Indication of circulatory problems

Colour	Circulatory problem
Pink or ruddy	Venous congestion
Mottled, dusky, pale	Inadequate arterial perfusion or arterial occlusion
Cyanotic	Inadequate arterial perfusion and/or insufficient venous return

Subsequently, although pulses may be present, perfusion is interrupted, muscle and nerve ischaemia ensues and, if untreated (usually via decompression fasciotomy), progresses to necrosis. Acute compartment syndrome is relatively infrequent in femoral fractures due to the capacity of the three compartments of the thigh to accommodate substantially higher blood volumes compared with those of the lower leg and the forearm. Severe bleeding into one or more compartments of the thigh is necessary to elevate the compartment pressure above the critical level (Brown and Sayers, 2007). That said, Paul is less than 35 years old and male, indicators which have been identified as important for the development of acute compartment syndrome (Shadgan et al., 2010; Shore et al., 2013), and therefore prompt recognition of symptoms at this stage is imperative. Paul's right leg should be elevated unless there are signs of arterial compromise.

Pain and Tenderness

The exact area of pain should be assessed and excessive movement of Paul's injured limb minimised. It is important to determine if his pain is increasing despite analgesia, as severe pain is a cardinal feature of acute compartment syndrome. Alternatively, in the initial assessment severe pain on passive motion may be a sign of neurological compromise. A variety of data to assess Paul's pain, including his subjective reports, objective signs of distress (e.g. physiological signs, behavioural indicators) and Pain Assessment Scales, could be used (Mano et al., 2013). Available scales include the Visual Analogue Scale (VAS), Verbal Numerical Rating Scales (VNRS) and Verbal Descriptor Scale (VDS). The Australian and New Zealand College of Anaesthetists (ANZCA) (2013) recommend that the practitioner's determination of the best scale to use is reliant on the nurses' clinical judgement and decision making. In Paul's case the VNRS is beneficial to facilitate this.

Neurological Assessment

Sensory Perception

Paul's ability to detect pain, light touch, deep touch, heat, cold, vibratory sense, proprioception (spatial awareness) and two-point discrimination should be assessed. Two-point discrimination is assessed by having Paul close his eyes while the nurse lightly touches the area distal (furthest away) from the injury. Paul will be asked to discern the difference between two distinct points (for example, can he determine the difference between one or two fingers being applied to his right calf). If Paul can feel pressure but cannot differentiate between one or two digits, this is a sign of decreasing neurovascular function and requires immediate medical notification.

Assessment for full sensation, abnormal sensation (paraesthesia), diminished sensation or numbness of Paul's right leg is tested using specialised equipment such as a touch test two-point discriminator. It is vital that the sensory status of Paul's limb is established and Paul reports full sensation with no loss of two-point discrimination. Sensory changes to Paul's right foot, for example, could indicate specific nerve injury or impending changes because of ischaemia (Greaves, 2008). As Paul is able to determine the difference between light applications of one or two digits by the nurse this is a clear indicator that the femoral nerve arising from the lumbar plexus is intact.

Motor Function

Motor function is assessed by asking Paul to move his leg if possible through a range of motion. When checking the motor response, paralysis or inability to move the extremity distal to the injury may indicate a peripheral nerve injury or ischaemic changes resulting from oedema. If any part of this assessment provokes Paul's pain it must be stopped. Table 12.9 lists some suggested methods of testing specific nerves.

After initial evaluation the open wound on Paul's right thigh should be sealed with sterile dressings and the limb immobilised in an air splint. Debridement and irrigation with sterile saline solution in the emergency room should be avoided in case of inoculation of the deeper tissues with nosocomial organisms (Committee ACoS, 2014). Only easily accessible foreign bodies should be removed before the application of sterile dressings in Paul's case. Nevertheless, irrigation of the open wound in the emergency room is advocated by many clinicians in the case of heavily contaminated wounds. The practical value of obtaining specimen cultures from the open wound in the emergency room has been questioned since they usually

Table 12.9 Testing specific nerve areas on the lower limb

Peroneal nerve
1. Sensory: touch lateral side of right great toe
2. Motor: ask Paul to wriggle the toes on his right foot

Femoral nerve
1. Sensory: touch anterior right thigh, medial aspect of right calf
2. Motor: loss of knee jerk

Tibial nerve
1. Sensory: touch each lateral and medial aspect on sole of foot
2. Motor: plantar flex ankle, flex great toe

---

isolate superficial contaminants or normal skin flora, while at the same time carrying the risk of causing wound contamination (Committee ACoS, 2014).

At this stage Paul should have a range of continuous non-invasive monitoring, including ECG, automated sphygmomanometer, core temperature probe and pulse oximeter, to aid frequent monitoring of vital physiological parameters. The core temperature probe will detect any potential for the development of hypothermia post trauma or pyrexia, suggesting infection.

Specific Investigations

X-ray is an essential method of determining the exact nature of the fracture and assists with providing a clinical and radiological classification that can be used in communication across the entire multidisciplinary team. Table 12.10 lists a range of venous blood samples that will be taken during the acute assessment period and Table 12.11 includes the usual secondary assessment details, which will be collected over the following hours.

Simple, repetitive instruction and explanation may help to alleviate some of Paul's anxiety, fear and uncertainty regarding his condition during the assessment phase. Equally, adequate ongoing pain assessment and relief are important methods of ensuring his comfort, compliance, understanding

Table 12.10   Routine venous blood sampling

1. Full blood count (FBC) – low Hb (anaemia), raised WBC (infection)
2. Clotting screen – if indicated by current medication, e.g. warfarin
3. Urea and electrolytes (U&E) – electrolyte balance and renal function
4. Capillary blood glucose if high or low glucose is suspected, e.g. diabetic patient
5. Blood group, save and cross match – for potential blood transfusion

Table 12.11   Secondary assessment

- Full clinical examination: peripheral pulses, jugular venous pressure (JVP), heart and lung sounds, ECG, systemic and musculo-skeletal examination
- Past medical history (PMH)
- Family (FH) and social history (SH)
- Systemic enquiry
- Drug history: prescribed, over-the-counter and recreational
- Chest/spinal/pelvic/limb X-ray

and consensual participation throughout the process. Words of reassurance, praise and comfort can go far to help to reassure Paul.

Neurological and vascular injuries can occur in any fracture and are more likely in cases with increasing fracture deformity. Peripheral nerve injury would be suspected if Paul were to report experiencing motor or sensory deficiencies. Management of neurological injury involves immediate reduction of the fracture and possible nerve exploration, with subsequent follow-up to assess whether or not neurological function returns.

The Case Scenario: Medical Management and Care Issues

Within an hour of arriving in the accident and emergency department, a full primary assessment has revealed that Paul is currently haemodynamically stable, fully conscious and alert and apyrexial. A series of investigations including X-ray images of his right limb have confirmed that he has a displaced, compound, comminuted fracture of the right shaft of femur, classification 3A on the Gustilo and Anderson scale. There is also a bony protrusion at the right thigh, external rotation of the lower leg and multiple abrasions on both legs. The wound has been sealed with a transparent occlusive dressing. He is not displaying any evidence of neurovascular impairment to his right extremity. A detailed secondary assessment has also revealed the following:

Head: lower lip abrasion
Neck: no tenderness
Chest: tender and painful
Abdomen: no tenderness and pelvis stable
Past medical history: nil
Medications: nil
Haemoglobin: 12.7 g/dL (normal 12 to 18 g/dL)
Toxicology screening: negative
Electrocardiograph: normal sinus rhythm – rate 92 beats per minute
Chest/pelvic X-ray: no abnormalities detected
Urinalysis: no abnormalities detected

He has given a detailed medical and social history. A decision is reached to take Paul to the operating theatre for further surgical intervention.

Consider the following:

1. What are the immediate priorities in Paul's management and care?
2. What surgical intervention would be the most appropriate in Paul's case?

Medical Management Strategies

Paul's immediate medical priorities include the assessment and management of potential life-threatening problems, limb-threatening conditions and coexistent conditions resulting from his accident. This includes:

1. Ongoing observation of vital signs repeated every 30 minutes until a stable trend is established.
2. High-flow oxygen therapy to maintain $SpO_2 > 95$ per cent.
3. IV access, fluid resuscitation and close fluid balance monitoring.
4. Regular pain assessment, analgesia and anti-emetic administration.
5. Entire body immobilisation until normal skull, spine and chest inspection is established.
6. Limb immobilisation.
7. Wound cleansing and occlusion.
8. Psychological support and reassurance.

Now that Paul's condition is stable, attention should be paid to the psychological aspects of management. Paul may feel threatened and liberal reassurance is needed because at this time Paul will not be able to evaluate the severity of his injury. Information and support for Paul and his family are important for their reassurance, cooperation and compliance in his management and care. The presence of familiar faces in an otherwise alien environment can help to orientate Paul and provide him with additional psychological support (Warren et al., 2013). Repeated simple explanations or instructions may become necessary if a deficit in recent memory is apparent.

Although he does not appear to have any immediate limb-threatening neurovascular conditions, the open and complex nature of Paul's fracture will necessitate surgical intervention. His fracture can be classified as type 3A according to the Gustilo and Anderson Score (Gustilo et al., 1984) (Table 12.12).

Table 12.12   Gustilo and Anderson classification of compound fractures

Type 1: low energy, wound < 1 cm
Type 2: wound > 1 cm with moderate soft tissue damage
Type 3: high energy wound > 1 cm with extensive soft tissue damage
Type 3A: adequate soft tissue cover
Type 3B: inadequate soft tissue cover
Type 3C: associated with arterial injury

The use of a classification system is important as it facilitates communication among medical and nursing clinicians regarding decision making, anticipating potential problems, suggesting treatment options and predicting patient and surgical outcomes (Ruedi et al., 2007). Various classification systems have been proposed in an effort to grade the extent of the initial musculoskeletal injury and to offer useful prognostic clues to help in deciding the optimal management (Sudkamp, 2000). The most widely used is that of Gustilo and Anderson (1984), which describes three groups of increasing severity based on the size of the open wound, the degree of its contamination and the extent of soft tissue injury (Table 12.12). Other classification systems include the Tscherne (Tscherne and Oestern, 1982) and Hanover Fracture Scales. However, the emphasis should be on appreciating the significance of the soft tissue injury more than committing to memory any of the scoring systems.

The five Rs summarise the main aims of fracture treatment and are summarised in Table 12.13.

The orthopaedic surgeon will manage the femoral fracture by inserting an intra-medullary nail into the femoral shaft in an effort to promote healing by callus formation. This tends to promote more rapid bone healing than that achieved by external fixation, which relies upon primary healing and so enables a more rapid rehabilitation. With this type of surgery, bone fragments are repositioned and/or reduced into their normal alignment and then held together by the insertion of rods through the marrow space in the centre of the bone. The surgeon is therefore able to reposition the fracture fragments exactly.

Table 12.13 The 5 Rs of fracture management

Resuscitation: shock may be related to pain and blood loss.

Reduction: realignment of fractured bone ends usually under general anaesthesia using an image intensifier.

Restriction: to prevent deformity and allow bone growth to proceed normally until bony union occurs. Methods used depend on bone affected and nature of injury, and include plaster cast, traction or internal or external fixation.

Restoration: limb immobilisation increases the risk of muscle and joint stiffness and loss of some function. Encourage to exercise all joints and muscles except those affected by the injury.

Rehabilitation: when the restriction is removed the limb must be exercised to restore normal ranges of movement.

Preparation for Surgical Intervention

Paul is likely to be placed on to the acute trauma list for intra-medullary nailing of the right femur as soon as an operating theatre, surgeon, anaesthetist and staff become available. This provides little time to ensure that the theatre preparation checklist (Chapter 9, Table 9.6) pertinent to Paul is completed.

The Case Scenario: Ongoing Care Issues

Paul is warded two hours later at 2 p.m. following wound debridement and reamed intra-medullary nailing of his right femoral fracture under general anaesthetic. The operating theatre notes record an uncomplicated procedure in the presence of continued physiological stability. An estimated blood loss of 1 litre is recorded. Paul received 3 litres of IV crystalloid and 4 units of blood. He is awake but drowsy and able to respond to verbal commands appropriately. A patient-controlled analgesia (PCA) device of IV morphine 1 mg with a lock-out dose of 10 minutes has been commenced. Paul has an IV infusion of Cephaloxin® and he has 100 per cent oxygen via venturi mask. Three small mepore dressings cover the wound at the intra-medullary nail insertion site and a medium-sized mepore covers the wound following wound debridement. Both dressings are clean. A urinary catheter remains in situ. The post anaesthetic care unit records show an uneventful initial recovery.

Nursing Care Issues
1. Consider what the immediate post-operative care would be.
2. What are the nursing responsibilities and underpinning rationale with regard to the PCA?
3. What potential complications may Paul develop following surgery with specific reference to the long bone surgery?

Ongoing Care Issues and the Role of the Nurse

Post-operative Observations

All patients require close observation of airway, breathing and circulation following a general anaesthetic. Assessment of vital signs should be clearly and accurately recorded every 30 minutes until a stable trend has been established and it is evident that potential complications have been avoided. Routine observations should include:

- Consciousness level: AVPU (see Chapter 1)
- Pulse: rate, regularity, depth

- BP
- Respiratory rate: rate, depth, noise
- SpO$_2$
- Skin colour
- Urine output: note the first urine void (urine retention can occur post anaesthesia) and continue to record output
- Temperature: four-hourly
- IV cannula site and intravenous fluid infusion
- Wound drainage

Any changes or abnormal findings must be reported to senior nursing and medical staff immediately. Post-operative complications following internal fixation of a fractured femur are reasonably rare; nevertheless, the initial injury, anaesthesia and surgery may all pose some potential risk to Paul's well-being. It is beyond the scope of this chapter to engage with more detailed routine post-operative care and management; however, it is important to note the principles of orthopaedic nursing management (Clarke and Santy-Tomlinson, 2014; Kneale and Davis, 2005). Specific management issues pertaining to Paul will be outlined.

Post-operative Pain Management

It is accepted that pain represents the fifth vital sign requiring assessment post operatively (Lorenz et al., 2009). The form of assessment tool used must reflect the fact that Paul is emerging from anaesthesia. The verbal numerical rating scale (VNRS) requires that Paul rate his perception of pain on a scale of 0 to 10, whereby 0 represents no pain and 10 the worst pain imaginable. This scale provides the nurse with an objective measure that may be re-evaluated as comfort measures are instituted. Paul is self-reporting a score of 3 at this time. Management of Paul's acute pain begins with the affirmation that he should have access to the best level of pain relief that may be provided safely.

It is the nurse's responsibility to ensure that Paul is aware of and understands how to use the PCA for pain relief. He should be clear that when he experiences pain he can self-administer a small bolus dose of morphine and that he should experience pain relief within a few minutes. PCA ensures that individuals can adjust the level of analgesic required according to the severity of pain. In theory, the plasma level of the analgesic will be relatively constant and side effects caused by fluctuations in plasma level will be eliminated.

Morphine is the most popular drug and will be considered here with reference to Paul. The ideal dose of morphine sulfate has been found to be 1 mg in 1 mL bolus (with a loading dose of 1–5 mg) in a PCA device

(Jarzyna et al., 2011); regular review by the nurse is needed in every case to ensure that pain relief is adequate. The aim of the lock-out period is to prevent over-dosage occurring because of over-enthusiastic demands for more analgesia. The lock-out time should be long enough for the previous dose to have an effect. In practice, lock-out times of between 5 and 10 minutes are enough for most opioids. A maximum dose can be programmed into most PCA devices to prevent overdose. In practice, it is more logical to accept that the analgesic requirements of patients will vary considerably and some patients may require large amounts to achieve adequate pain relief. Paul appears to be successfully titrating his analgesia to a point where he is comfortable rather than pain free, stating that he 'expects some pain after surgery'. It would be expected that Paul would progress to oral analgesia the day following surgery. The nurse should take special notice of Paul developing pain that appears to be out of proportion to the injury and surgery and be suspicious of impending acute compartment syndrome. The orthopaedic surgical team should be updated regarding pain control.

Neurovascular Limb Assessment

Neurovascular inspection of Paul's right limb should be performed in the same way as the pre-operative assessment. Additional observation of the site of surgery, the type of dressing, the presence of drains and/or drainage and the status of the distal extremities is equally important. Ongoing monitoring of extremity colour, capillary refill, sensation and mobility will be maintained every 15 minutes for the first 2 hours, every 30 minutes for the following 2 hours, hourly for the following 2 hours and thereafter every 2 hours for the following 18 hours. Acute compartment syndrome remains a potential complication in the post-operative phase (Weinstein and Buckwalter, 2005), and so neurovascular observation is aimed at recognising and addressing concerns early. Paul does not appear to have any unexpected changes in neurovascular status.

Monitor Wound Areas

Sutures or clips are usually used to close the wound and will be removed at approximately 10 days post operation. The mepore dressings provide a sterile, self-adhesive absorbent barrier and should be left intact unless the surgeon authorises otherwise. The nurse should maintain a high level of suspicion for infection given that Paul's injury was an open fracture. Prophylactic intravenous antibiotics may be used for longer durations with open fractures as compared to closed fractures (Schenker et al., 2012; Buckholz et al., 2014). The nurse should assess for infection and report if pyrexia, increased pain, redness, swelling or discharge from the wound is noted and documented. Excessive blood loss should be measured and recorded on the fluid balance chart and in rare cases may necessitate a return to theatre for further exploration. If a small drain is inserted near the wound site, blood loss should be recorded and the drain removed 24 to 48 hours later once bleeding has ceased. MRSA prophylaxis treatment will continue with anti-bacterial agents such as Octenidine® 0.3 per cent lotion applied to the body for three minutes every day and 2 per cent Mupirocin® nasal ointment three times a day for five days.

Monitor Potential Development of Complications

Deep vein thrombosis (DVT) and pulmonary embolism (PE) are important complications to recognise and prevent (Autar, 2007). DVT prophylaxis with subcutaneous injection of weight-adjusted low molecular weight heparin (LMWH) should be medically prescribed once the post-operative bleeding risk is acceptable, usually 12 to 24 hours later (Lucassen et al., 2011). Gentle distal limb movement to exercise limb muscles may also be encouraged and full length anti-embolism stockings (AES) measured and fitted to both limbs (NICE, 2010). Vigilant observation of all pressure areas and regular pressure relief is essential to prevent pressure sore development. Early mobilisation is encouraged, but according to Barker and Marval (2010) and Wells and Anderson (2013) venous thrombo-embolism (VTE) risks may extend up to 12 weeks post surgery.

Emotional Support

Paul may experience many painful and frightening events before, during and after the operation. These experiences give rise to emotions that range from anxiety to sheer terror. Nurses can provide comfort and emotional support to the individual at this time of crisis. A calm, reassuring voice, clear explanation, time for listening and an approachable visibility can all provide Paul with some sense of security. Honesty with respect to pain, discomfort and issues related to enforced immobility should help. The acute care inpatient stay is brief, but it is the insightful nurse who can balance the issues discussed in this chapter with thoughtful consideration of the challenges ahead for Paul and his family. Family members should be encouraged to participate in Paul's care wherever possible.

Early Mobilisation

Paul will be able to get out of bed the following day once his observations are stable and the PCA has been removed. Physiotherapists will help Paul to learn to walk with the aid of crutches for the following five or six weeks. At this stage

Paul should regain independence with his usual daily activities, including personal hygiene, and a healthy diet and fluid intake should have resumed.

Monitor Complications Specific to Intra-medullary Nailing

Early complications following operative fracture management include visceral injury, vascular injury, acute compartment syndrome and nerve injury. Fat embolism syndrome (FES) is a rare but recognised complication of long bone fractures, such as in Paul's case, with a reported incidence of 2 to 23 per cent in this patient group (Powers and Talbot, 2011). FES usually occurs 24 to 72 hours after a fracture or following surgery. Bone marrow from the fractured bone or other injured adipose tissue releases fatty globules that enter the bloodstream through torn veins at the injury site (Akoh et al., 2014; Shaikhr, 2009). Fatty globules may travel to the lungs, where they become entangled in the microvasculature of the lung to form an embolus with subsequent occlusion of the pulmonary circulation. They can also become trapped and cause occlusion of the small vessels of the brain and the kidneys. Lipase breaks down the trapped fat emboli into free fatty acids. Fat embolism can be prevented or reduced by moving the fractured extremity as little as possible prior to fixation, proper splinting and early surgical fixation of the fracture, which prevents the globules being released into the bone marrow. It is therefore imperative to monitor the patient's neurological and respiratory status carefully for any sign of confusion and hypoxaemia.

Summary

The importance of musculoskeletal trauma management cannot be overstated. A systematic approach to assessment and intervention improves patient outcomes through early recognition of potentially life-threatening injuries and intervention for identified problems. Priorities in trauma management are to ensure adequate oxygenation and ventilation, control haemorrhage, and maintain tissue perfusion to vital organs. The management of any patient who has sustained a fracture must take into account not just the fracture but the whole patient. Patients require immediate assessment of their respiration, level of consciousness and circulation. Once care has been paid to these vital factors, nursing attention can be directed towards the injured limb, the vertebral column or the pelvis. The role of the nurse is of utmost importance and can have a profound impact on the patient's outcome.

This chapter has considered trauma of the femur, which is a potentially serious and life-threatening event. It has provided insight into the importance of understanding the mechanism of injury, the extent of injury and one possible fixation technique. Potential complications and considerations have been outlined with a specific focus on priorities of assessment and management throughout the initial acute phase. The goal of treatment is alignment and function and the nursing role can significantly impact upon the quality of care and promote positive outcomes. By discussing the rationale for timely, appropriate interventions it has been shown that life- and limb-saving challenges can be overcome and a positive outcome attained.

Further Reading

Dandy, J. D. and D. J. Edwards. *Essential Orthopaedics and Trauma*, 5th edn (London: Churchill Livingstone, 2009).

Eliott, M., R. Tate and K. Page. 'Do Clinicians Know How to Use Pulse Oximetry? A Literature and Clinical Implications', *Australian Critical Care*, 19(4) (2006), 139–44.

Epstein, O., G. D. Perkin, J. Cookson, I. S. Watt, R. Rakhit, A. W. Robbins and G. A. W. Hornett. *Clinical Examination*, 4th edn (London: Mosby International Ltd, 2008).

O'Reilly, M. 'Major Trauma Management', in G. Jones (ed.), *Emergency Nursing Care: Principles and Practice* (London: Greenwich Medical Media, 2003).

References

Akoh, C. C, C. Schick, J. Otero and M. Karam 'Fat Embolism Syndrome after Femur Fracture Fixation: A Case Report', *Iowa Orthopaedic Journal*, 34 (2014), 55–62.

Anderson, P. A., R. D. Murchow, A. Munoz, W. L. Tontz and D. K. Resnick. 'Clearance of the Asymptomatic Cervical Spine: A Meta-Analysis', *Journal of Orthopaedic Trauma*, 24 (2) (2010), 100–6.

Australian and New Zealand College of Anaesthetists (ANZCA) and Faculty of Pain Medicine. *Acute Pain Management: Scientific Evidence*, 3rd edn (Melbourne: Australian and New Zealand College of Anaesthetists and Faculty of Pain Medicine, 2010).

Autar, R. 'NICE Guidelines on Reducing the Risk of Venous Thromboembolism (Deep Veined Thrombosis and Pulmonary Embolism) in Patients Undergoing Surgery', *Journal of Orthopaedic Nursing*, 11(3/4) (2007), 169–76.

Barker, R. C. and P. Marval. 'Venous Thromboembolism: Risks and Prevention', *Critical Care and Pain*, 11(1) (2010), 18–23.

Brown, M. and R. Sayers. 'Compartment Syndromes', in R. Fitridge and M. Thompson (eds), *Mechanism of Vascular Disease: A Textbook for Vascular Surgeons* (Cambridge: Cambridge University Press, 2007).

Buckholz, R. W., J. D. Heckman and C. Court-Brown. *Rockwood and Green's Fractures in Adults*, 8th edn (Philadelphia: Lippincott Williams and Wilkins, 2014).

Bulstrode, C. *Oxford Textbook of Trauma and Orthopaedics* (Oxford: Oxford University Press, 2015).

Committee American College of Surgeons (ACoS). *Advanced Trauma Life Support (ATLS) for Doctors*, 8th edn (Chicago: Committee ACoS, 2014) [Online]. Available from: www.facs.org/trauma/atls/index.html (accessed 15 April 2015).

Clarke, S., and J. Santy-Tomlinson. 'Orthopaedic and Trauma Nursing: An Evidence-based Approach to Musculo-Skeletal Care', (Chichester: Wiley-Blackwell, 2014).

Dandy, J. D. and D. J. Edwards. *Essential Orthopaedics and Trauma*, 5th edn (London: Churchill Livingstone, 2009).

Davis, J. W., M. J. Sise, R. Albrecht and D. A. Kuhls. 'ACoS Trauma Prevention Committee. Topical Updates: Getting Started, Fall Prevention, Domestic Violence and Suicide', *Journal of Trauma*, 70(4) (2011), 996–1001.

Department for Transport. *Reported Road Casualties in Great Britain: Quarterly Provisional Estimates Q2* (2015) [Online]. Available from: www.gov.uk/government/uploads/system/uploads/attachment_data/file/473850/quarterly-estimates-april-to-june-2015.pdf (accessed 31 January 2016).

Duggan, M. and B. P. Kavanagh. 'Pulmonary Atelectasis: A Pathogenic Perioperative Entity', *Anaesthesiology*, 102(4) (2005), 838–54.

Eckes-Roper, J. *Trauma Nursing Secrets* (Philadelphia: Hanley & Belfus Inc., 2003).

Epstein, G., G. Perkin, J. Cookson, I. Watt, R. Rakhit, A. Robins and G. Hornett. *Clinical Examination*, 4th edn (London: Mosby, 2008).

Greaves, I. *Trauma Care Manual* (London: Arnold, 2008).

Gustilo, R. B., R. M. Mendoza and D. N. Williams. 'Problems in the Management of Type III (Severe) Open Fractures: A New Classification of Type III Open Fractures', *Journal of Trauma*, 24 (1984), 742–6.

Humbyrd, C. J., P. Benjamin, A. S Chanmungan and D. M. Laporte. *Orthopaedic Emergencies* (Oxford: Oxford University Press, 2012).

Jarzyna, D., C. R. Jungquist, C. Pasero, J. Willens, A. Nisbet, L. Oakes, S. J. Dempsey, D. Santangelo and R. C. Polomano. 'American Society for Pain Management Nursing Guidelines on Monitoring for Opioid-induced Sedation and Respiratory Depression', *Pain Management Nursing*, 12(3) (2011), 118–45.

Kneale, D. and P. S. Davis. *Orthopaedic and Trauma Nursing*, 2nd edn (London: Churchill Livingstone, 2005).

Licina, P. and A. M. Nowitzke. 'Approach and Considerations Regarding the Patient with Spinal Injury', *International Journal of the Care of the Injured*, 36 (2005), SB 2–12.

Lorenz, K. A., C. D. Sherbourne and L. R. Shugarman. 'How Reliable Is Pain as the Fifth Vital Sign', *American Board of Family Medicine*, 22(3) (2009), 291–8.

Lucassen, W., G. J. Geersing and P. M. Erkens. 'Clinical Decision Rules for Excluding Pulmonary Embolism: A Meta-Analysis', *Annals of Internal Medicine*, 155(7) (2011), 448–60.

Lui, B. C., R. Ivers and R. Norton. 'Helmets for Preventing Injury in Motorcycle Riders', *Cochrane Database Systematic Review* 28(1) (2008), CD 004333.

Lumley, J. S. P. *Surface Anatomy: The Anatomical Basis Of Clinical Examination*, 4th edn (London: Churchill Livingstone, 2008).

Magee, D. J. *Orthopaedic Physical Assessment*, 4th edn (Philadelphia: Saunders Elsevier, 2005).

Mano, C. A., W. Kanitz and M. Jolly, M. 2013. Pain scores among Emergency Department patients: Comparisons by Emergency Department Diagnosis, *Journal of Emergency Medicine*, 44(1) (2013), 46–52.

Marieb, E. N. *Essentials of Human Anatomy and Physiology*, 11th edn (London: Pearson, 2015).

Mikhail, J. 'The Trauma Triad of Death: Hypothermia, Acidosis and Coagulopathy', *AACN Clinical Issues* 10(1) (1999), 85–94.

National Association of Emergency Medicine and Surgery Physicians and ACoS. 'Spinal Precautions and the Use of the Long Backboard', *Prehospital Emergency Care*, 17(3) (2013), 392–3.

National Institute of Clinical Excellence (NICE). *Venous Thromboembolism: Reducing the Risk of Venous Thromboembolism in Patients Admitted to Hospital, Clinical Guideline 92* (National Institute of Clinical Excellence, 2010).

National Institute of Clinical Excellence (NICE). *Intravenous Fluid Therapy in Adults in Hospital, Clinical Guideline 174* (National Institute of Clinical Excellence, 2013).

Powers, K. A. and L. A. Talbot. 'Fat Embolism Syndrome after Femur Fracture with Intra-medullary Nailing: Case Report', *American Journal of Critical Care*, **20**(3) (2011), 263–7.

Rodrigues, M. and B. M. Qureshi. *The Unofficial Guide to Radiology: Chest, Abdomen and Orthopaedic X Rays, Plus CTs, MRIs and Other Important Modalities.* (Cambrian, UK: Zeshan Qureshi Publication, 2014).

Ruedi, T. P., R. Buckley and C. Moran (eds). *AO Principles of Fracture Management* (New York: Thieme Medical Publishers, 2007).

Sasser, S. M, R. C. Hunt and M. Faul. 'Guidelines for Field Triage of Injured Patients' (2011) [Online]. Available from: www.facs.org/quality-programs/trauma/vrc/resources (accessed 15 April 2015).

Schenker, M. L, S. Yannascoll, K. D. Baldwin, J. Ahn and S. Mehta 'Does Timing to Operative Debridement Affect Infectious Complications in Open Long Bone Fractures? A Systematic Review' (2012). *American Journal of Bone and Joint Surgery*, **94**(12) (2012), 1057–64.

Shadgan, B., D. Menon and D. Sanders. 'Current Thinking About Acute Compartment Syndrome of the Lower Extremity', *Canadian Journal of Surgery*, **53**(5) (2010) 329–34.

Shaikhr, N. 'Emergency Management of Fat Embolism Syndrome', *Journal of Emergencies, Trauma and Shock*, **2**(1) (2009), 29–33.

Shore, B. J., M. P. Glotzbecker and D. Zurakowski. 'Acute Compartment Syndrome in Children and Teenagers with Tibial Shaft Fracture: Incidence and Multivariable Risk Factors', *Journal of Orthopaedic Trauma*, **27** (2013), 616.

Spinks, A., C. Turner, J. Nixon and R. J. McClure. '"The WHO Safe Communities" Model for the Prevention of Injury in Whole Populations', *Cochrane Database Systematic Review*, **8**(3) (2009), CD004445.

Stahal, P. F., C. E. Hayde, W. Wyrwich and W. Ertal. 'Current Concepts of Polytrauma Management: From ATLS to "Damage Control"', *Orthopade*, **34** (2005), 823–36.

Sudkamp, N. *Soft Tissue Injury: Pathophysiology and its Influences on Fracture Management – Evaluation of Closed and Open Injuries. AO Principles of Fracture Management* (Stuttgart: Thieme, 2000).

Tscherne, H. and H. J. Oestern. 'A New Classification of Soft-tissue Damage in Open and Closed Fractures', *Unfalheilkunde*, **85**(3) (1982), 111–15.

Warren, A. M., K. Stucky and J. J. Sherman. 'Rehabilitation Psychology's role in the Level 1 Trauma Center', *Journal of Trauma and Acute Care Surgery*, **74**(5) (2013), 1357–62.

Weinstein, S. L. and J. A. Buckwalter. *Turek's Orthopaedics Principles and Their Application*, 6th edn (Philadelphia: Lippincott, Williams and Wilkins, 2005).

Wells, P. and D. Anderson. 'The Diagnosis and Treatment of Venous Thrombo-embolism', *Haematology*, **1** (2013), 457–63.

Woodrow, P. *Intensive Care Nursing: A Framework for Practice* (London: Routledge, 2012).

World Health Organization (WHO). *Global Status Report on Road Safety: Supporting a Decade of Action* (WHO: Geneva, 2013).

Conclusion

The preceding chapters have provided a comprehensive review of the assessment and management required by acutely ill adults presenting with a range of common but serious illnesses. The authors' brief was to identify and discuss the knowledge and skills required to recognise and respond rapidly and effectively to the needs of the acutely ill adults, particularly where there is evidence of deterioration in clinical status. This concluding section will briefly review issues which need to be considered by acute care services providers and educators in order to ensure healthcare professionals can deliver appropriate care to acutely ill adults.

Teaching and learning about acute and critical illness

The National Patient Safety Agency (NPSA) (2007) report, the National Institute for Health and Clinical Excellence (NICE) (2007) guideline (CG:50) and the Department of Health's (2008c) competencies *Recognising and Responding to Acutely Ill Patients in Hospital* all highlighted the importance of ensuring that nurses in all settings are able to recognise, interpret the significance of, and act upon data which indicates deterioration in at-risk patients and which requires urgent reassessment by specialist nursing or medical staff. Similar concerns were raised in the National Confidential Enquiry into Patient Outcome and Death (NCEPOD) in 2009. Since the first edition of this book was written there have been three more significant reports published: the Francis Report (Report of the Mid Staffordshire NHS Foundation Trust Public Inquiry (Francis, 2013)), the Cavendish Review (Department of Health (DH), 2013) and the Keogh Report (NHS England, 2013). These reports look much more widely at issues of patient safety, quality of care, the role and training of healthcare support staff, and the need to better provide and manage urgent and emergency care services in the NHS. However, all of these reports drew attention, directly or indirectly, to the need to ensure a high level of competence in areas of acute care assessment, monitoring and specialist intervention where required. For nurses and the healthcare support staff with whom they routinely work, these competences include the ability to accurately record routine observations and ensure the information gathered is transmitted in a timely manner to monitor progress and identify change which may require urgent intervention by other members of the health professional team. The broader findings and recommendations contained in these reports underlined the central importance of the knowledge and understanding of assessment, monitoring, and referral in acute illness which have been the focus of this book.

Initial and continuing education plays an important role in ensuring nurses and increasingly, through assistant practitioner programmes, health-care support staff, have the competence to carry out these important activities in all settings (Manley and Hardy, 2006; Giddens, 2007; Higginson and Jones, 2009; Nursing and Midwifery Council (NMC), 2010; DH, 2013). Nurse education programmes have been delivered in universities for more than 20 years now. The increased emphasis on developing skills in assessment, problem solving and critical thinking has been welcomed overall but there remain some concerns that students exiting undergraduate nursing programmes may not possess the necessary knowledge, understanding and skills required for effective provision of comprehensive acute care support (Armitage et al., 2007; Chapman and Blackman, 2010). Such knowledge and skill deficits are not confined to new nursing graduates; concerns are also evident in medicine with junior doctors subject to similar pressures to develop competence in assessment and management of the acutely ill adult (Frost and Wise, 2012).

In common with other authors, we have found that both pre- and post-registration students have developed a basic knowledge of the mechanisms of disease and have some competence in measuring a core set of vital signs and completing related assessments, including conducting a primary survey and simple analyses of urine and blood (Garside and Prescott; 2008; Steen and Costello, 2008). However, we have also consistently found that the majority of student nurses at undergraduate level and up to one year after initial registration have only limited knowledge and understanding of normal physiological parameters (for example, the normal range of blood glucose in a healthy adult). In addition, whilst most students can obtain and report on the vital signs they have assessed, their ability to interpret and recognise the significance of these vital signs, whether normal or abnormal, is frequently limited. This has important repercussions for patient safety; in the absence of knowledge of normal parameters, abnormal assessment findings are unlikely to be recognised and acted upon appropriately. Such findings have been identified elsewhere in the United Kingdom (UK) and in other countries (Lofmark et al., 2003; Chapple and Aston, 2004; Mole et al., 2007; Steen and Costello, 2008; Liaw et al., 2011). Different explanations have been proposed; these include the lack of structured educational preparation and limited opportunities for learning within clinical place-ments, together with variable support from managers in provider organi-sations. However, in practice no single explanation can account for this observed deficit in knowledge and understanding.

A review of 26 studies by Liaw et al. (2011) concluded that various educational strategies, including standardised tools for assessment and management of clinical deterioration, clinical decision making models and inclusion of clinical deterioration training as a core competence in pre-registration nurse education could improve the skills of nurses in recognis-ing and responding to acutely ill patients and so address important aspects of patient safety. There is also evidence that structured problem-orientated or problem-based learning approaches in both initial and continuing education programmes can increase students' engagement with learning, can develop critical thinking skills and can help integrate knowledge and understanding of more complex concepts such as those required to be understood when working with pathophysiology and disease (Ehrenberg and Häggblom, 2006; Murray et al., 2008; Shin and Kim, 2013). The use of real and hypothetical case studies draws on the problem-based approach and has been used successfully in medicine and in nursing to develop knowledge, understanding and clinical competence in acute and critical care settings (Cioffi, 2000; Alinier et al., 2006; Garside and Prescott, 2008; McCaughey and Traynor, 2010). We endorse the use of case studies in teach-ing and learning and have drawn upon this approach within the book to introduce and develop explanations of common signs, symptoms, responses and interventions in acute and critical illness. This approach has also been used effectively in clinical practice settings and can contribute directly to helping students to apply knowledge directly to practice situations.

Objective structured clinical examinations/assessments (OSCE/OSCAs) can also be used alongside problem-based learning as a means to develop and then test assessment and other clinical skills (Lofmark et al., 2003; Mole et al., 2007; Murray et al., 2008). More recently computer-driven simulations and critical incident techniques have also been used to develop skills in assessment and management of acute and critical illness (Buckley and Gordon, 2011; Flo et al., 2013). These approaches challenge students to apply their knowledge in the context of practice and to use critical think-ing skills to make decisions on the course of action required in response to a particular problem scenario. However, the importance of engaging in structured learning opportunities in actual clinical practice settings can-not be underestimated. In the UK, the Nursing and Midwifery Council (NMC) requires clinical practice assessment in pre- and post-qualifying programmes to be competency based and encourages the use of skills work-books to ensure a defined range of clinical assessment and management skills (essential skill clusters) are demonstrated by experienced nurses in practice settings and then practised by students under supervision (NMC, 2010). The competency-based approach also underpins the Department of Health's (2008c) report *Recognising and Responding to Acutely Ill Patients in Hospital*; these competencies should now be informing skills development and assessment for nurses and other healthcare practitioners working in all clinical areas. The importance of maintaining post-registration clinical competence is further endorsed by the NMC's plans to introduce mandatory revalidation in 2016.

We continue to hold the view that working with experienced registered nurses and alongside medical staff in assessing and managing patients in hospital and primary care settings is an effective development opportunity. Participating in the provision of acute and critical care will help consolidate learning and enable nurses and other healthcare professionals to apply their theoretical knowledge in practice. Where these learning opportunities are jointly planned by experienced nurses providing acute and critical care services in NHS or primary care trusts and colleagues in higher education, there is evidence that nurses can develop appropriate knowledge, understanding and skills (Anderson et al., 2006; Garside and Prescott, 2008; Steen and Costello, 2008; Chapman and Blackman, 2010). In turn, patients and other health professionals will benefit as safe and appropriate care is provided. Such teaching and learning approaches can be focused on single disciplines such as nursing or medicine but the value of these and other professional groups learning together in interprofessional groups is now well established (Young et al., 2007; Anderson et al., 2006; Bandali et al., 2008; Shin and Kim, 2013).

The NPSA (2007) report and NICE (2007) guidance recognised the need for focused training and improved communication between healthcare professionals to achieve early recognition and appropriate response to acute illness in adults in hospital. These remain important areas of focus in an NHS where patient acuity and level of dependency is consistently high. In support of this the Department of Health (DH, 2008a, 2008b) defined programmes of training and specific competencies for assistant critical care practitioners (an advanced support worker role at level 4 on the NHS Career Framework) and advanced practitioners in critical care. Most registered nurses working in acute and critical care will function at a level in between these two important roles, but the competencies developed for patient assessment, monitoring vital signs and observation of the patient, together with basic airway management should now be informing educational programmes in acute and critical care.

There are examples of service providers and higher education providers working together to prepare pre-registration and continuing education students to develop competence in early recognition and response to acute illness in hospitals and primary care settings (Garside and Prescott, 2008; Steen and Costello, 2008; Chapman and Blackman, 2010). The resources provided by Skills for Health, the Sector Skills Council for the UK health sector and the *Knowledge and Skills Framework* (DH, 2004) can be utilised by healthcare provider organisations and higher education partners to develop training programmes similar to those identified by Garside and Prescott (2008) and the Derby NHS Foundation Trust (2015). If the recommendations of the NPSA (2007) and the Department of Health (2008c) are to be achieved and the NICE (2007) clinical guidelines are to be consistently applied in practice, teaching and learning should be jointly planned by education and service providers, should be problem orientated, and actively engage students in providing a rationale for their assessment of the actions required in a given situation.

Links to online resources

Skills for Health website
www.skillsforhealth.org.uk See, for example, the Core Skills Training Framework.

The Knowledge and Skills Framework (KSF) (Department of Health, 2004)
www.dh.gov.uk/en/Publicationsandstatistics/Publications/Publications PolicyAndGuidance/DH_4090843. The full KSF document is still available via the Department of Health web archives. However, a simplified KSF is now available and is promoted by NHS Employers at: www.nhsemployers.org/SimplifiedKSF

NHS Employers provide online examples of case studies and linked resources. These typically highlight innovation and good practice in staff development and training in in line with national policy directives or acute care priorities such as the Surviving Sepsis Campaign. These resources can be accessed at: www.nhsemployers .org/case-studies-and-resources?sort=date_desc.

References

Alinier, G., B. Hunt, R. Gordon and C. Harwood. 'Effectiveness of Intermediate-fidelity Simulation Training Technology in Undergraduate Nursing Education', *Journal of Advanced Nursing*, **54**(3) (2006), 359–69.

Anderson, E., N. Manek and A. Davidson. 'Evaluation of a Model for Maximising Interprofessional Education in an Acute Hospital', *Journal of Interprofessional Care*, **20**(2) (2006), 182–94.

Armitage, M. J. Eddlestone and T. Stokes. 'Recognising and Responding to Acute Illness in Adults in Hospital: Summary of NICE Guidance', *British Medical Journal*, **335** (2007), 258–9.

Bandali, K., K. Parker, M. Mummery and M. Preece. 'Skills Integration in a Simulated and Interprofessional Environment: An Innovative Undergraduate Applied Health Curriculum', *Journal of Interprofessional Care*, **22**(2) (2008), 179–89.

Buckley, T. and C. Gordon. 'The Effectiveness of High Fidelity Simulation on Medical–Surgical Registered Nurses' Ability to Recognize and Respond to Clinical Emergencies', *Nurse Education Today*, **31**(7) (2011), 716–21.

Chapman, L and J. Blackman. 'Using Supported Learning to Ensure Nurse Recruits are Skilled to Care for Acutely Ill Patients', *Nursing Times*, 106 (11) (2010), 10–11.

Chapple, M. and E. S. Aston. 'Practice Learning Teams: A Partnership Approach to Supporting Students' Clinical Learning', *Nurse Education in Practice*, **4** (2) (2004), 143–9.

Cioffi, J. 'Nurses' Experiences of Making Decisions to Call Emergency Assistance to their Patients', *Journal of Advanced Nursing*, **32**(1) (2000), 108–14.

Department of Health (DH). *The NHS Knowledge and Skills Framework (NHS KSF) and the Development Review Process* (London: Department of Health, 2004).

Department of Health (DH). *The National Education and Competence Framework for Advanced Critical Care Practitioners* (London: Department of Health, 2008a).

Department of Health (DH). *The National Education and Competence Framework for Assistant Critical Care Practitioners* (London: Department of Health, 2008b).

Department of Health (DH). *Competencies for Recognising and Responding to Acutely Ill Patients in Hospital* (London: Department of Health, 2008c).

Department of Health (DH). *The Cavendish Review: An Independent Review into Healthcare Assistants and Support Workers in the NHS and Social Care Settings* (London: Department of Health, 2013) [Online]. Available from: www.gov.uk/government/publications/review-of-healthcare-assistants-and-support-workers-in-nhs-and-social-care (accessed 30 May 2015).

Ehrenberg, A. C. and M. Häggblom. 'Problem-based Learning in Clinical Nursing Education: Integrating Theory and Practice', *Nurse Education in Practice*, **7** (2006), 67–74.

Flo, J., E. K. Flaathen and L. Fagerstrom. 'Simulation as a Learning Method in Nursing Education – A Case Study of Students' Learning Experiences During Use of Computer-driven Patient Simulators in Preclinical Studies', *Journal of Nursing Education and Practice*, **3**(8) (2013), p. 138.

Francis, R. 'Report of the Mid Staffordshire NHS Foundation Trust Public Inquiry. HC 947', (London: The Stationery Office, 2013). Available from: www.midstaffspublicinquiry.com (accessed 13 April 2015). 3(8) (2013), 138–147.

Frost, P. J and M. P. Wise 'Early Management of Acutely Ill Ward Patients: How Junior Doctors can Develop a Systematic Approach to Managing Patients with Acute Illness in Hospital', *British Medical Journal*, **345** (2012), e5677. doi: 10.1136/bmj.e5677.

Garside, J. and S. Prescott. 'Improving the Care of Acutely Ill Patients Outside ICU Settings', *Nursing Times*, **104**(22) (2008), 25–6.

Giddens, J. F. 'A Survey of Physical Assessment Techniques Performed by RNs: Lessons for Nursing Education', *Journal of Nurse Education*, 46(2) (2007), 83–7.

Higginson, R., and B. Jones. 'Respiratory Assessment in Critically Ill Patients: Airway and Breathing', *British Journal of Nursing*, 18(8) (2009), 456, 458–61.

Liaw, S. Y., A. Scherbier, P. Klainin-Yobas and J. J. Rethans. 'A Review of Educational Strategies to Improve Nurses' Role in Recognizing and Responding to Deteriorating Patients', *International Nursing Review*, 58 (3), (2011), 296–303.

Lofmark, A., C. Gustavsson and K. Wikblad. 'Student Nurses' Ability to Perform Pain Assessment', *Nurse Education Practice*, 3 (2003), 133–43.

Manley, K. and S. Hardy. *Improving Services to Patients Through Ongoing Development of Critical Care Teams*. A Report Commissioned by the Department of Health (England). (London: Department of Health, 2006).

McCaughey, C. S. and M. K. Traynor. 'The Role of Simulation in Nurse Education', *Nurse Education Today*, 30(8) (2010), 827–32.

Mole, L. J., G. Hogg and S. Benvie. 'Evaluation of the Teaching Pack Designed for Nursing Students to Acquire the Essential Knowledge for Competent Practice in Blood Transfusion Administration', *Nurse Education in Practice*, 7 (2007), 228–37.

Murray, C., M. Grant, M. Howarth and J. Leigh. 'The Use of Simulation as a Teaching and Learning Approach to Support Practice Learning', *Nurse Education in Practice*, 8 (2008), 5–8.

National Confidential Enquiry into Patient Outcome and Death (NCEPOD) *Caring to the End? A Review of the Care of Patients who Died in Hospital Within Four Days of Admission* (NCEPOD, 2009). Available from: www.ncepod.org.uk/2009dah.htm (accessed 16 June 2015).

National Institute for Health and Clinical Excellence (NICE). *Acutely Ill Patients in Hospital: Recognition of and Response to Acute Illness in Adults in Hospital. NICE Clinical Guideline 50* (London: National Institute for Health and Clinical Excellence, 2007).

National Patient Safety Agency (NPSA). *Safer Care for the Acutely Ill Patient: Learning From Serious Incidents*, Fifth Report from the Patient Safety Observatory (London: NHS National Patient Safety Agency, 2007).

NHS England. *High Quality Care for All, Now and for Future Generations: Transforming Urgent and Emergency Care Services in England – Urgent and Emergency Care Review End of Phase 1 Report* (Leeds: NHS England, 2013).

Nursing and Midwifery Council (NMC). *Standards for Pre-registration Nursing Education.* (London: Nursing and Midwifery Council, 2010).

Shin, I. S. and J. H. Kim. 'The Effect of Problem-based Learning in Nursing Education: A Meta-Analysis', *Advances In Health Sciences Education: Theory And Practice*, 18(5) (2013), 1103–20.

Steen, C. D. and J. Costello. 'Teaching Pre-registration Student Nurses to Assess Acutely Ill Patients: An Evaluation of Acute Illness Management Programme', *Nurse Education in Practice*, 8 (2008), 343–51.

Young, L., P. Baker, S. Waller, L. Hodgson and M. Moor. 'Knowing Your Allies: Medical Education and Interprofessional Exposure'. *Journal of Interprofessional Care*, 21(2) (2007), 155–63.

Index

CPSIA information can be obtained
at www.ICGtesting.com
Printed in the USA
LVOW13s1955190518
577817LV00009B/70/P